# Networking Technologies in Smart Healthcare

This text provides novel smart network systems, wireless telecommunications infrastructures, and computing capabilities to help healthcare systems using computing techniques like IoT, cloud computing, machine and deep learning Big Data along with smart wireless networks. It discusses important topics, including robotics manipulation and analysis in smart healthcare industries, smart telemedicine framework using machine learning and deep learning, role of UAV and drones in smart hospitals, virtual reality based on 5G/6G and augmented reality in healthcare systems, data privacy and security, nanomedicine, and cloud-based artificial intelligence in healthcare systems.

**The book:**
- Discusses intelligent computing through IoT and Big Data in secure and smart healthcare systems.
- Covers algorithms, including deterministic algorithms, randomized algorithms, iterative algorithms, and recursive algorithms.
- Discusses remote sensing devices in hospitals and local health facilities for patient evaluation and care.
- Covers wearable technology applications such as weight control and physical activity tracking for disease prevention and smart healthcare.

This book will be useful for senior undergraduate, graduate students, and academic researchers in areas such as electrical engineering, electronics and communication engineering, computer science, and information technology. Discussing concepts of smart networks, advanced wireless communication, and technologies in setting up smart healthcare services, this text will be useful for senior undergraduate, graduate students, and academic researchers in areas such as electrical engineering, electronics and communication engineering, computer science, and information technology. It covers internet of things (IoT) implementation and challenges in healthcare industries, wireless network, and communication-based optimization algorithms for smart healthcare devices.

## Wireless Communications and Networking Technologies: Classifications, Advancement and Applications
*Series Editor: D.K. Lobiyal, R.S. Rao and Vishal Jain*

The series addresses different algorithms, architecture, standards and pro-tocols, tools and methodologies which could be beneficial in implementing next generation mobile network for the communication. Aimed at senior undergraduate students, graduate students, academic researchers and pro-fessionals, the proposed series will focus on the fundamentals and advances of wireless communication and networking, and their such as mobile ad-hoc network (MANET), wireless sensor network (WSN), wireless mess network (WMN), vehicular ad-hoc networks (VANET), vehicular cloud network (VCN), vehicular sensor network (VSN), reliable cooperative network (RCN), mobile opportunistic network (MON), delay tolerant networks (DTN), flying ad-hoc network (FANET) and wireless body sensor network (WBSN).

**Wireless Communication**
Advancements and Challenges
*Prashant Ranjan, Ram Shringar Rao, Krishna Kumar and Pankaj Sharma*

**Wireless Communication with Artificial Intelligence**
Emerging Trends and Applications
*Anuj Singal, Sandeep Kumar, Sajjan Singh and
Ashish Kr. Luhach*

**Computational Intelligent Security in Wireless Communications**
*Suhel Ahmad Khan, Rajeev Kumar, Omprakash Kaiwartya,
Raees Ahmad Khan and Mohammad Faisal*

**Networking Technologies in Smart Healthcare: Innovations and Analytical Approaches**
*Pooja Singh, Omprakash Kaiwartya, Nidhi Sindhwani, Vishal Jain and
Rohit Anand*

**Artificial Intelligence in Cyber Physical Systems: Principles and Applications**
*Anil Kumar Sagar, Parma Nand, Neetesh Kumar, Sanjoy Das and
Subrata Sahana*

For more information about this series, please visit: https://www.routledge.com/Wireless%20Communications%20and%20Networking%20Technologies/book-series/WCANT

# Networking Technologies in Smart Healthcare
## Innovations and Analytical Approaches

Edited by
Pooja Singh
Omprakash Kaiwartya
Nidhi Sindhwani
Vishal Jain
Rohit Anand

**CRC Press**
Taylor & Francis Group
Boca Raton  New York  London

CRC Press is an imprint of the
Taylor & Francis Group, an **informa** business

Front cover image: Birth Brand/Shutterstock

First edition published 2023
by CRC Press
6000 Broken Sound Parkway NW, Suite 300, Boca Raton,
FL 33487-2742

and by CRC Press
4 Park Square, Milton Park, Abingdon, Oxon, OX14 4RN

*CRC Press is an imprint of Taylor & Francis Group, LLC*

© 2023 selection and editorial matter, Pooja Singh, Omprakash
Kaiwartya, Nidhi Sindhwani, Vishal Jain and Rohit Anand
individual chapters, the contributors

ISBN: 978-1-032-14545-7 (hbk)
ISBN: 978-1-032-14548-8 (pbk)
ISBN: 978-1-003-23988-8 (ebk)

DOI: 10.1201/9781003239888

Typeset in Sabon
by SPi Technologies India Pvt Ltd (Straive)

# Contents

# About the book

This reference text covers intelligent computing through internet of things (IoT) and Big Data in smart healthcare systems. The text covers important topics, including 5G, wireless body area networks, fuzzy logic optimization of medical data analytics, communication and detection of sanitation solutions during epidemics, and security and privacy on the internet of medical things. It is aimed at graduate students and academic researchers in the fields of electrical engineering, electronics and communication engineering, and computer science and engineering. This text covers the applications of internet of medical things and cloud-based artificial intelligence in healthcare systems and discusses the use of intelligent model for coronary heart disease diagnosis and IoT approach of managing smart healthcare services. The title of this book is intended to provide academic and business researchers with a platform to introduce their new ideas on how current wireless communication, networking, and detection technologies can quickly address the present epidemic situation toward healthcare sector caused by COVID-19 to get better solutions.

# Preface

This book is written for the healthcare professionals who wish to understand the principles and applications of information and communication technologies in healthcare. The text is presented in a way that should make it accessible to anyone and independent of prior technology knowledge. It is suitable as a textbook for undergraduate and postgraduate training in the clinical aspects of informatics and as an introductory textbook for those pursuing a postgraduate career in health and biomedical informatics. The text is designed to be used by all the healthcare professionals, including nurses and allied health professionals and not just medical practitioners. When I use the term "clinician" in this book, I am referring to any healthcare practitioner directly involved in health monitoring and patient care. Those with a background in information and communication technology should find the book a valuable introduction to the diverse applications of technology in health and to summarize the unique challenges of this domain.

With this edition, we have kept the essential backbone of the informatics story. Part 1 contains foundational chapters that explain simply the abstract concepts that are core to the informatics. The subsequent chapters then are built upon those foundations. Part 2 contains a set of chapters that explore all the main themes of the book from the perspective of informatics skills. Practicing clinicians must understand how to communicate effectively, structure information, ask questions, search for answers, and make robust decisions. Informatics is as much about doing as it is about the tools we use and these chapters make clear why the study of health informatics is the foundation of all other clinical activities. We return to each of these information and communication system themes in later chapters, taking a more technological focus. The book has a strong emphasis on demonstrating what works and what does not work in informatics. We have created a new evaluative framework based on the value of information that runs through the book, to help in understanding why some classes of intervention appear to work so much better than others. Each chapter ends with the content intended to test the reader's understanding of the chapter or stimulated discussion of the material.

Health informatics has undergone many changes since the appearance of the second edition in 2003. New themes have emerged, and new methods and technologies have also been adopted. Old ideas have fallen by the wayside. The chapters cover Implementation, Information System Safety, Social Networks and Social Media Interventions, Model Building for Decision Support, Data Analysis and Scientific Discovery, Clinical Bioinformatics and Personalized Medicine, and Consumer Informatics. The chapters are extensive and focus as much as possible on the basic concepts and principles, rather than simple narrative descriptions of the topics. There are many new concepts within the chapters, covering diverse topics, including health information exchanges, M-health, patient consent models, natural language processing, and even augmented reality. The research base of our discipline grows rapidly, and it is very easy to create chapters that date quickly. The main focus is on creating an introductory work that has some longevity and explores the core concepts needed to understand our discipline with a single and unified voice, or writing an encyclopaedic multiauthor work that tries to do everything. At least for this book, we think we have still managed to keep the book to a "single voice" overview – although we have had many expert colleagues help us with sourcing, writing and structuring the material, and checking what has been written. I hope that the clarity of this text makes up for any limitations in its comprehensiveness.

# About the editors

**Dr. Pooja Singh** is presently working as an Associate Professor in the Department of Computer Science and Engineering at Galgotias University, Greater Noida, India. Previously she worked with GL Bajaj Institute of Technology and Management, affiliated to AKTU, Greater Noida, India. Dr. Singh has also been appointed for her postdoctoral program at the Federal Institute of Education, Science and Technology of Ceara (IFCA), Brazil, Latin America, USA, from Feb'22. She has 14 years of working experience; previously she was associated with Amity University, Noida, as Assistant Professor for 13 years.

Dr. Pooja Singh was awarded the Best Researcher Award 2022, Nomination Winner by INSO Awards: International Research Awards on Science, Technology and Management, Chennai, India, and Best Faculty Award 2020–21 by the Ministry of Corporate Affairs, Government of India. She is also an Honorary member of the Indian Engineering Teacher Association, with USA and Indo-UK technology and research, confederation of science.

She received her doctorate (CSE) and MTech (CSE) degree from Banasthali Vidyapith, Rajasthan (NIRF Rank 61, 2021) and BTech (IT) degree from Government College of Purvanchal University, Jaunpur, Uttar Pradesh.

Dr. Singh has published numerous (40 research papers in international peer-reviewed journals and conferences, including SCI, Scopus indexed, Springer, Elsevier, IEEE with good impact factor, and many other papers published in the IEEE national conference and some research work presented at IIT-Delhi).

She has also published various patents and some are granted in the field of AI and ML at national and international level.

Dr. Singh is an author of the book titled "Machine Learning Technique," she is also a book-editor for Taylor & Francis, and she has also published many book chapters for Springer, CRC, and IGI global publications. Dr. Singh has organized various workshops and conferences as TCP member at the university and college level. She has delivered various seminars and attended more than 50 FDP/STP from reputed institutes like IIT-Kharagpur,

IIT-Delhi, IIT-Roorkee, and NITTTR-Chandigarh. She is a professional member with IEEE, IRED, UACEE, ACEEE, IAENG, IACSIT, etc. She is also a reviewer for many reputed journals like Springer, IEEE, Wireless personal communication (Scimago Journal), and IGI Global Book Chapter Peer Reviews, Springer. Dr. Singh is also an advisory committee member Advisory Board/Committee member, RSRI DAAI'2022, Editorial Board member of IJCSSCA, Journal, Editorial Board member of *Journal of Research and Reviews: Machine Learning and Cloud Computing* under MAT Journal and Editorial Board member of *Journal of IoT Security and Smart Technology*, under MAT Journal. Her areas of interest are AI, WSN, ML, IoT, Biomedical image analysis, and AIoT.

**Dr. Omprakash Kaiwartya** is currently working at the School of Science and Technology, Nottingham Trent University (NTU), UK, as a Senior Lecturer and Course Leader for MSc Engineering (Electronics, Cybernetics and Communications). Previously, he was a Research Associate (equivalent to Senior Lecturer) in the Department of Computer and Information Science at Northumbria University, Newcastle, UK, where he was involved in the gLINK, European Union project. Prior to this, he was a Post-Doctoral Fellow (equivalent to Lecturer) in the Faculty of Computing, University of Technology (UTM), Malaysia. Before moving to Malaysia, he completed his BSc in Computer Science from Guru Ghansidas Central University, Bilaspur Chhattisgarh, India, and Master combined PhD degree from the School of Computer and Systems Science, Jawaharlal Nehru University (JNU), New Delhi, India. Overall, he has authored/co-authored over 100 international publications, including journal articles, conference proceedings, book chapters, and books. Dr. Omprakash's research interest focuses on IoT-centric smart environment for diverse domain areas, including Transport, Healthcare, and Industrial Production. His recent scientific contributions are in Internet of Connected Vehicles (IoV), E-Mobility, Electronic Vehicles Charging Management (EV), Internet of Healthcare Things (IoHT), Smart use case implementation of Sensor Networks, and Next Generation Wireless Communication Technologies (6G and Beyond). Furthermore, Omprakash is a Fellow of Higher Education Academy (FHEA), IEEE Senior member, and BCS Professional member. He has served as a TPC member or Reviewer in 100+ International Conferences and Workshops, including IEEE Globecom, IEEE ICC, IEEE CCNC, IEEE ICNC, IEEE VTC, IEEE INFOCOM, ACM CoNEXT, ACM MobiHoc, ACM SAC, and many more. Furthermore, he has been reviewing papers for 30+ international journals, including IEEE magazines on Wireless Communications, Networks, Communications, IEEE Communications Letters, IEEE Sensors Letters, IEEE Transactions on Industrial Informatics, Vehicular Technologies, Intelligent Transportation Systems, Big Data, and Mobile Computing. Moreover, Omprakash has been an editorial member of various Special Issues with top-ranked journals in Communication Society and serving as an Associate Editor of IET Intelligent Transport Systems, IEEE Internet of Things Journal, Springer, EURASIP Journal on Wireless Communication and Networking, MDPI Electronics, Ad-Hoc and Sensor Wireless Networks, and KSII Transactions on Internet and Information Systems.

**Dr. Nidhi Sindhwani** is currently working as an Assistant Professor in the Department of Electronics and Communication Engineering, at the Amity School of Engineering and Technology, Amity University, India. She has teaching experience of more than 15 years. She has received her BE degree in Electronics and Communication Engineering in 2004 and ME degree in Signal Processing in 2008, both from Mahrishi Dayanand University, Rohtak. She has received her PhD (ECE) from UCOE, Punjabi University Patiala in 2018. Her current research interest includes Wireless Networks and Communication, IOT, Machine learning, and Signal Processing. Dr. Sindhwani has published numerous papers with good impact factor in reputed international journals and conferences, including Springer, Taylor & Francis, Inderscience, IEEE, and IGI Global. She is also the lifetime member of Indian Society of Technical Education (ISTE).

**Dr. Vishal Jain** is presently working as an Associate Professor at the Department of Computer Science and Engineering, School of Engineering and Technology, Sharda University, Greater Noida, UP, India. Before that, he worked for several years as an Associate Professor at Bharati Vidyapeeth's Institute of Computer Applications and Management (BVICAM), New Delhi. He has more than 14 years of experience in academics. He has earned several degrees: PhD (CSE), MTech (CSE), MBA (HR), MCA, MCP, and CCNA. He has more than 550 research citations with Google Scholar (h-index score 13 and i-10 index 19) and has authored more than 95 research papers in professional journals and conferences. He has authored and edited more than 25 books with various reputed publishers, including Springer, Apple Academic Press, CRC, Taylor and Francis Group, Scrivener, Wiley, Emerald, and IGI-Global. His research areas include information retrieval, semantic web, ontology engineering, data mining, ad hoc networks, and sensor networks. He received a Young Active Member award for the year 2012–13 from the Computer Society of India, Best Faculty Award for the year 2017, and Best Researcher Award for the year 2019 from BVICAM, New Delhi.

**Dr. Rohit Anand** is currently working as an Assistant Professor in the Department of Electronics and Communication Engineering at G. B. Pant DSEU Okhla-1 Campus (formerly G. B. Pant Engineering College), Government of NCT of Delhi, New Delhi, India. He has teaching experience of more than 20 years, including UG and PG Courses. He is a Life member of Indian Society for Technical Education (ISTE) and a Member of IEEE. He has published 12 book chapters in reputed books and 19 research papers in Scopus/SCI indexed journals. He has chaired a special session in 13 International Conferences and presented more than 20 papers in National and International Conferences. He has got the Best Paper Presentation award in an international conference held in Gwalior, India. He is presently a reviewer in many highly indexed journals like IEEE Transactions on Industrial Informatics, International Journal of Microwave and Wireless Technologies, Journal of Optical Communications, KSII Transactions on Internet and Information Systems and Journal of Integrative Bioinformatics. He has guided 12 students in M.Tech. Dissertation. He has got awards such as Indian and Asian Record holder, Integral Humanism award, and Best Teacher award. His research areas include Electromagnetic Field Theory, Antenna Theory and Design, Wireless Communication, Optimization, Image Processing, Optical Fiber Communication, IoT, etc.

# Contributors

**Badraddine Aghoutane**
FS My Ismail University
Morocco

**Tarik Ahajjam**
LSTI-IDMS My Ismail University
  Faculty of Sciences and Technics
Morocco

**Rohit Anand**
G.B. Pant DSEU Okhla-1 Campus
  (formerly GBPEC)
New Delhi, India

**C. Ashwini**
SRM Institute of Science and
  Technology
Ramapuram, India

**Younes Balboul**
Artificial Intelligence and Data
  Science and Emerging Systems
  Laboratory
Sidi Mohamed Ben Abdellah
  University of FES
Morocco

**Benaissa Bernoussi**
Artificial Intelligence and Data
  Science and Emerging Systems
  Laboratory
Sidi Mohamed Ben Abdellah
  University of FES
Morocco

**Sahithi Bommareddy**
Delhi Technological University
Delhi, India

**Pankaj Dadeech**
Swami Keshvanand Institute of
  Technology, Management and
  Gramothan
Jaipur, India

**Aman Dahiya**
Maharaja Surajmal Institute
  of Technology
New Delhi, India

**Shiela David**
SRM Institute of Science and
  Technology
Ramapuram, India

**Vijaypal Singh Dhaka**
Manipal University
Jaipur, India

**Moulhime Elbekkali**
Artificial Intelligence
  and Data Science and
  Emerging Systems
  Laboratory
Sidi Mohamed Ben Abdellah
  University of FES
Morocco

Youssef Farhaoui
LSTI-IDMS My Ismail University
  Faculty of Sciences and Technics
Morocco

Mohammed Fattah
EST My Ismail University
Morocco

K. Gunasekaran
Muthayammal Engineering College
  (Autonomous)
Namakkal, India

Deena Nath Gupta
Jamia Millia Islamia
New Delhi, India

Yogesh Gupta
BML Munjal University
Gurgaon, India

Jaspinder Kaur
Chandigarh University
Mohali, India

Javed Ahmad Khan
Department of IT
Govt. Girls Polytechnic Ballia
UP, India

Ajay Kumar
Meerut Institute of Engineering and
  Technology
Meerut, India

Rajendra Kumar
Jamia Millia Islamia
New Delhi, India

Mohammed Mahfoudi
Artificial Intelligence and Data
  Science and Emerging Systems
  Laboratory
Sidi Mohamed Ben Abdellah
  University of FES
Morocco

P. M. Manohar
Raghu Engineering College
  (Autonomous)
Visakhapatnam, India

Said Mazer
Artificial Intelligence and Data
  Science and Emerging Systems
  Laboratory
Sidi Mohamed Ben Abdellah
  University of FES
Morocco

Ridhima Mehta
School of Computer and Systems
  Sciences
Jawaharlal Nehru University
New Delhi, India

Shweta Mogre
Prestige Institute of Management
  and Research
Indore, India

Monika
Shaheed Rajguru College of Applied
  Sciences for Women
University of Delhi
Delhi, India

Mohammed Moutaib
EST My Ismail University
Morocco

Rekha Narang
Geeta University
Panipat, India

Neelam Nehra
Maharaja Surajmal Institute of
  Technology
New Delhi, India

Binay Kumar Pandey
Govind Ballabh Pant University of
  Agriculture and Technology
Uttarakhand, India

Digvijay Pandey
Department of Technical Education
Dr. A. P. J. Abdul Kalam Technical
   University
UP, India

Sanjay S. Pawar
UMIT, SNDT Women's University
Mumbai, India

K. Radhika
Muthayammal Engineering College
   (Autonomous)
Namakkal, India

Ghanshyam Raghuwanshi
Manipal University
Jaipur, India

Rahul
Delhi Technological University
Delhi, India

Yahya Rbah
Artificial Intelligence and Data
   Science and Emerging Systems
   Laboratory
Sidi Mohamed Ben Abdellah
   University of FES
Morocco

T. K. Revathi
Sona College of Technology
Salem, India

Saarthak
Chandigarh University
Mohali, India

Gitimayee Sahu
UMIT, SNDT Women's University
Mumbai, India

S. Sankar
Sona College of Technology,
Salem, India

G. Saranya
SRM Institute of Science and
   Technology
Ramapuram, India

B. Sathiyabhama
Sona College of Technology
Salem, India

T. Shankar
GCE
Trichy, Tamil Nadu, India

Geetanjali Sharma
Maharaja Surajmal Institute of
   Technology
New Delhi, India

Nidhi Sindhwani
Amity University
Noida, India

Man Mohan Singh
Meerut Institute of Engineering and
   Technology
Meerut, India

Pooja Singh
University Institute of Engineering
   (UIE)-Computer Science and
   Engineering (CSE)
Chandigarh University
Gharuan, Mohali, Punjab, India

Deepak Sinwar
Manipal University
Jaipur, India

N. Srikanth
Annamalai University
Chidambaram, Tamil Nadu, India

P. Suresh
Muthayammal Engineering College
   (Autonomous)
Namakkal, India

**Subodh Kumar Tripathi**
Meerut Institute of Engineering and
    Technology
Meerut, India

**Ankit Trivedi**
Comp-Feeder Group of Institutions
Indore, India

**N. Suthanthira Vanitha**
Muthayammal Engineering College
    (Autonomous)
Namakkal, India

**Ramesh Kumar Verma**
Bundelkhand Institute of
    Engineering and Technology
Jhansi, India

**G. Yamuna**
Annamalai University
Chidambaram, Tamil Nadu, India

**Sumit Zokarkar**
Prestige Institute of Management
    and Research
Indore, India

Chapter 1

# Smart healthcare in smart city using wireless body area network and 5G

*Gitimayee Sahu and Sanjay S. Pawar*
UMIT, SNDT Women's University, Mumbai, India

## CONTENTS

## 1.1 INTRODUCTION

Smart healthcare plays an important role in the smart cities using 5G technology. Smart gadgets like a smart thermometer, smart watch, wireless glucometer for blood sugar monitoring, sphygmomanometer, electrocardiogram (ECG), and electroencephalogram (EEG) monitoring devices are connected to the patient's body. All these sensors evaluate various parameters of the body, process, and store in internet of things (IoT) cloud storage. They use the networks such as wireless body area network (WBAN), wireless local area network (WLAN), femtocell, or Home eNodeB (HeNB) for communication purposes. The intelligent gadgets process the data from various sensors and biomedical systems. They access the right information and provide the accurate solutions and minimize the medical errors and improve the efficiency of the system in an economical way. Femtocell is a low power base station (BS) typically used indoors to provide coverage for short-range communication like homes, theaters, stadiums, malls, offices, and small businesses. Femtocell and macro base station (MBS) constitute a heterogeneous cellular network (HetNet) of the 5G technology. The next-generation 5G technology provides enhanced capabilities, scalability, and high-speed services to the end-users. The essential use cases of 5G are eMBB (enhanced mobile broadband), URLLC (ultra-reliable low latency communications), and mMTC (massive machine type communications). It also supports enhanced applications like augmented and virtual reality (AR/VR), highly secure connectivity, and guaranteed QoS. eMBB supports a high data rate across a wide coverage area. URLLC provides ultralow latency of nearly 1 msec, which is essential for remote surgery, autonomous vehicles, and tactile internet services. There are many growth and complexity in signal processing and multiplexing methods in the air interface. The listed advancements in technologies are (i) universal filtered multicarrier (UFMC), (ii) filter bank multicarrier (FBMC), (iii) generalized frequency division multiplexing (GFDM), (iv) new radio waveforms such as 5G new radio (NR), and (v) non-orthogonal multiple access (NOMA) [1].

The 5G enhanced performance parameter requirements as per International Mobile Telecommunications (IMT) Advanced are shown in Table 1.1.

The applications of 5G include smart city, smart agriculture, internet of drones (IoD), industrial automation, smart home building, IoT and cloud computing, industrial IoT (IIoT; Industry 4.0), digital twin, and mobile

*Table 1.1* 5G performance requirements of IMT 2020

| Parameters | Value |
| --- | --- |
| Highest peak data rate | 20 Gbit/s |
| Area traffic capacity | 10 Mbit/s/square m |
| Network energy efficiency | 100 times more than IMT Advanced (IMT-A) |
| Connection density | $10^6$ devices/square km. |
| Mobility | 500 km/hr |
| Spectrum efficiency | Three times more compared with IMT Advanced (IMT-A) |
| User experienced data rate | 100 Mbit/s |
| Service density | 10 Gbps/square km.s |
| End-to-end latency | Order of millisecond |

internet mission-critical applications, viz. self-driving cars, eHealth services, and remote surgeries. 5G and IoT become the important drivers of next-generation smart healthcare. The key technologies of 5G, i.e., device-to-device communication (D to D), augmented and virtual reality (AR/VR), massive multiple input multiple output (MIMO) and fractal antennas for C and X bands [2–5], millimeter wave (mmWave) and beam-forming, and heterogeneous network (HetNet) are the main building blocks of the smart home. The HetNet is a multi-tier network that consists of a macro cell and small cells (femto, micro, and picocell). Femtocell or, HeNB is an indoor solution that provides broadband application, high data rate, and ultralow latency to nomadic users. These technologies specify the main service requirements of the upcoming 5G wireless network.

There are many challenges of 5G smart healthcare. First is the ultra-densification of the network due to a large number of sensors and devices in an area (nearly $10^6$ number of devices per sq. km.). Second is the high energy consumption due to IoT applications due to a wireless sensor network. These sensors empower the devices in the network to sense and communicate the data between them. For exchanging information, these devices need to perform monitoring, sensing, processing, and communicating with each other. Moreover, data transmission between devices requires more energy. Hence, at least 10 years of battery life is required for specific applications.

For smart healthcare, different network-layer optimizations such as scheduling, routing, congestion control, resource allocation, and QoS enhancement along interference mitigation are required. The energy-efficient mechanisms have been proposed in 5G and IoT to address these main challenges for smart healthcare solutions. The proposed solutions have been shown to increase throughput (e.g., via high data rate and bandwidth), reliability, energy efficiency, transmission coverage as well as reduce end-to-end delay.

## 1.2 LITERATURE REVIEW

The major contributions of the proposed chapter include:

- **5G smart healthcare architecture** includes key enabling technologies, specifically small cells, D2D communication, mmWaves, software-defined network (SDN), and network function virtualization (NFV).
- A glossary of 5G smart healthcare considering communication technologies, requirements, objectives, and performance measure is presented.
- Challenges and future research works in 5G and IoT-based smart healthcare are also discussed.

Table 1.2 Literature survey on smart healthcare using wireless body area network (WBAN)

| References | Contribution of the authors |
| --- | --- |
| Dhafer Ben et al. [6] | • Explains wearable antennas to establish human and machine interaction. There are three different types of communications.<br>  i.  Intra-body<br>  ii.  Inter-body (i.e., body to body)<br>  iii.  Off body communication.<br>• Intra-body and inter-body communication are challenging due to minimum power consumption, storage, and processing capability. Hence, there is impact on throughput, packet reception ratio, and latency. |
| Elham M. et al. [7] | • Wearable radio frequency identification (RFID) tag is used for body-centric communication.<br>• It does healthcare, enhances security, and biomedical applications.<br>• It is flexible, integral, and light weight.<br>• The performance of RFID tags on body dipole antenna is investigated.<br>• It is designed and implemented with an embroidered dipole tag which provides a range of 2.5 m when differentiated by 1-mm thick layer of cotton fabric on the human arm |
| Zhonglin Cao et al. [8] | • Explains near-field communication using low-cost sensors |
| Farhana et al. [9] | • Combination of energy-efficient, portable, and computer processing elements with clothing results in wearable format, which is composed of tiny interactive devices.<br>• A WBAN is a developing technology that emerged for wearable monitoring applications.<br>• WBAN is remodeled as a wearable computer that communicates with the users and I/O devices.<br>• It is integrated by using a large number of miniature wireless sensors specifically kept on the human body, which generates real-time data to users by observing different critical parameters with limited energy storage. |
| Qi et al. [10] | • First, analysis of different applications of IoT in smart healthcare from diverse aspects (i.e., measuring blood pressure, diabetics, oxygen saturation, heartbeat, and EEG) is done.<br>• Second, the author reviewed the existing work of IoT that enables technologies for smart healthcare applications using the various perceptions such as infrastructure and current technologies (i.e., networking, sensing, and data processing) |
| Islam et al. [11] | • First, it is focused on IoT-based real-time healthcare, network architecture, platforms and empowered with medical transmission and reception.<br>• Second, the research work supervises chronic diseases, care of elderly, pediatric patients, and fitness management with IoT. |

| Baker et al. [12] | • It discusses advanced architecture for next-generation smart healthcare.<br>• It provides review on short-range and long-range communication standards.<br>• It discusses special condition monitoring (i.e., wearables and nonintrusive sensors measuring blood pressure, blood oxygen level, and vital signs) |
|---|---|
| Mahmoud et al. [13] | • Survey on cloud of things (CoT), platforms, and how to implement it in smart healthcare applications.<br>• Energy efficiency in smart healthcare applications |
| Dhanvijay et al. [14] | • IoT-based healthcare systems for WBAN<br>• Review of resource allocation power management, energy efficiency, security and privacy related to IoT-based smart healthcare. |
| Gang Zhou [15] | • Explains the concept of BodyQoS for radio-agnostic which allocates radio resources with media access control (MAC) layer channel sharing. When the bandwidth of the channel reduces due to path loss, fading, and interference, body QoS dynamically assigns channels for adequate communication-guaranteed QoS. |
| Shuo Tian [16] | • Explains healthcare in an intelligent manner with diagnosis of the diseases with required treatments, virtual assistants, managing health-related services, preventing the chronic diseases, monitoring the risk factor of the patient, and research related to drugs. |
| Zeadally S. [17] | • Explains the issues and challenges related to smart healthcare. The authors have emphasized on collection of data using various sensors, storage of the data in appropriate servers using IoT and big data theory, and classification of data and suggestion by medical experts on real-time basis as per priority. |
| Mahashreveta C. [18] | • Healthcare in smart city is challenging and highly significant. In urban areas, industries and offices are located at the center of the city and residential areas are far from the city. Hence, elderly peoples for emergency medical assistance need to go to hospital which will take more time. If the patients can be monitored on real-time basis and they are provided with required virtual assistance and tele-medicines immediately, it will fulfill the objective of smart city with smart healthcare. |
| Sindhwani N. et al. [19, 20] | • MIMO antenna for personal communication can also be used with WBAN for high-speed data communication. |

## 1.3 SMART HEALTHCARE SOLUTION USING 5G NETWORK ARCHITECTURE

5G network is characterized as ultra-dense heterogeneous architecture. It includes Small cells under the wide coverage of the high-powered macrocell. The small cells are low-powered BSs having a transmission range of few meters to few miles in diameter. It provides flexible coverage and enhances spectral and energy efficiency. The different types of small cells play an important role in many operations of 5G smart healthcare. It demands a high data rate (e.g., remote surgery requires a data rate up to 137 Mbps to 1.6 Gbps), which is feasible due to its low transmitting power and millimeter wave front hauls HeNB. Small cells are of three different types (Femto, Pico, microcells) depending on the transmission power, which varies from shorter coverage to larger coverage area. Femtocells or HeNB are used to expand the coverage and capacity within small proximity, such as mall, stadium, auditorium, hospital, and home. They reinforce up to 30 users over a range of 0.1 km. The description of small cells is indicated in Table 1.3.

The BAN will be attached with various sensors for monitoring the vital parameters of the patient. All the measured parameters will be communicated wirelessly using femtocell to store in IoT and cloud database of smart city. As urban cities are converting into smart cities with technologies, with increase in infrastructure, the data and information also rise with applications. The smart city provides significant improvement in resources like electricity and water, smart parking with traffic management, eco-friendly environment by proper waste management, and using green energy (solar panel, wind mills, and wave energy). By proper video surveillance, criminal activity can be tracked and security measures can be taken to protect senior citizen, women, and children. But the main significant sector is the health sector which should be developed with (i) remote monitoring of the patients, (ii) storing the data on real-time basis at IoT and cloud storage, (iii) differentiating the data as per priority of the patient, and (iv) providing instant medical support by remotely monitoring through WBAN. Through telemedicine, the required medicine should reach the patient's doorstep with minimum amount of time. The entire process should be optimized with artificial intelligence and machine learning technique. With this technique, the

*Table 1.3* Summary of small cells

| Cell types | Cell radius | Users | Location |
| --- | --- | --- | --- |
| Femto cell (HeNB) | 0.01–0.1 km | 1–30 | Indoor |
| Pico cell | 0.25–1 km | 30–100 | Indoor/outdoor |
| Micro cell | 0.2–2 km | 100–2000 | Indoor/outdoor |
| Macro cell | 8–30 km | More than 2,000 | Outdoor |

accuracy of the system enhances with appropriate treatment and minimum error. With the integration of 5G technique, the mechanism becomes advanced because it provides broad bandwidth, high throughput, minimum delay, massive connection of sensors and devices, high reliability, low latency, and advanced security.

## 1.4 5G SMART HEALTHCARE USING WIRELESS BODY AREA NETWORK (WBAN)

WBAN is a promising technology for remote healthcare monitoring (HCM) using domestic electronics gadgets, such as wearable sensors and smart phones, around the human body. WBANs are described by many features, which are low cost, noninvasive, and promptly measures vital body parameters with high reliability. They are beneficial to hospital fraternity such as medical experts, patients, and health workers. To measure the physical activity of the patient, sensors like accelerometer was used, and for diabetes, blood pressure checkup, glucometer along with insulin pump and sphygmomanometer (blood pressure cuff) was used. The physiological vital signs of the patients were tracked and recorded by monitoring the patient remotely. The medical experts then treated with necessary medicine and precautions. The patients' emotional reactions were observed, and if abnormality was detected, it was immediately intimated to the health workers and experts. A multisensor data-fusion scheme was recommended to dynamically detect the handshakes of two people and captivate the heartbeat of patients based on their emotions. It does signal processing in the node environment (C-SPINE). SPINE is a software architecture that uses programmable sensor devices for designing collaborative WBAN networking. Specifically, the TinyOS version of SPINE stiffens the Bluetooth, as well as the IEEE 802.15.4 standard, including the framework of the ZigBee technology. The WBAN can communicate with other BAN, HeNB, and MBS using mm-wave backhaul and D to D communication as shown in Figure 1.1.

Using small cells, the area spectrum efficiency of the network can be enhanced by reusing the higher frequencies spatially. Moreover, in small cells, the control plane and user plane are able to function separately. The connectivity and mobility of the user equipment (UE) are supported by the control plane while transportation of the data between different UEs was managed by the user plane. Hence, the UE must attach to the MBS for outdoor scenarios and SBS for the indoor scenarios. MBS uses a control plane for user mobility and handover. MBS generally uses lower frequency for a broad range and wide coverage area. SBS uses higher frequencies for indoor and line of sight communication for high throughput and broadband application. Generally, higher frequencies in the millimeter-wave range are used for indoor scenario in order to transmit data between the devices.

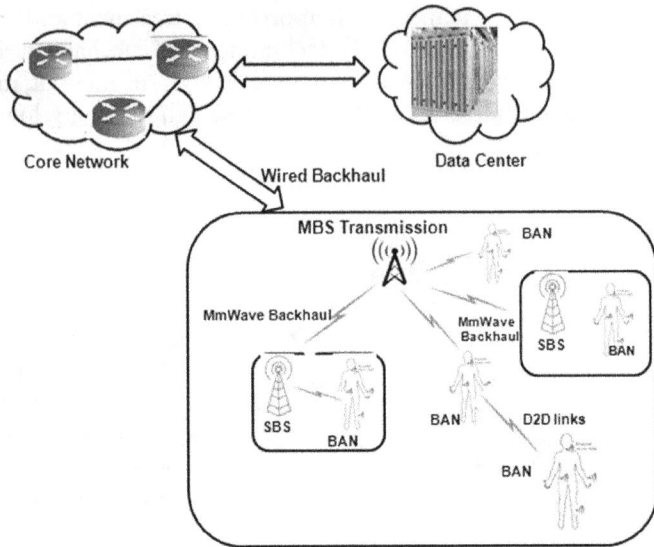

*Figure 1.1* 5G smart healthcare architecture.

WBAN consists of tiny biomedical sensors of the finite size that have defined energy resource capacities, small memory size, and limited computation capability. To efficiently manage and control, a large number of WBANs carrying information about the health in large-scale deployment for remote HCM becomes a challenging task [21]. IoT and cloud computing are the upcoming technologies that provide high data storage, computing and analysis, and processing of utilities at a lower cost. It will be integrated with the WBAN system and facilities for remote communication.

The WBAN technology includes Category I which is composed of intra WBAN-based IOT communication. It consists of different sensors like retina sensor, asthma sensor, EEG monitoring ECG, and muscle pressure monitoring using pressure sensors. All these data are accumulated and stored in personal server. Category II describes inter WBAN-based IoT and cloud computing. It includes WBAN to WBAN communication (D to D), i.e., inter WBAN and ad hoc network based on communication between WBAN and BSs. Category III is beyond WBAN-based IOT communication. It accumulates all the data available from various WBANs and stores in the cloud data center so that the data can be permeated easily to the medical expert and to the nearby persons of the patient by authenticated login and password.

Cloud-enabled body software as a service (BCSaaS) [22] is an enhanced technique for BANs using sensors. BCSaaS network measures and processes the heartbeat of the cardiac patients on a real-time basis. Due to the significant applications, this is deployed on a large-scale manner, especially for continuous monitoring of patients with heart disease.

## 1.5 ALLOCATED FREQUENCY BANDS FOR WBAN

The frequency band 402–405 MHz has been allocated for sensor-to-sensor, sensor-to-body surface, and sensor-to-external communication purposes. The spectrum bands 13.5 MHz, 50 MHz, 400 MHz, 600 MHz, 900 MHz, and 2.4 GHz, 3.1–10.6 GHz have been allocated for body surface-to-body surface communication scenarios. The spectrum bands 900 MHz, 2.4, 3.1–10.6 GHz are allocated for body surface-to-external communication scenarios. Figure 1.2 shows the different allocated frequency bands for WBAN for different countries. Table 1.4 presents the channel models used for WBAN. Different channels are used for communication between sensors, sensors-to-body surface for line of sight (LoS), and nonline-of-sight (NLoS) communication.

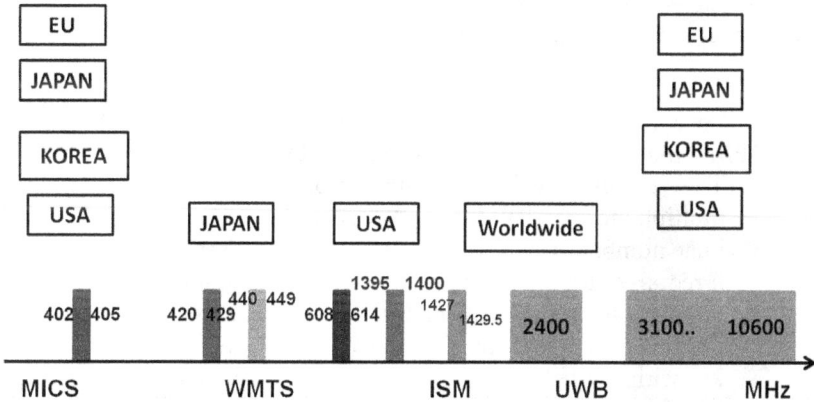

Figure 1.2 Frequency allocation for WBAN worldwide.

Table 1.4 Channel model for WBAN

| Scenario | Description | Frequency band | Channel |
|---|---|---|---|
| S1 | Sensor to sensor | 402–405 MHz | CM1 |
| S2 | Sensor to body surface | 402–405 MHz | CM2 |
| S3 | Sensor to external | 402–405 MHz | CM2 |
| S4 | Body surface to body surface (LoS) | 13.5, 50, 400, 600, 900 MHz, 2.4, 3.1–10.6 GHz | CM3 |
| S5 | Body surface to body surface (NLoS) | 13.5, 50, 400, 600, 900 MHz, 2.4, 3.1–10.6 GHz | CM3 |
| S6 | Body surface to external (LoS) | 900MHz, 2.4, 3.1–10.6 GHz | CM4 |
| S7 | Body surface to external (NLoS) | 900MHz, 2.4, 3.1–10.6 GHz | CM4 |

## 1.6 LOW-POWER WIDE AREA NETWORK COMMUNICATION SYSTEMS IN WBANS

Low-power wide area network (LPWAN) technique is upcoming and attaining recognition over the traditional short-distance wireless communication. It is due to its competence to challenge long-distance economic connectivity and large-scale information exchange at low power level [23].

The WBAN systems usually use short-range and cellular technologies for patient's health-related communication, which utilizes a large amount of energy during uninterrupted monitoring of patients' health conditions. It's due to the sensors in WBANs mostly depending on battery power. Hence, to achieve the long-range, low power, cost effective, and real-time data communication, an energy-efficient WBAN system is needed. The LPWAN systems are contemplated to be feasible for accomplishing the above-mentioned WBAN QoS prerequisites.

### 1.6.1 Description of LPWAN communication systems

A. The **proprietary-based** LPWAN communication systems include (i) RPMA Ingenu, (ii) SIGFOX, and (iii) LoRa.
   i. The various LPWAN communication systems are random phase multiple access (RPMA) and Ingenu access point (AP). Because huge number of sensors and devices are connected with each other, it requires large amount of capacity and scalability. RPMA has low pathloss, it can pass through the concrete, massive buildings and provide coverage in rural places up to 10 km and in rural up to 3 km with limited mobility support. It is highly energy efficient but interference level is also high.
   ii. **SIGFOX** is a software-based communication solution where the network and computing complexity are handled in the cloud rather than in the device. It decreases energy consumption and cost of operation is also low. It provides wide area rural coverage up to 50 km and urban coverage up to 10 km which is more compared with RPMA. It uses differential binary phase shift keying (DBPSK) and Gaussian frequency shift keying (GFSK) modulation scheme. The main issue is high interference, nonsupport of mobility, low reliability, and sustainability.
   iii. The ultra **long-range radio (LoRa)** is a low-power, low-cost, and high-performance both way semiduplex module which has 15 dBm transmission power and operates at frequency 169/433/915MHz. It has a data rate of 50 kbps which is high compared with RPMA and SIGFOX. It supports rural coverage up to 15 km and urban coverage up to 5 km. It uses FDMA at downlink and SC-FDMA at uplink. It provides long-range communication with high interference level.

B. The **nonproprietary**-based LPWAN communication system consists of (i) long-term evolution category M1 (LTE-M1), (ii) extended coverage GSM(EC-GSM), and (iii) narrowband (NB-IoT).

    i. **LTE-M1 (4G)** has a transmission power of 20 dBm. It has rural coverage area of 15 km, battery life span of 10 years, and urban coverage up to 10 km. It can connect up to 20,000 sensors, supports mobility of the devices, supports remote monitoring of healthcare, and is highly energy efficient. It has limited network capacity and minimum 10 years of battery life span.

    ii. **EC-GSM** has transmission power up to 33 dBm, data rate up to 10 kbps. It can connect up to 50,000 sensor devices. It has TDMA, FDMA, GMSK, and 8 PSK modulation schemes. It supports remote HCM and is highly energy efficient but the limitation is extremely low data rate.

    iii. **NB-IoT Technology**: Narrow band-IoT (NB-IoT) technology is also known as the LTE Cat-NB1. This technology is a propitious standard in the 3GPP specification that was devised to accomplish low-power communication. Hence, it will enhance the battery lifetime of the connected sensor devices, increase the signal coverage, and will also adopt the dynamic deployment and flexible architecture.

For cloud IoT devices with small packet transmissions, smaller RF bandwidth operation is sufficient. Hence, complexity is reduced further. The system with 200 kHz operating bandwidth is ideal to achieve the low-cost objective of cloud IoT (CIoT) [24]. NB IoT is an LTE based air interface designed for low complexity IoT devices. LTE operates within single physical resource block (PRB) compared to six PRB operations of LTE-M. With single tone transmission, support uplink transmission can be further simplified. With the support of single tone with 3.75 kHz carrier spacing, the uplink operation is simplified which allows extended coverage with minimum repetitions.

The key concept of NB-IoT includes OFDM with 15 kHz single carrier subcarrier (SCS) which is equivalent to the operation of PRB. The fame, subframe, and slot structure are similar to LTE. Normal cyclic prefix is supported in downlink. The uplink transmission includes single carrier FDMA (SC-FDMA). Single carrier transmission is possible with 15 kHz at 3.75 kHz subcarrier spacing. Sub-PRB allocation with less than single carrier allocation is possible for multitone operation. The 3.75 kHz operation uses 2 msec of slot duration. For in-band deployment, one of the PRB of LTE can be replaced by NB-IoT carrier using the air interface timing. The NB-IoT PRB power is boosted for extended coverage. For guard band deployment, the carriers are used from outside the operating PRB but within the LTE bandwidth which is used for NB-IoT. The NB-IoT power is boosted for extended coverage. In standalone deployment, dedicated carrier is assigned for NB-IoT outside the LTE operating bandwidth, which is used to replace the GSM carrier and is of 200 kHz. The transmission power is used by NB-IoT PRB [25].

NB-IoT could be used in a broad range of IoT applications, for example, wireless networks that consist of wireless sensors [26], WBANs such as smart healthcare, eHealth services, monitoring and diagnosing abnormalities and deceases. It also includes IIoT, digital twin, smart machineries attached with sensors, interconnected devices, smart home, smart city, and smart agriculture, including mobile edge computing [27, 28].

Moreover, NB-IoT supports GSM, GPRS, 3G (WCDMA). and LTE technologies for compatibility and very good performance. During uplink, it uses single carrier frequency division multiple access (SC-FDMA) technique with data rate ranging from 0.3 to 180 kbps [29], whereas in the downlink communication, it uses orthogonal frequency division multiple access (OFDMA) modulation technique and transmits at a data rate of 0.5–200 kbps. Generally, it uses MAC layer for uplink transmission which uses channel sharing and physical layer for downlink transmission [30]. NB-IoT provides low latency, i.e., 10 s or less for uplink data communication and supports wider area coverage with distance up to 35 km. NB-IoT devices have transmission power of about 20–23 dBm, and large amount of battery lifespan, i.e., more than 10 years by utilizing battery-power-saving methods. NB-IoT has high energy efficiency, because it has the capability of extended discontinuous reception (eDRX) and power saving scheme. The power saving scheme boosts for optimizing the power consumption, by moving the sensors into sleep mode when they are not used. Furthermore, eDRX extends the sleeping cycles during idle modes of the system.

The architecture of WBAN using NB-IoT is as shown in Figure 1.3. It consists of next-generation NB-IoT healthcare sensor devices, radio access network (RAN), an internet cloud platform, various WBAN usages, and remote HCM centers. The biomedical sensor devices are equipped to transmit health-related information to the NB-IoT cellular RAN, and, thereafter, the BS transmits to an internet cloud platform, where the health data would deliver to the remote healthcare centers.

Considering the capabilities of the NB-IoT technology, it guarantees to next-generation WBANs in HCM in terms of satisfying critical WBAN QoS requirements, along with high energy efficiency, long-range communications, the capability of connecting many sensor devices, and higher data reliability.

Table 1.5 shows the comparison between enhanced machine type communication (eMTC) and narrowband IoT (NB-IOT).

## 1.7 CLASSIFICATION OF 5G SMART HEALTHCARE

Figure 1.4 explains the classification of the upcoming 5G smart healthcare. The presented terminologies are based on the following parameters: data transmission methodologies, prerequisites, purposes, performance measures, and avenues.

## Health Care Monitoring Using WBAN & NB-IoT Communication

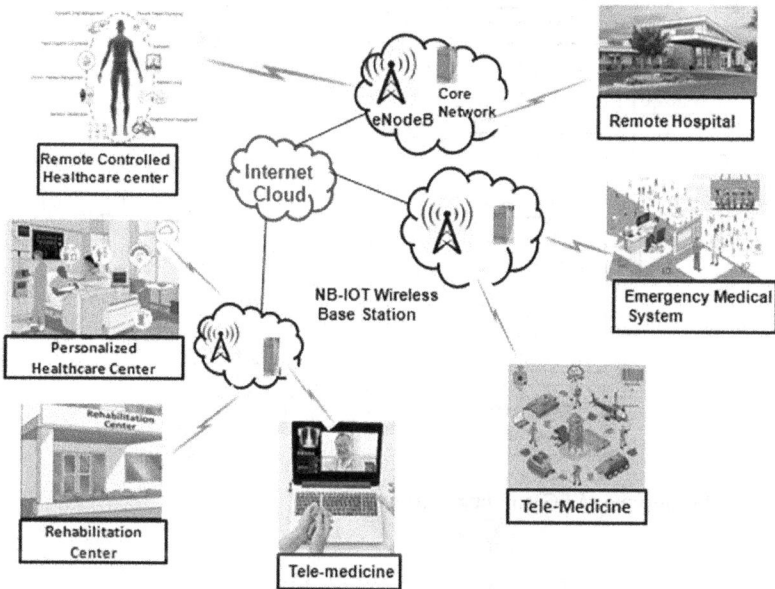

*Figure 1.3* NB-IoT communication for WBANs in HCM.

*Table 1.5* Technology comparison between eMTC and NB-IoT

| | Release 15 | | | | |
| --- | --- | --- | --- | --- | --- |
| | eMTC | | | NB-IoT | |
| | Cat. M1 | Car. M2 | Non BLUE in CE | Cat. NB1 | Cat. NB2 |
| Downlink Peak data rate | ~1 Mbps | ~4 Mbps | ~27 Mbps | | |
| Uplink peak data rate | ~3 or ~1 Mbps | ~7 Mbps | ~7 Mbps | | |
| UE receive bandwidth | 1.4 MHz | 5 MHz | 20 MHz | | |
| MCL | 164 dB | | | | |
| Maximum cell size | 100 km. | | | 300 ms in normal coverage area 8.3 s in extreme coverage | |
| Latency (Max. 10 s) | 200 ms in normal coverage 8.5 s in extreme coverage | | | 35.6 years in normal coverage 11.4 years in extreme coverage | |
| Battery life | 36.2 years in normal coverage 8.8 years in extreme coverage | | | | |
| Reliability | 90 to 99.9% | | | | |
| UE transmit power | 14/20/23 dBm | | | | |

Ref. Nokia solutions and network 2016

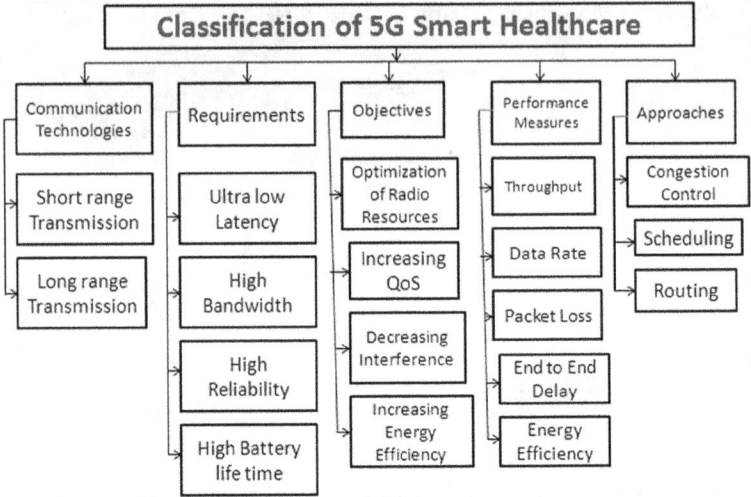

*Figure 1.4* Taxonomy of 5G smart healthcare.

## 1.8 DATA TRANSMISSION METHODOLOGIES FOR SMART HEALTHCARE

Smart healthcare is based on different short-range and long-range data transmission methodologies to transmit the data among devices and servers. Many short-distance wireless technologies include Wi-Fi, Bluetooth, ZigBee, and wireless metropolitan area network (WMAN) and WiMAX which are mainly used for small distance data transmission in BAN. Longer range data transmission technologies, like GSM, GPRS, 3G-WCDMA, 4G long-term evolution (LTE), and LTE-A are used for the transmission of data from local server to RAN in smart healthcare [31]. Moreover, LTE-machine type communication (LTE-M) is suggested to accomplish the requirement of IoT devices and sensors [32, 33] in wireless networks. In release 13, 3GPP requires additional enhancement of battery lifetime, device complexity, and coverage area.

In addition to the existing technologies and protocols, LoRa association systematizes the long range wide area network (LoRaWAN) protocol to reinforce smart healthcare operations to assure the intractability among different operators. In addition, SIGFOX is a compact radio band technology consisting of a star topology–based framework that provides a highly dynamic and adaptive global network for the smart healthcare applications with minimum power consumption. A comparative analysis of suggestive data transmission technologies is represented in Table 1.5.

## 1.8.1 Specifications of smart healthcare

- Ultralow latency
- High bandwidth
- Ultrahigh reliability
- High battery life time

## 1.8.2 Purposes of smart healthcare

1. **Utilization of resources:**
   Maximum utilization of resources is done to have low power/energy consummation while increasing the network capacity and lifetime. Resource optimization methods [34, 35] play a significant role in smart healthcare network based on 5G technology. A large number of sensors and IoT devices in smart healthcare generate a huge amount of data and utilize bandwidth and more capacity of the network. Network resource utilization must be able to guarantee maximum usage of system resources, to enhance network efficiency without considering additional hardware and software.

2. **Increasing QoS:**
   Quality of service (QoS) refers to the capability of the network to obtain broad bandwidth and regulate more network performance parameters such as bit error rate (BER), end-to-end latency, and uptime. QoS also comprises of regulating the network resources on high preference for a specified data (audio, video, and text files) in the network. The main objective is to prioritize the QoS of the network, which consists of low latency, high dedicated end-to-end bandwidth, jitter in a regulated way, and loss characteristics.

3. **Decreasing interference:**
   The approach of frequency reuse can be utilized in the smart healthcare system to obtain optimized resource allocation. In addition, user throughput and traffic capacity can be increased in the network. Hence, with the densification of the network and frequency reuse, there will be load sharing among MBS and local access networks which enhances network efficiency. Higher co-channel interference degrades QoS, user experience, and capacity reduction of healthcare system. Hence, efficient interference minimization methods such as absolute blank subframe (ABS), fractional frequency reuse (FFR), coordinated multipoint (CoMP), and dynamic power allocation methods need to be adopted.

4. **Increasing energy efficiency:**
   Energy efficiency is one of the main objectives for implementing smart healthcare network, because many sensors and IoT devices arc used for monitoring the data in real time and store in IoT cloud. Due to

densification of the APs, energy consumption of the network increases. Hence, to decrease cost of operation, the network entities should be functional with minimum energy expenditure. Though the capacity of the battery increases but it may not be sufficient to fulfill the user demands. Hence, energy-efficient methods are required to improve the lifetime of the sensors and devices used in the network.

### 1.8.3  List of parameters to enhance the performance

a. **Data rate:** It is the rate at which data is transmitted from source node to the destination node of the network [36].
b. **Throughput:** It is the number of packets transmitted per unit time. It is the measure of amount of time required to complete the assigned task in a specific time by the network.
c. **Packet loss ratio:** It is the amount of loss of packets during transfer of information from source node to the destination node of the network.
d. **End-to-end delay:** It is the total amount of time required for delivery of the data packet from source to destination across the entire network.
e. **Energy efficiency:** It is the amount of energy required by the source and destination node to transmit and receive data. Therefore, adequate routing and protocols are needed for enhancing energy efficiency.

### 1.8.4  Open concerns and claims of 5G smart healthcare using WBAN

The features, importance, challenges, and requirements for 5G smart healthcare are shown in Table 1.6.

### 1.8.5  Security challenges in WBAN

Consider the inter WBAN–based D2D communication between the sensors, where privacy and security of the medical data of individuals are highly essential. A robust security D2D data communication protocol must be used for medical health monitoring WBAN system.

Figure 1.5 shows the WBAN security model. The inter WBAN network can be established, where one node will act as server and other nodes will relay the information. Both way authentication and authorization should happen between the patient and the doctor to secure and maintain the confidentiality of the information. The network management entity will generate confidential key for each information exchange between the patron and the recipient for security.

Table 1.6 Features, importance, challenges, and requirements for 5G smart healthcare

| Features | Importance | Research challenges | Major requirements |
|---|---|---|---|
| Connectivity | Guaranteeing that IoT devices from different domains can communicate. | • How to collaborate and integrate massive number of sensors and IoT devices in a broad range during high mobility?<br>• How to manage resource allocation and manage accurately with low delay in ultra-dense network?<br>• How to regulate energy of IoT devices to achieve higher energy efficiency? | • Efficient use of resource blocks (RBs) and frequency channels for communication between the sensors and IoT devices.<br>• Smart usage of technology (i.e., LTE, LTE advanced [LTE-A], WiMAX, WLAN, etc.)<br>• Development of intelligent algorithms to connect and communicate large number of devices attached to the network.<br>• Development of clustering services to increase resource availability and support mixed workload. |
| Interoperability | Provides communication platform for IoT devices referring to different standards | • Associating devices for operator locked-in services. | • Globally, integrated and flexible architecture for IoT devices to incorporate and communicate (i.e., coordinated access point [CoAP] and IP). |
| Energy-efficient and cost-efficient communication | Provides smart healthcare application on large scale, if communication is of low cost | • How to extend IoT devices' battery life? | • Next-generation wireless communication and micro-electronics to deliver cost-efficient communication and prolonged battery life.<br>• Development of artificial intelligence–based routing protocols. |
| Big data | Enhancing performance of IoT network by processing effective information recognized from valid sources (i.e., analyzing patient data can minimize network congestion process) | • Requirement of tools to process huge amount of generated data and information<br>• Resourceful data acquisition and information in centralized manner. | • Centralized processing of big data center.<br>• Usage of IoT network resources in a secured manner. |
| Security | Secure environment (attack free) to deploy the services | • Integration and installation of cloud-based software's and hardware's both devices and network level in a secured way<br>• Early prediction of both inner and outer faults and threats.<br>• Data integrity between the devices with high security and minimum delay | • Finding the security threats and vulnerabilities of the network at different levels that work as initial points for various attacks. |

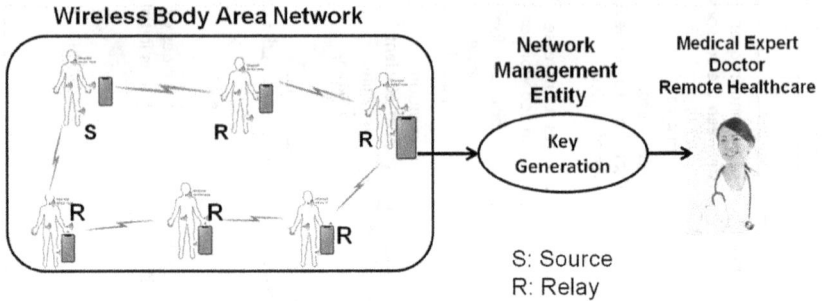

*Figure 1.5* WBAN security system model.

## 1.9 CONCLUSION

In this research work, we have presented a cloud-based continuous remote monitoring system for patients using WBAN and 5G technology. The network architecture of IoT-based 5G smart healthcare and the essentials to enable cloud-based healthcare is discussed. Then, LPWAN and comparison between different technologies, Narrowband IoT, comparison of 5G smart healthcare, different wireless technologies, necessities, and objectives of smart healthcare were discussed. The challenges related to smart healthcare include energy efficiency and authenticity of data transmission to remote healthcare centers. It attributes to the small distance of communication system associated with WBAN. To enhance energy efficiency, mainly the LPWAN devices are being used in smart healthcare which has longer battery life, medium data rate, and provides wide area coverage. It operates at a free-licensed ISM band at 2.4 GHz. The deployment cost for nonproprietary-based LPWAN Communication Systems (mainly for 5G technology) such as LTE-machine to machine, i.e., LTE-M1, extended coverage-GSM (EC-GSM), and NB-IoT is very less but it is able to support nearly 50,000 sensor devices in the network. The LPWAN architecture can be contemplated as a useful candidate for cloud-based remote HCM using WBAN systems in order to accomplish adequate data communications with high energy efficiency, ultrareliable, and low latency [37]. Because the WBAN carries health-related information, proper modulation technique should be used to carry more data per bandwidth. The modulation techniques must be reliable, energy efficient, and highly secure. Hence, proper encryption, authentication, and key agreement should be done which will make real-time signal processing faster with security.

## REFERENCES

[1] Series, M. (2015). IMT Vision–Framework and overall objectives of the future development of IMT for 2020 and beyond. Recommendation ITU, 2083, 0.

[2] Anand, R., & Chawla, P. (2020). Optimization of Inscribed Hexagonal Fractal Slotted Microstrip Antenna using Modified Lightning Attachment Procedure Optimization. *International Journal of Microwave and Wireless Technologies*, 12(6), 519–530.

[3] Chibber, A., Anand, R., & Arora, S. (2021, September). A Staircase Microstrip Patch Antenna for UWB Applications. In *2021 9th International Conference on Reliability, Infocom Technologies and Optimization (Trends and Future Directions) (ICRITO)* (pp. 1–5). IEEE.

[4] Chawla, P., & Anand, R. (2017). Micro-Switch Design and its Optimization using Pattern Search Algorithm for Applications in Reconfigurable Antenna. *Modern Antenna Systems*, 10, 189–210.

[5] Dahiya, A., Anand, R., Sindhwani, N., & Deshwal, D. (2021). Design and Construction of a Low Loss Substrate Integrated Waveguide (SIW) for S Band and C Band Applications. *MAPAN*, 36, 355–363.

[6] Arbia, D. B., Alam, M. M., Moullec, Y. L., & Hamida, E. B. (2017). Communication Challenges in On-Body and Body-to-Body Wearable Wireless Networks—A Connectivity Perspective. *Technologies*, 5(3), 43.

[7] Moradi, E., Koski, K., Ukkonen, L., Rahmat-Samii, Y., Björninen, T., & Sydänheimo, L. (2013, March). Embroidered RFID Tags in Body-Centric Communication. In *2013 International Workshop on Antenna Technology (iWAT)* (pp. 367–370). IEEE.

[8] Cao, Z., Chen, P., Ma, Z., Li, S., Gao, X., Wu, R. X., ... & Shi, Y. (2019). Near-Field Communication Sensors. *Sensors*, 19(18), 3947.

[9] Tufail, F., & Islam, M. H. (2009, April). Wearable Wireless Body Area Networks. In *2009 International Conference on Information Management and Engineering* (pp. 656–660). IEEE.

[10] Qi, J., Yang, P., Min, G., Amft, O., Dong, F., & Xu, L. (2017). Advanced Internet of Things for Personalised Healthcare Systems: A Survey. *Pervasive and Mobile Computing*, 41, 132–149.

[11] Islam, S. R., Kwak, D., Kabir, M. H., Hossain, M., & Kwak, K. S. (2015). The Internet of Things for Health Care: A Comprehensive Survey. *IEEE Access*, 3, 678–708.

[12] Baker, S. B., Xiang, W., & Atkinson, I. (2017). Internet of Things for Smart Healthcare: Technologies, Challenges, and Opportunities. *IEEE Access*, 5, 26521–26544.

[13] Mahmoud, M. M., Rodrigues, J. J., Ahmed, S. H., Shah, S. C., Al-Muhtadi, J. F., Korotaev, V. V., & De Albuquerque, V. H. C. (2018). Enabling Technologies on Cloud of Things for Smart Healthcare. *IEEE Access*, 6, 31950–31967.

[14] Dhanvijay, M. M., & Patil, S. C. (2019). Internet of Things: A Survey of Enabling Technologies in Healthcare and Its Applications. *Computer Networks*, 153, 113–131.

[15] Zhou, G., Li, Q., Li, J., Wu, Y., Lin, S., Lu, J., ... & Stankovic, J. A. (2011). Adaptive and Radio-Agnostic QoS for Body Sensor Networks. *ACM Transactions on Embedded Computing Systems (TECS)*, 10(4), 1–34.

[16] Tian, S., Yang, W., Le Grange, J. M., Wang, P., Huang, W., & Ye, Z. (2019). Smart Healthcare: Making Medical Care More Intelligent. *Global Health Journal*, 3(3), 62–65.

[17] Zeadally, S., Siddiqui, F., Baig, Z., & Ibrahim, A. (2019). Smart Healthcare: Challenges and Potential Solutions Using Internet of Things (IoT) and Big Data Analytics. *PSU Research Review*, 4(2), 149–168. https://doi.org/10.1108/PRR-08-2019-0027

[18] Mahashreveta Choudhary. Smart Healthcare for a healthy smart city. https://www.geospatialworld.net/blogs/smart-healthcare-for-a-healthy-smart-city/

[19] Sindhwani, N., & Singh, M. (2020). A Joint Optimization Based Sub-band Expediency Scheduling Technique for MIMO Communication System. *Wireless Personal Communications*, 115 (3), 2437–2455.

[20] Sindhwani, N., & Singh, M. (2016). FFOAS: Antenna Selection for MIMO Wireless Communication System using Firefly Optimization Algorithm and Scheduling. *International Journal of Wireless and Mobile Computing*, 10(1), 48–55.

[21] Singh, P., Raw, R. S., Khan, S. A., Mohammed, M. A., Aly, A. A., & Le, D. N. (2021). W-Geo R: Weighted Geographical Routing for VANET's Health Monitoring Applications in Urban Traffic Networks. *IEEE Access*, 10, 38850–38869.

[22] Fortino, G., Parisi, D., Pirrone, V., & Di Fatta, G. (2014). Body Cloud: A SaaS Approach for Community Body Sensor Networks. *Future Generation Computer Systems*, 35, 62–79.

[23] Mekki, K., Bajic, E., Chaxel, F., & Meyer, F. (2019). A Comparative Study of LPWAN Technologies for Large-Scale IoT Deployment. *ICT Express*, 5(1), 1–7.

[24] Anand, R., Sinha, A., Bhardwaj, A., & Sreeraj, A. (2018). Flawed Security of Social Network of Things. In *Handbook of Research on Network Forensics and Analysis Techniques* (pp. 65–86). IGI Global.

[25] Gupta, A., Srivastava, A., Anand, R., & Tomažič, T. (2020). Business Application Analytics and the Internet of Things: The Connecting Link. Inc. In *New Age Analytics* (pp. 249–273). Florida, FL: Apple Academic Press.

[26] Meelu, R., & Anand, R. (2010, November). Energy Efficiency of Cluster-based Routing Protocols used in Wireless Sensor Networks. In *AIP Conference Proceedings* (Vol. 1324, No. 1, pp. 109–113). American Institute of Physics.

[27] NB-IOT-Enabling new business opportunity. www.huawei.com/minisite/4-5g/img/NB-IOT.pdf

[28] Juneja, S., Juneja, A., & Anand, R. (2020). Healthcare 4.0-Digitizing Healthcare Using Big Data for Performance Improvisation. *Journal of Computational and Theoretical Nanoscience*, 17(9–10), 4408–4410.

[29] Anand S., Routray S. K. (2017) Issues and Challenges in Healthcare Narrowband IoT. In *Proceedings of the IEEE 2017 International Conference Inventive Communication and Computational Technologies (ICICCT)*, Coimbatore, India, March 2017

[30] Durand, T. G., Visagie, L., & Booysen, M. J. (2019). Evaluation of Next-Generation Low-Power Communication Technology to Replace GSM in IoT-Applications. *IET Communications*, 13(16), 2533–2540.

[31] Ramli, S. N., & Ahmad, R. (2011, December). Surveying the Wireless Body Area Network in the Realm of Wireless Communication. In *2011 7th International Conference on Information Assurance and Security (IAS)* (pp. 58–61). IEEE.

[32] Kohli, L., Saurabh, M., Bhatia, I., Sindhwani, N., & Vijh, M. (2021). Design and Development of Modular and Multifunctional UAV with Amphibious Landing. In *Processing and Surround Sense Module. Unmanned Aerial Vehicles for Internet of Things (IoT): Concepts, Techniques, and Applications*, 207.

[33] Kohli, L., Saurabh, M., Bhatia, I., Shekhawat, U. S., Vijh, M., & Sindhwani, N. (2021). Design and Development of Modular and Multifunctional UAV with Amphibious Landing Module. In *Data Driven Approach towards Disruptive Technologies: Proceedings of MIDAS 2020* (pp. 405–421). Singapore: Springer.

[34] Sindhwani, N., Bhamrah, M. S., Garg, A., & Kumar, D. (2017, July). Performance Analysis Of Particle Swarm Optimization and Genetic Algorithm in MIMO Systems. In *2017 8th International Conference on Computing, Communication and Networking Technologies (ICCCNT)* (pp. 1–6). IEEE.

[35] Sindhwani, N. (2017). Performance Analysis of Optimal Scheduling Based Firefly Algorithm in MIMO System. *Optimization*, 2(12), 19–26.

[36] Kirubasri, G., Sankar, S., Pandey, D., Pandey, B. K., Singh, H., & Anand, R. (2021, September). A Recent Survey on 6G Vehicular Technology, Applications and Challenges. In *2021 9th International Conference on Reliability, Infocom Technologies and Optimization (Trends and Future Directions)(ICRITO)* (pp. 1–5). IEEE.

[37] Juneja, S., Juneja, A., & Anand, R. (2019, April). Reliability Modeling for Embedded System Environment Compared To Available Software Reliability Growth Models. In *2019 International Conference on Automation, Computational and Technology Management (ICACTM)* (pp. 379–382). IEEE.

Chapter 2

# Information theory-based fuzzy logic optimization of medical data analytics during the COVID-19 pandemic

*Ridhima Mehta*

Jawaharlal Nehru University, New Delhi, India

## CONTENTS

## 2.1 INTRODUCTION

The most widespread chronic illnesses of heart failure and the ongoing pandemic of coronavirus disease are the main causes of death in the world nowadays. One of the most prevalent cardiovascular disorders have been considerably affected during the current outbreak of COVID-19 pandemic. Specifically, the face-to-face health expert consultancy at the hospitals and medical centers for providing healthcare services to critical patients at the initial stage has been curtailed and restricted to only the emergency situations. To implement better health monitoring system for cardiac patients through the severely ongoing global coronavirus syndrome, advanced artificial intelligence strategy incorporating the multivariable fuzzy decision-making is emerging as a potential scheme. Based on the natural language processing method, the flexible fuzzy logic technique [1, 2] can conveniently model arbitrarily complex nonlinear systems by representing the semantics of implicitly vague linguistic terms. It is capable of effective handling of the inherent data ambiguities through persuasive knowledge representation and automated information transformation processes. This learning methodology emerges as a key problem-solving strategy to derive precise conclusions from the approximate system information. This technique based on the algebraic framework of vagueness is predominantly robust because it does not require the specification of precise values of the system inputs and outputs. The computationally intelligent fuzzy logic approach is employed for modeling and assessing the performance of smart healthcare technology. This novel methodology of implementing the adaptive patient-centric healthcare service model with fewer medical facilities uses the efficient soft computing design structure.

The machine learning-based fuzzy logic reasoning based on the fuzzy set theory and partial membership concept was originally introduced by Lotfi A. Zadeh [3]. In this context, the imprecise and dynamic data is inherently modeled by the vague and qualitative expressions that cannot be directly correlated with any quantification like numerical values. Multiple-valued fuzzy logic architecture provides an effective scheme for handling the uncertain and ambiguous data formulation to optimize the large multivariate database analysis and the performance in disparate practical applications of the medical world. It is based on the acquisition and forwarding of the vital medical parameters associated with the specific patients' information to the concerned artificial intelligence expert with the medical background. This facilitates the virtual monitoring of the patients' health status through the knowledge of the certain medical health database of particular individuals for the optimal evaluation of the unseen COVID-19 cases suffering earlier from the serious heart ailments.

### 2.1.1 Motivation

The significant development of healthcare information technology and electronic infrastructure services is essential for assessing and reviewing the users' health status data from anywhere in this ongoing pandemic dissemination across the whole globe. According to the recent health statistics, the two widespread diseases of cardiac arrest and COVID-19 epidemics have emerged as the biggest causes of deaths worldwide. In particular, the current health conditions of the heart patients suffering simultaneously from the coronavirus disease can be evaluated through the smart medical systems based on fuzzy control architecture. This fuzzy logic-based healthcare monitoring model employs the optimization [4–6] of multiple physiological characteristics related to the considered two types of illnesses. A more reliable and accurate estimation of the risk factors associated with the prevailing health conditions of cardiovascular disease and COVID-19 patients can be observed through the sample real-time medical dataset. It is aimed at contributing the desired training reliability to the developed health system with improved precision performance. The simulation experiments are designed and implemented such that the proposed smart healthcare management system integrated with the data analytical structure accomplishes enhanced accuracy by substantiating through the information-theoretical and error prediction metrics.

## 2.1.2  Organization of the chapter

The remainder of this chapter is organized as follows. First, we introduce a survey of the related works in section 2.2. The proposed fuzzy design model is discussed in section 2.3. In section 2.4, we provide and analyze the simulation results for the developed healthcare protocol based on the fuzzy logic controller. Finally, the whole work is concluded in section 2.5 with the possible future research directions.

## 2.2  RELATED WORKS

Numerous research studies have been carried out in the recent past that focused on the performance analysis of generalized medical system model. For instance, the presented system architecture is designed with the wearable biosensors at the patient's end, Android handheld devices and the web-based application interface [7]. In this work, the instantaneous monitoring and treatment of cardiac patients is effectuated through the remote ubiquitous social networking system analyzing the critical heart data under the expert medical facilities. Common machine learning approaches including the support vector machines (SVM), artificial neural networks, and deep learning techniques [8] are employed to operationalize the speedy prognosis of chronic illness through the electronic medical health applications [9]. The healthcare data collection and processing, accompanied with the smart information security and privacy issues relating to the patient testing records is maintained for assessing the performance analysis of the developed system. The authors in Ref. [10] studied the association between the global COVID-19 pandemic and the cardiovascular disease from the medical service prospects. Detection of chronic heart disease based on the electrocardiogram (ECG) beat type tests is addressed using the SVM classification strategy [11]. These beat signals are mapped to the corresponding images, which are explored for the feature extraction phase, together with the deployment of linear, quadratic, cubic, and Gaussian kernel classifier functions. Real-time diagnosis of COVID-19 symptoms and the supervised treatment measures are implemented through the internet of things (IoTs) paradigm [12]. In this framework, the conglomeration of diversified machine learning algorithms incorporating the neural network, naïve bayes, k-nearest neighbor, decision table, etc. is applied on the concrete dataset for the enhanced accuracy prediction.

Dynamic spectrum assignment among the massive population of humans infected by the ongoing coronavirus pandemic is explored through the cognitive radio-based IoT network [13]. This structure supports the early diagnosis of critical medical conditions via remote clinical monitoring and test screening procedures for better prevention and restrained rapid spreading of the disease. The application of the Industry 4.0 technology for the advanced management and treatment of COVID-19 patients is conducted [14] to deal with the global healthcare emergency situation by the appropriate surveillance detection system. The proposed healthcare system model in Ref. [15] based on the IoT implementation technology enables the remote monitoring of patients through the autonomous assessment of various biological human health-related parameters. The authors in Ref. [16] developed a mathematical analysis framework together with the multidimensional machine learning approach for dealing with the spread of COVID-19 crises in smart cities environment equipped with the smart health security and infrastructure facilities around the globe. In Ref. [17], the authors explored the clinical decision support system and risk modeling estimation associated with the COVID-19 emergency situation for remote patient monitoring through the virtual consultation analyses and artificial intelligence strategies in Southern American regions. The IoT framework for fog-based real-time prediction of developing the infectious COVID-19 exposure risk is presented in Ref. [18]. The user health characteristics are assessed through the fuzzy computing paradigm by employing the distance tracking function among the individuals by means of short-range Bluetooth wireless interface. The telemedicine strategy is developed in Ref. [19] to provide medical treatment to the cardiovascular patients during lockdown enforcement in COVID-19 pandemic with limited in-hospital care and practical visits for the direct clinical assessment. Furthermore, the authors in Ref. [20] introduced the long-range ECG signal monitoring system in the dual temporal and frequency domain for detection of the cardiovascular disease risk factors on the basis of the integrated fog layer computing and deep learning techniques.

Moreover, another study conducted the cooperative distant patient health monitoring by employing the technique of end-to-end deep neural network for control and prevention of COVID-19 infection among the individuals [21]. This scheme utilized wireless body area network composed of the wearable embedded sensing devices for the collection of substantial body measurements consolidated with the fog and cloud computing architecture. Digital health controlling and management system is developed by Seshadri et al. [22] for the emerging COVID-19 outbreak to synchronously treat the cardiac and respiratory disorders through the wearable sensing devices. Preliminary prognosis and inspection of the asymptotic COVID-19 patients is implemented in Ref. [23] based on the smart IoT interlinked web information configuration by using sensors and actuators. In a similar way, Valsalan et al. [24] proposed a distant patients' health status evaluation scheme by employing the IoT database server infrastructure and the application of the microcontroller sensing devices. These sensors are designed to measure the body temperature, pulse rate, and room humidity parameters with the rapid emergence and subsequent dealing with the novel coronavirus disease.

More recently, the spread of epidemic COVID-19 trend and risk evaluation of the community transmission in Ireland is examined in Ref. [25] using the medical data hub for the hospitalized surveillance system. Cognitive computing and deep learning techniques are applied to evaluate the cardiac abnormality conditions and health status prediction during the progressive worldwide COVID-19 pandemic [26]. For this, the advanced drug medication and enhanced proficiency of the healthcare personnels are established through the complex system of artificial intelligence methodology. Work in Ref. [27] reviewed the heart monitoring technologies through the machine learning-based biosignal detection system with multiple modalities. In this context, technical and remote medical impediments related to crucial personal health information of reprocurement, security, and privacy issues are determined to devise the scalable cardiovascular observational tools. The body of work in Ref. [28] identified the emergent area of optimal patient care and management in critical cardiac illness of heart failure through the error-prone wearable sensing technology, including the global positioning system (GPS), barometers, and heart rate and rhythm sensor devices. The authors in Ref. [29] discussed the patient-oriented home monitoring system for the continuous cardiac disease management in the current era of elevated COVID-19 mortality cases via the implantable medical devices.

To this end, the current study is aimed at analyzing the proposed healthcare system under the diverse human physical conditions based on fuzzy logic theory for enhancing the accuracy and reliability of the developed adaptive model on the subsequent unseen medical diagnosis data. The presented mathematical system model employs fuzzy multiple-attribute decision-making incorporated in the fuzzy inference control unit. Because these attributes characterizing the physiological symptoms and states of the person's general health typically have distinctive units and range of values, fuzzy logic is trivially adopted to consider their simultaneous effect on the patient's health assessment and associated risk estimation. The fuzzy logic modeling captures the human expert knowledge and real-world experience by specifying a predefined list of fuzzy control rules determining the dynamic behavior of the complex health monitoring [30]. Nonlinear and time-varying fuzzy logic systems with the underlying inconstancy apply these linguistic fuzzy specification rules with synchronous execution to identify the relationship between the input and the output fuzzy variables [31]. Such rule-based fuzzy methodology representing the subjective human ideas is employed to compute the updated and optimized parameter values for the employed output fuzzy variables through the uncertain reasoning mechanism. The extensive simulation experiments for performance efficiency of the proposed computationally intelligent smart healthcare system are implemented and validated using the MATLAB Fuzzy Logic Toolbox simulator.

## 2.3 PROPOSED FUZZY LOGIC SYSTEM

In the proposed work, the design of fuzzy logic controller is aimed at dynamically computing the output fuzzy variables with adaptive parameter setting technique. The key components of a generic fuzzy logic system include the fuzzification module, the knowledge rule database, the fuzzy inference engine, and the defuzzification module [32]. The fuzzification interface transforms the space of crisp inputs into the analogous fuzzy values through the input membership functions that are fed into the core inference unit. The knowledge rule-base module executed using the human expertise experience or autonomic information generation comprises of the linguistic control rules stipulating the behavior of the system. These rules are designed and implemented using the membership functions of the fuzzy sets and the numerical input–output relationship necessary for the MIMO decision-making procedure. The inference engine unit encompassing the knowledge database and the fuzzy reasoning mechanism deploys the linguistic rule-base for the deduction operation on the specified rules to generate the corresponding fuzzy outputs. Subsequently, these fuzzy outputs are applied to the defuzzification interface, which performs the inverse operation of fuzzification component by converting the fuzzy output values back into the space of crisp control values. The fuzzification and defuzzification modules [33, 34] correspond to the coding and decoding of the healthcare data records comprising of the patients' subjective symptoms and the generalized physical fitness conditions.

Figure 2.1 represents the general architecture model of the proposed fuzzy logic-based healthcare system protocol. This scheme employs five fuzzy input parameters, viz., blood oxygen level, body temperature, serum triglycerides, systolic blood pressure, and age. The input variable of blood oxygen level is classified into hypoxemia (lower than normal oxygen level), normal, and hyperoxemia (surplus supply of oxygen to the body organs and cells causing oxygen toxicity in each tissue). The body temperature is measured to be normal and high fever conditions, whereas the age parameter is typically categorized into youth, adult, and seniors. Likewise, the input dimension of the

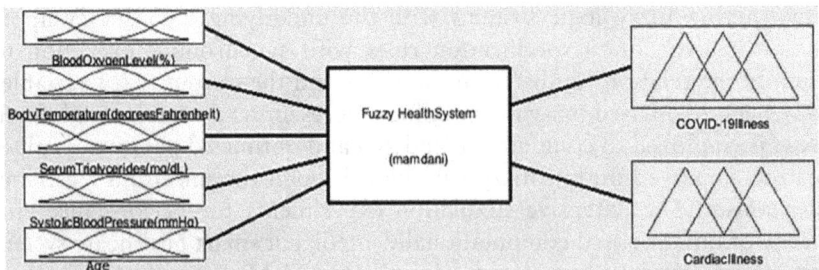

*Figure 2.1* Basic architecture of the proposed fuzzy logic-based healthcare system.

serum triglycerides fat in the blood elevating the risk of heart attack is designated by normal, high, and very high linguistic labels. Finally, the systolic blood pressure input variable assessing the amount of force exerted against the walls of the cardiovascular arteries during each heart beat is labeled according to the normal and hypertension (high blood pressure in circulation of the blood through the heart pumping vessels) categories. There have been various optimization techniques designed so far [35–39]. The two output variables associated with the presented fuzzy optimization technique implementing the medical data analysis include the most prevalent disease risks associated with the COVID-19 and cardiac illness patients. Each of these attributes is classified into low, moderate, high, and very high-risk factors concerning the two chronic life-threatening ailments. The values of these fuzzy output parameters are estimated and analyzed using the fuzzy inference system (FIS) editor execution in the MATLAB simulator. Disparate categories of the linguistic terms for each of the input and output fuzzy variables are employed to implement the fuzzification phase of the fuzzy control procedure. This categorization enables the qualitative interpretation of the information usage and the subjective formulation of the expert knowledge database.

Figures 2.2 and 2.3 graphically represent the fuzzy membership functions for the above-deployed input and output attributes assessing the health status of the persons suffering from the chronic disease conditions. These functions are elucidated by the widely applied triangular, trapezoidal, Gaussian, Gaussian combination, and generalized bell-shaped membership curves. The interrelation among the input and output variables is illustrated in Table 2.1. For instance, the fuzzy output of COVID-19 illness is determined by the three inputs of blood oxygen level, human body temperature, and age. The second fuzzy output of cardiac disease risk depends on the input variables of serum triglycerides, systolic blood pressure, and age. Table 2.2 enumerates the various linguistic labels corresponding to the deployed fuzzy input and output variables, together with their associated membership functions and the analogous fuzzy numbers.

The characteristic membership functions deployed in the fuzzification and defuzzification phases of the fuzzy control system are represented by the graphical structures that certainly categorize the fuzzy input and output variables, respectively. These indicator functions are mathematically formulated as shown in the generic Equations (2.1)–(2.4). These membership functions are specified for a vector $\chi$ and regulated by the scalar parameters $\alpha_1$, $\alpha_2, \alpha_3, \alpha_4$, such that $\alpha_1 < \alpha_2 < \alpha_3 < \alpha_4$. Here, $\chi$ is the vector of numerical input variables for which the related membership values are computed using the suitable membership function. Triangular and trapezoidal fuzzy sets belonging to the linear membership functions and nonsmooth points of intersection are specified using three $(\alpha_1, \alpha_2, \alpha_3)$ and four $(\alpha_1, \alpha_2, \alpha_3, \alpha_4)$ parameters, respectively. The three parameters determining the triangular membership function denote the lower limit, peak, and upper limit specifications of the graphical curve. For the trapezoidal membership function, the stated four

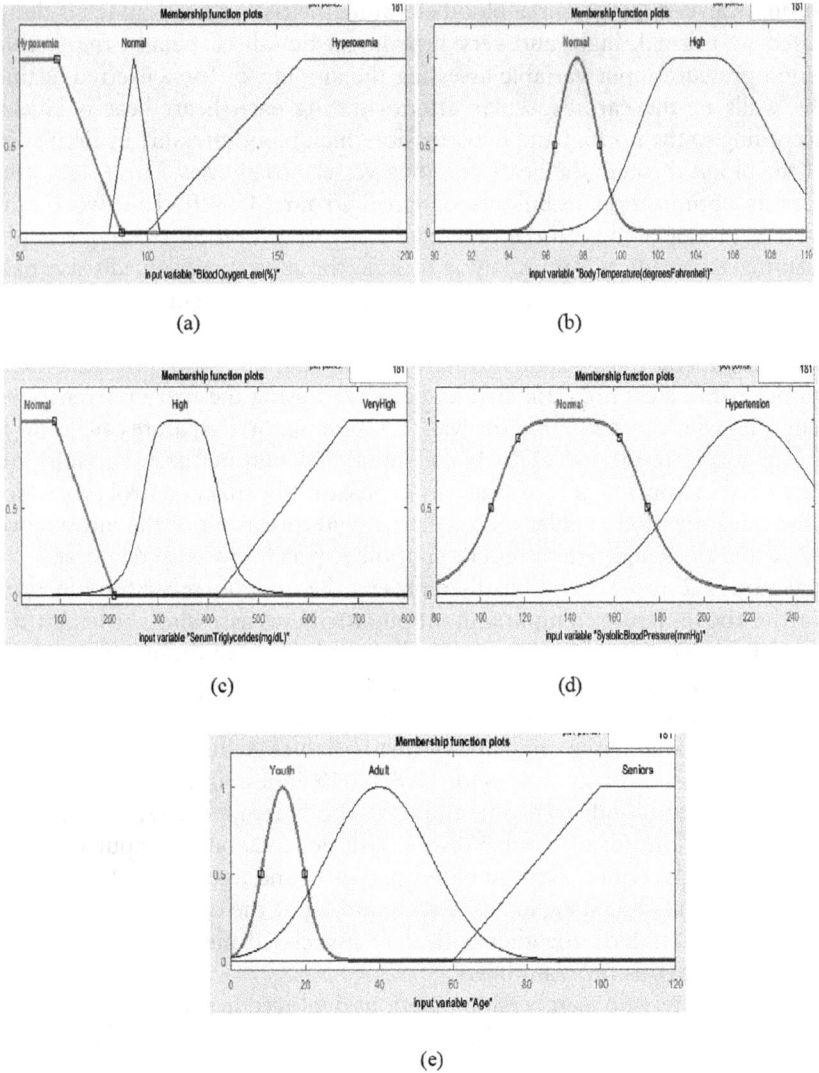

(a)

(b)

(c)

(d)

(e)

Figure 2.2 Fuzzy membership functions associated with the five input variables of (a) blood oxygen level, (b) body temperature, (c) serum triglycerides, (d) systolic blood pressure, and (e) age.

parameters demonstrating the trapezoidal curve relatively describe the lower limit, lower support limit, upper support limit, and upper limit of the trapezoid. The triangular membership function can be explicated as a special instance of the trapezoidal one. In addition, the nonlinear generalized bell-shaped membership function defined in Equation (2.3) is described in terms of the adaptable parameters of the breadth $\alpha_1$, the center $\alpha_3$, and the non-negative parameter $\alpha_2$ modulating the slope of this particular distribution.

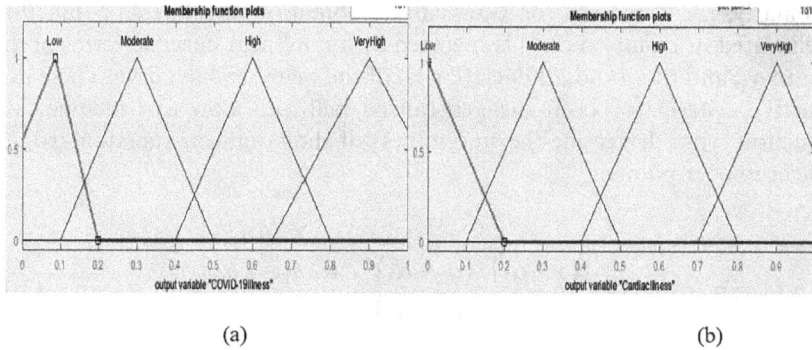

(a)

(b)

*Figure 2.3* Fuzzy membership functions associated with the output variables of (a) COVID-19 illness and (b) cardiac illness.

*Table 2.1* Relationship between input and output variables

| Output variable | Input variables |
|---|---|
| COVID-19 illness | Blood oxygen level, body temperature, age |
| Cardiac illness | Serum triglycerides, systolic blood pressure, age |

*Table 2.2* Fuzzy linguistic terms and their corresponding membership functions and fuzzy numbers for different input and output variables

| Variable | Linguistic term | Membership function | Fuzzy numbers |
|---|---|---|---|
| Blood oxygen level | Hypoxemia | Trapezoidal | [5 35 65 90] |
|  | Normal | Triangular | [85 95 105] |
|  | Hyperoxemia | Trapezoidal | [100 160 220 250] |
| Body temperature | Normal | Gaussian | [1.032 97.7] |
|  | High | Gaussian combination | [2 103.03 2.8 105.03] |
| Serum triglycerides | Normal | Trapezoidal | [-20 0 90 210] |
|  | High | Generalized bell-shaped | [80 2.5 345] |
|  | Very high | Trapezoidal | [420 680 920 1200] |
| Systolic blood pressure | Normal | Generalized bell-shaped | [35 2.5 140] |
|  | Hypertension | Gaussian | [30 220] |
| Age | Youth | Gaussian | [5 14] |
|  | Adult | Gaussian | [14 40] |
|  | Seniors | Trapezoidal | [60 100 150 195] |
| COVID-19 illness (output) | Low | Triangular | [-0.104 0.08597 0.2] |
|  | Moderate | Triangular | [0.1 0.3 0.5] |
|  | High | Triangular | [0.4 0.6 0.8] |
|  | Very high | Triangular | [0.65 0.9 1.15] |
| Cardiac illness (output) | Low | Triangular | [-0.2 0 0.2] |
|  | Moderate | Triangular | [0.1 0.3 0.5] |
|  | High | Triangular | [0.4 0.6 0.8] |
|  | Very high | Triangular | [0.7 0.9 1.1] |

Similarly, the Gaussian (or Gaussian combination) membership function delineated in Equation (2.4) is specified by a nonlinear curve in terms of the mean $\alpha_1$, and the standard deviation $\alpha_2$ of the membership curve. These distinctive criteria for both the generalized bell and Gaussian membership function types determine the smoothness of the nonlinear function around the crossover points.

$$f\left(\chi;\alpha_1,\alpha_2,\alpha_3\right)=\begin{cases} 0 & \chi \leq \alpha_1 \\ (\chi-\alpha_1)/(\alpha_2-\alpha_1) & \alpha_1 \leq \chi \leq \alpha_2 \\ (\alpha_3-\chi)/(\alpha_3-\alpha_2) & \alpha_2 \leq \chi \leq \alpha_3 \\ 0 & \alpha_3 \leq \chi \end{cases} \tag{2.1}$$

$$f\left(\chi;\alpha_1,\alpha_2,\alpha_3,\alpha_4\right)=\begin{cases} 0 & \chi \leq \alpha_1 \\ (\chi-\alpha_1)/(\alpha_2-\alpha_1) & \alpha_1 \leq \chi \leq \alpha_2 \\ 1 & \alpha_2 \leq \chi \leq \alpha_3 \\ (\alpha_4-\chi)/(\alpha_4-\alpha_3) & \alpha_3 \leq \chi \leq \alpha_4 \\ 0 & \alpha_4 \leq \chi \end{cases} \tag{2.2}$$

$$f\left(\chi;\alpha_1,\alpha_2,\alpha_3\right)=\frac{1}{1+\left|\dfrac{\chi-\alpha_3}{\alpha_1}\right|^{2\alpha_2}} \tag{2.3}$$

$$f\left(\chi;\alpha_1,\alpha_2\right)=e^{\frac{-(\chi-\alpha_1)^2}{2\alpha_2^2}} \tag{2.4}$$

In addition, in spite of several different methods of defuzzification available in the literature, our model uses the most commonly employed center of mass or centroid approach of defuzzification. In this scheme, the overall crisp control action is computed such that the quantifiable defuzzified output value $\delta^\bullet$ in crisp logic is expressed as follows:

$$\delta^\bullet=\frac{\displaystyle\int_{\delta^{\min}}^{\delta^{\max}} f\left(\delta\right)*\delta\, d\delta}{\displaystyle\int_{\delta^{\min}}^{\delta^{\max}} f\left(\delta\right) d\delta} \tag{2.5}$$

This defuzzification technique discretely evaluates the optimal point representing the center of gravity for the considered area under the curve to an arbitrary accuracy. It exhibits the essential property of continuous data distribution, making it appropriate for the efficient design of adaptive fuzzy controller. The defuzzified value is the x-coordinate of the centroid of the fuzzy set $f$ defined over the universe of discourse $\delta$ of the fuzzy output variables. Here, the denominator $\int_{\delta^{\min}}^{\delta^{\max}} f(\delta)d\delta$ denotes the area of the region bounded by the aggregated membership curve over the interval $(\delta^{\min}, \delta^{\max})$. The fuzzy inference strategy exploited in this analytical approach is Mamdani's model. This inference technique incorporates the decision-making methodology with respect to parameter classification, rules specification, and synchronous intelligent data-processing format. In the direct Mamdani fuzzy reasoning system, the output variables are represented by fuzzy sets, which subsequently require defuzzification to convert these fuzzy output variables obtained by the inference engine back into the space of analogous precise output variables. This approach used for modeling the proposed system through the scale transformation of the fuzzy inputs to the associated fuzzy output set is implemented in the Fuzzy Logic Toolbox [40].

Furthermore, we assume that $N = \{n_1, n_2, n_3, ..., n_i\}$ is the vector comprising of the total number of fuzzy input variables, with each variable labeled relatively by $\Lambda = \{\lambda_1, \lambda_2, \lambda_3, ..., \lambda_i\}$ linguistic values' vector. Then, if $o$ is the overall number of fuzzy output variables, the average-case complexity of the knowledge rule-base is given by the expression $\Omega\left(\sum_o \Lambda^N\right)$. In the developed fuzzy logic algorithm for health monitoring system applications, there are five fuzzy input variables, each with $\{3, 2, 3, 2, 3\}$ linguistic terms. This indicates that there are $3 * 2 * 3$ combinations of rules for each of the COVID-19 illness and cardiac illness output variables, contributing a total of 36 fuzzy logical rules. These linguistic fuzzy inference rules that provide a basis for the approximate reasoning are shown in Table 2.3, where each row is used to map the certain combination of the specific fuzzy input variables to the corresponding fuzzy output variable. This rule-base is acquired from the cognition of expert experience and facilitates the simulation of the human-like decision-making and reasoning process of the flexible fuzzy controller. The performance of the fuzzy control system is particularly affected by the proper design and selection of fuzzy production rules and membership functions.

## 2.4 SIMULATION RESULTS AND DISCUSSION

In this section, the performance parameters for the given fuzzy system are dynamically estimated through the various simulation experiments and rigorous assessments. In our simulation analysis, the performance evaluation of the proposed fuzzy-based health model is implemented using the MATLAB simulation software. The rule-viewer implementation comprising of the 36 fuzzy control rules for the proposed FIS is demonstrated in Figure 2.4. The particular screenshot of the rule-explorer window can be outlined as follows: for the given system inputs, blood oxygen level = 109%, body temperature = 98.2 Fahrenheit, serum triglycerides = 480 mg/dL, systolic

Table 2.3 Fuzzy logic inference rules for the proposed healthcare model

| Rule No. | Oxygen level | Body temperature | Serum triglycerides | Blood pressure | Age | COVID-19 illness | Cardiac illness |
|---|---|---|---|---|---|---|---|
| 1 | Hypoxemia | Normal | — | — | Youth | High | — |
| 2 | Hypoxemia | Normal | — | — | Adult | Moderate | — |
| 3 | Hypoxemia | Normal | — | — | Seniors | High | — |
| 4 | Hypoxemia | High | — | — | Youth | High | — |
| 5 | Hypoxemia | High | — | — | Adult | High | — |
| 6 | Hypoxemia | High | — | — | Seniors | Very high | — |
| 7 | Normal | Normal | — | — | Youth | Low | — |
| 8 | Normal | Normal | — | — | Adult | Low | — |
| 9 | Normal | Normal | — | — | Seniors | Low | — |
| 10 | Normal | High | — | — | Youth | Moderate | — |
| 11 | Normal | High | — | — | Adult | Low | — |
| 12 | Normal | High | — | — | Seniors | High | — |
| 13 | Hyperoxemia | Normal | — | — | Youth | Moderate | — |
| 14 | Hyperoxemia | Normal | — | — | Adult | Moderate | — |
| 15 | Hyperoxemia | Normal | — | — | Seniors | High | — |
| 16 | Hyperoxemia | High | — | — | Youth | High | — |
| 17 | Hyperoxemia | High | — | — | Adult | Moderate | — |
| 18 | Hyperoxemia | High | — | — | Seniors | Very high | — |
| 19 | — | — | Normal | Normal | Youth | — | Low |
| 20 | — | — | Normal | Normal | Adult | — | Low |
| 21 | — | — | Normal | Normal | Seniors | — | Moderate |
| 22 | — | — | Normal | Hypertension | Youth | — | Moderate |
| 23 | — | — | Normal | Hypertension | Adult | — | Moderate |

| | | | | | | | |
|---|---|---|---|---|---|---|---|
| 24 | — | — | Normal | Hypertension | Seniors | — | High |
| 25 | — | — | High | Normal | Youth | — | Moderate |
| 26 | — | — | High | Normal | Adult | — | High |
| 27 | — | — | High | Normal | Seniors | — | Very high |
| 28 | — | — | High | Hypertension | Youth | — | High |
| 29 | — | — | High | Hypertension | Adult | — | High |
| 30 | — | — | High | Hypertension | Seniors | — | Very high |
| 31 | — | — | Very High | Normal | Youth | — | Moderate |
| 32 | — | — | Very High | Normal | Adult | — | High |
| 33 | — | — | Very High | Normal | Seniors | — | Very high |
| 34 | — | — | Very High | Hypertension | Youth | — | Very high |
| 35 | — | — | Very High | Hypertension | Adult | — | Very high |
| 36 | — | — | Very High | Hypertension | Seniors | — | Very high |

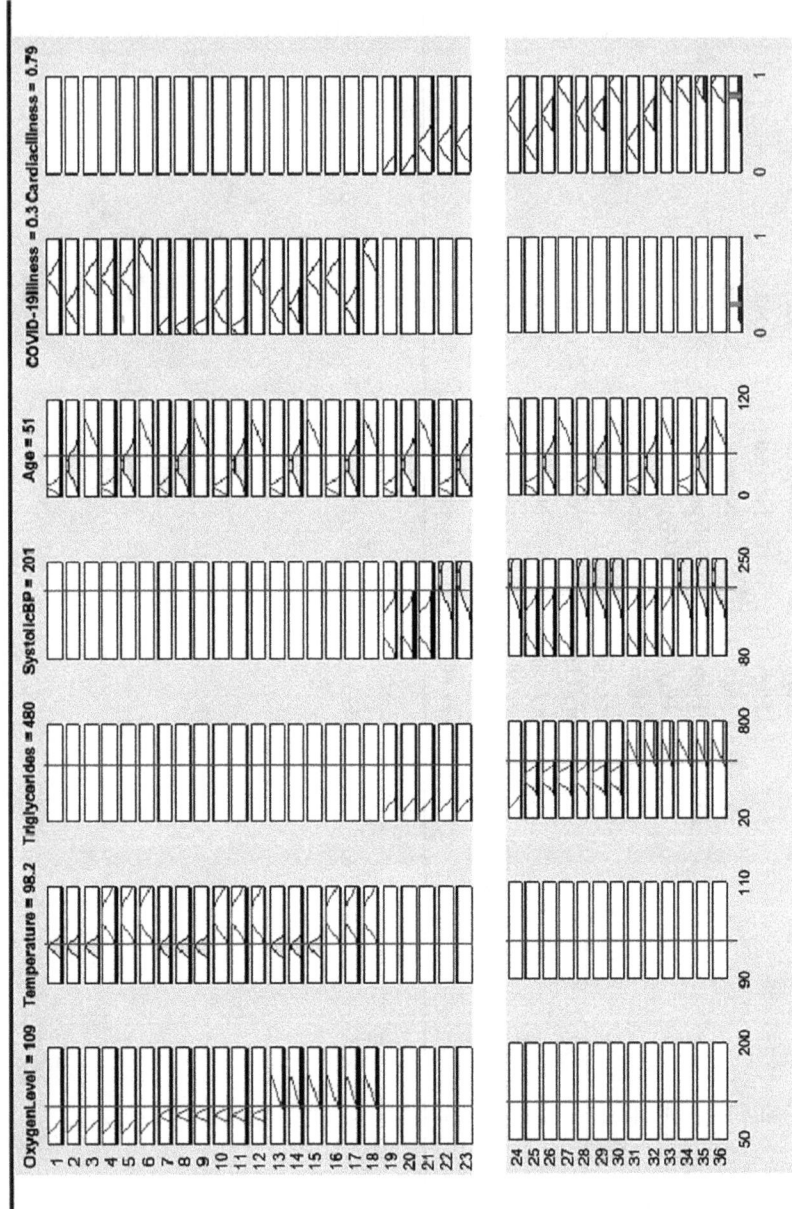

*Figure 2.4* Fuzzy inference rule-viewer in Fuzzy Logic Toolbox.

blood pressure = 201 mmHg, and age = 51, and then the corresponding system outputs, COVID-19 illness risk probability = 0.3 and cardiac illness risk probability = 0.79. Moreover, Figure 2.5 shows the three-dimensional decision control surfaces for the two fuzzy outputs of the COVID-19 illness and cardiac illness illustrating the dependency correlation between the employed fuzzy input and output variables.

The designed fuzzy healthcare system model is trained with a sample medical dataset corresponding to the particular diagnostic record of the heart patients' health status suffering from the current COVID-19 pandemic. This data modeling framework is corroborated by varying the size of medical data informatics from 1 to 25. The surveyed health data samples [41] related to the human heart functioning concatenated with the specific COVID-19 symptoms comprising the real-time data simulated over a given period are exemplified in Table 2.4. This data collection instance constituting the medicative analytical health outcomes in terms of the prevalence of chronic risk factors is used to build a model for assessing the system performance accuracy on the consecutive unknown clinical data. Figure 2.6 depicts the actual and the fuzzy predicted values of COVID-19 risk factor metric for each dataset instance. On an average, the risk level associated with the COVID-19 disease evaluated using the proposed fuzzy model is 13.66% lower than the conventional modeling mechanism. Likewise, the histogram indicating the estimated and the corresponding measured values of the cardiac disease risk output is plotted in Figure 2.7. It can be computed that the presented optimal health model implemented with the given medical database exhibits 10.93% higher cardiac failure risk compared with the standard technique.

In Figure 2.8, the median absolute deviation is graphically represented as a function of the increasing number of data instances assessed for a group of COVID-19 patients with preexisting cardiovascular disease. For the given sample clinical dataset $\Psi$ with each individual data instance denoted by $\Psi_k$, the median absolute deviation metric is measured as given in the Equations (2.6) and (2.7). This robust residual statistical measure in our proposed heuristic optimization model for COVID-19 illness fuzzy output is higher by a factor of 1.0987 compared with the nonfuzzy approach. In the same way, cardiac illness output through the fuzzy computation technique demonstrates 2.586 increased proportion of the average median absolute deviation metric.

$$\text{Median Absolute Deviation} = \text{Median}\left( \left| \Psi_k - \acute{\Psi} \right| \right) \tag{2.6}$$

$$\acute{\Psi} = \text{Median}(\Psi) \tag{2.7}$$

Furthermore, we evaluate the performance of the proposed fuzzy-based health monitoring model using various accuracy metrics. These include the

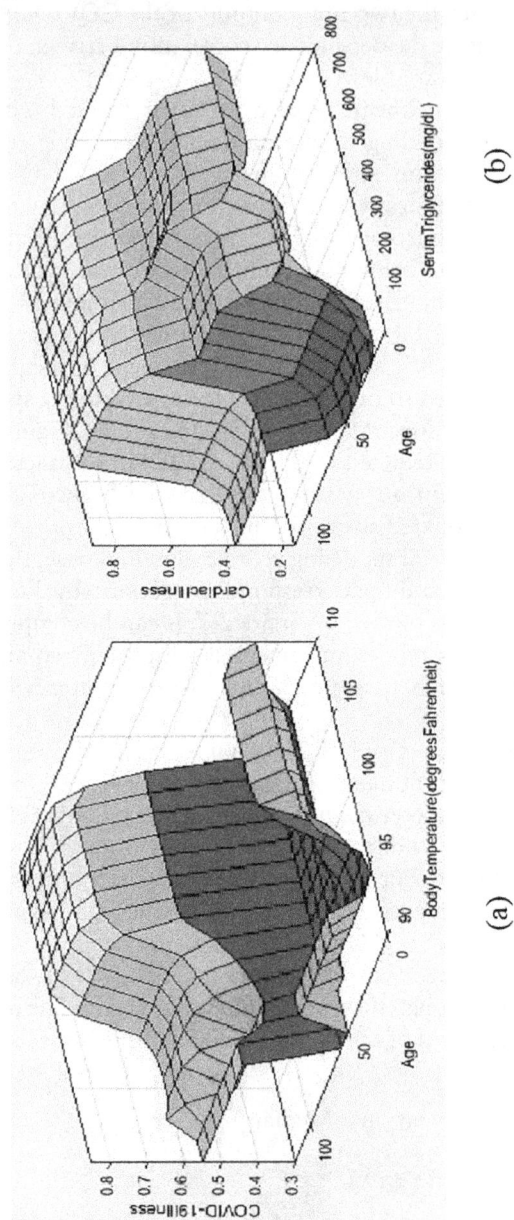

*Figure 2.5* Three-dimensional decision surface control viewer for (a) COVID-19 illness and (b) cardiac illness outputs of the proposed fuzzy inference system.

Table 2.4 Sample dataset for accuracy assessment of the proposed smart health model

| Rule no. | Blood oxygen level | Body temperature | Serum triglycerides | Systolic blood pressure | Age | Actual COVID-19 illness | Predicted COVID-19 illness | Actual cardiac illness | Predicted cardiac illness |
|---|---|---|---|---|---|---|---|---|---|
| 1 | 98.1 | 98.2 | 200 | 145 | 62 | 0.4157 | 0.211 | 0.376 | 0.452 |
| 2 | 89.2 | 99.1 | 224 | 137 | 44 | 0.361 | 0.174 | 0.321 | 0.6 |
| 3 | 80.2 | 97.6 | 445 | 150 | 33 | 0.2854 | 0.32 | 0.4105 | 0.64 |
| 4 | 95.9 | 101 | 480 | 122 | 65.4 | 0.467 | 0.382 | 0.4606 | 0.687 |
| 5 | 123 | 97.6 | 247 | 147 | 31.3 | 0.3758 | 0.302 | 0.3153 | 0.597 |
| 6 | 104.9 | 98.5 | 153.9 | 134.6 | 60 | 0.4303 | 0.287 | 0.3309 | 0.131 |
| 7 | 80.2 | 100 | 340.1 | 192.9 | 29.5 | 0.3157 | 0.535 | 0.4401 | 0.595 |
| 8 | 125 | 98.2 | 154 | 170.1 | 27.8 | 0.3805 | 0.317 | 0.31 | 0.213 |
| 9 | 109.3 | 97.01 | 188.8 | 162.5 | 15.2 | 0.2908 | 0.319 | 0.276 | 0.28 |
| 10 | 100.4 | 98.5 | 119 | 220.8 | 26 | 0.3258 | 0.139 | 0.3906 | 0.301 |
| 11 | 75.75 | 97.9 | 177.2 | 192.9 | 34.9 | 0.2858 | 0.322 | 0.38549 | 0.293 |
| 12 | 64.6 | 99.7 | 153.9 | 180.2 | 52.8 | 0.3407 | 0.485 | 0.4 | 0.248 |
| 13 | 62.3 | 101.5 | 188.8 | 192.9 | 17 | 0.266 | 0.599 | 0.3407 | 0.303 |
| 14 | 69.03 | 98.5 | 142.2 | 167.5 | 40.3 | 0.2959 | 0.338 | 0.3357 | 0.193 |
| 15 | 78 | 98.8 | 165.5 | 180.2 | 33 | 0.3 | 0.361 | 0.3503 | 0.248 |
| 16 | 91.4 | 99.4 | 130.6 | 172.6 | 29.5 | 0.3306 | 0.102 | 0.3107 | 0.202 |
| 17 | 95.9 | 100.9 | 200.4 | 192.9 | 27.8 | 0.3608 | 0.0996 | 0.37568 | 0.353 |
| 18 | 142.9 | 99.1 | 456.6 | 152.3 | 58.2 | 0.5197 | 0.3 | 0.49 | 0.666 |
| 19 | 165.3 | 98.8 | 258.7 | 159.9 | 20.6 | 0.46 | 0.366 | 0.3158 | 0.446 |
| 20 | 118.3 | 97.9 | 142.2 | 142.2 | 8.06 | 0.3058 | 0.334 | 0.1965 | 0.124 |
| 21 | 107.1 | 99.4 | 188.8 | 154.9 | 31.3 | 0.3706 | 0.306 | 0.306 | 0.268 |
| 22 | 95.9 | 102.1 | 165.5 | 144.7 | 34.9 | 0.4006 | 0.0808 | 0.2859 | 0.159 |
| 23 | 78 | 100.6 | 223.7 | 129.5 | 17 | 0.286 | 0.587 | 0.2313 | 0.45 |
| 24 | 89.2 | 103 | 281.9 | 139.6 | 26 | 0.376 | 0.183 | 0.301 | 0.568 |
| 25 | 195.3 | 97.01 | 538.1 | 162.5 | 70.7 | 0.45847 | 0.502 | 0.5797 | 0.785 |

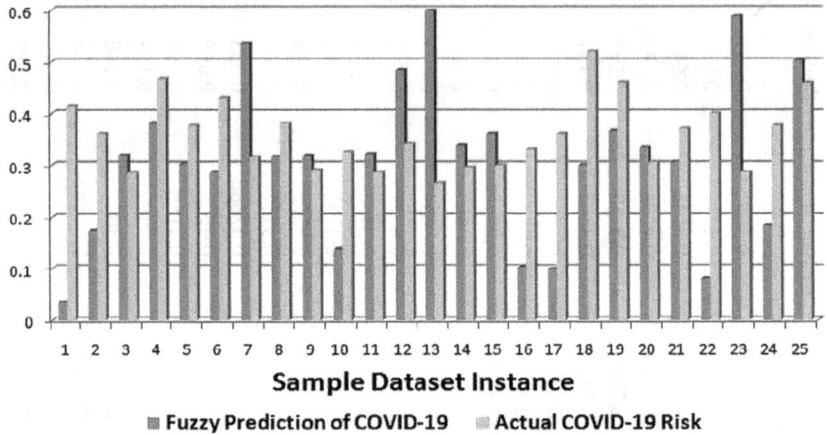

Figure 2.6 Fuzzy predicted and actual values of COVID-19 risk factor for each dataset instance.

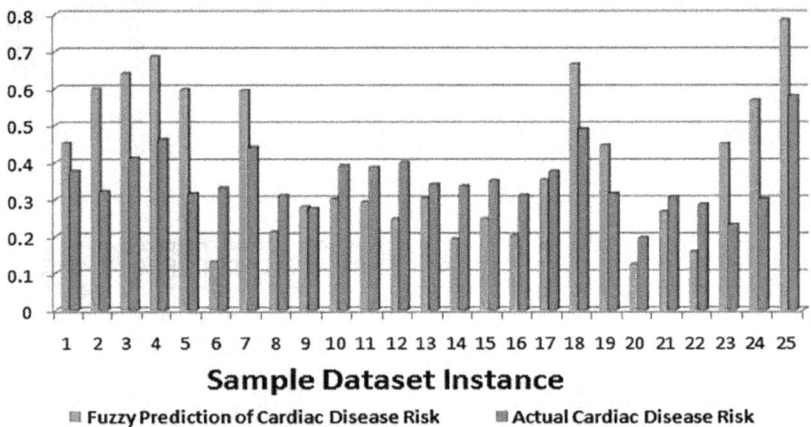

Figure 2.7 Fuzzy predicted and actual values of cardiac disease risk factor for each dataset instance.

mean gamma deviance, R-squared, Chi-square, and Pearson correlation coefficient statistics. These diverse precision assessment parameters are mathematically expressed as given in the respective Equations (2.8)–(2.11). Here, $\tau$ represents the total number of dataset instances considered for the presented model analysis and verification, $\Psi_k$ is the actual output value of the $k$-th data instance, $\ddot{\Psi}_k$ is the corresponding fuzzified prediction value of the output estimated using the developed model, $\tilde{\Psi}$ is the mean of the observed values acquired via the standard data analysis scheme, and $\ddot{\tilde{\Psi}}$ is the mean of the fuzzy prediction values retrieved through the simulation experiments. Figure 2.9 shows the evolution of the measured mean gamma

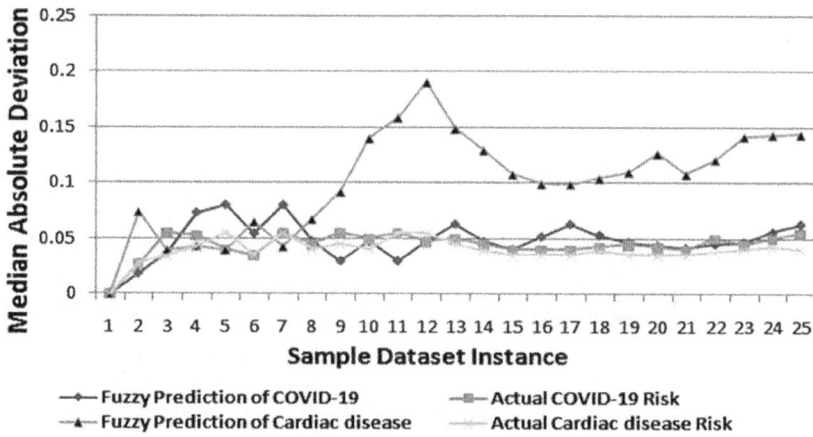

*Figure 2.8* Evolution of median absolute deviation with the number of sample values for the fuzzy estimation and observed values of the two fuzzy outputs.

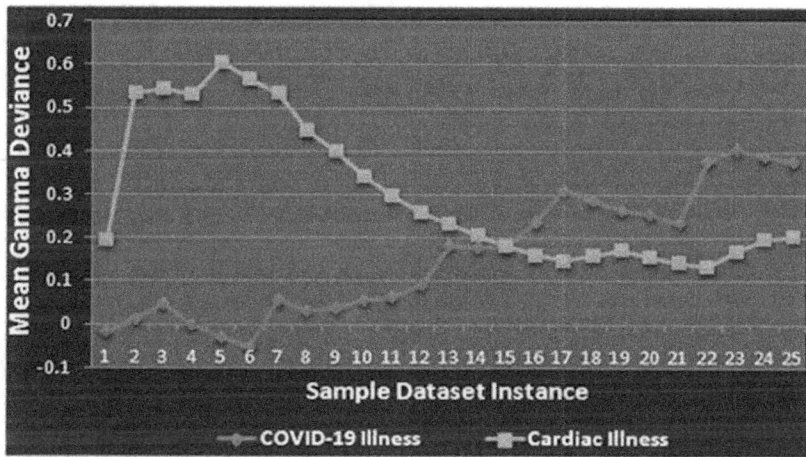

*Figure 2.9* Evolution of mean gamma deviance metric versus the number of sample data instances for the two fuzzy outputs.

deviance with the increasing number of data instances that is evaluated for the anticipated output parameters. It can be noticed that this metric exhibiting an average value of 0.16 for COVID-19 illness output augments with the progression in the contemplated dataset records. On the contrary, the cardiac illness risk output demonstrates an average value of 0.302 for the mean gamma deviance performance measure, which gradually declines and converges to approximately 0.205. The coefficient of determination, indicated by the R-squared statistics estimation for the two examined fuzzy outputs

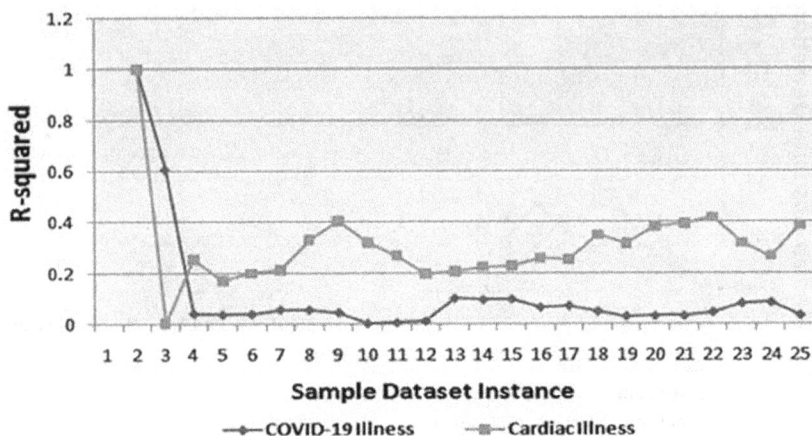

*Figure 2.10* Evolution of R-squared metric versus the number of sample data instances for the two fuzzy outputs.

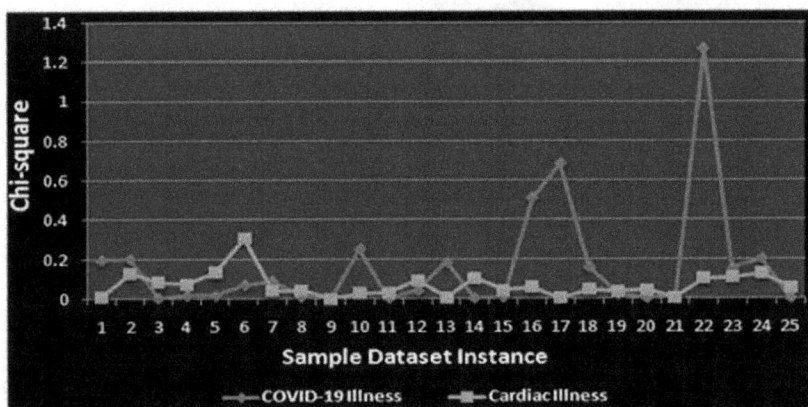

*Figure 2.11* Evolution of Chi-square statistic with the increasing number of sample data instances for the two employed fuzzy outputs.

assessing the risk factor associated with the prevailing global chronic diseases, is plotted in Figure 2.10. The expected value of this metric is 62.45% higher for cardiac illness than for COVID-19 illness output, signifying greater efficiency of the developed optimization model in computing the noncontagious heart disease. Figure 2.11 illustrates the evolvement of the Chi-square statistical measure versus the number of sample data instances for the two deployed healthcare system outputs. This metric is defined as the normalized aggregate of the squared deviations between the fuzzy estimated and the correlated theoretical output attributes. The average value of this metric is 58.9% higher for the COVID-19 risk output compared with the

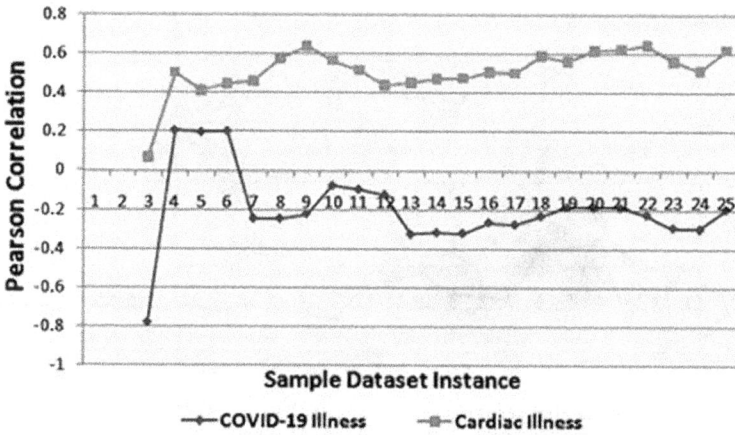

*Figure 2.12* Evolution of Pearson correlation coefficient with the number of sample values for the two fuzzy outputs.

cardiac disease risk output. In addition, Figure 2.12 depicts the Pearson correlation coefficient for the given output bi-variate dataset. This symmetric measure interpreting the strength of the linear relationship between two random variables is defined as the ratio of the covariance of the two variables to the product of their corresponding standard deviations. Ranging from −1 to +1, it can be observed that this metric is mostly negative for COVID-19 illness output with an average value of −0.192. For cardiac illness fuzzy output, the Pearson correlation coefficient is enhanced by 62.714%, with the mean value of 0.5148, indicating the stronger relationship between the heart-related output variables.

$$\text{Mean Gamma Deviance} = \frac{1}{\tau}\sum_{k=1}^{\tau}2\left(\log\left(\frac{\ddot{\Psi}_k}{\Psi_k}\right)+\left(\frac{\Psi_k}{\ddot{\Psi}_k}\right)-1\right) \qquad (2.8)$$

$$R-\text{Squared} = 1 - \frac{\sum_{k=1}^{\tau}\left(\Psi_k - \ddot{\Psi}_k\right)^2}{\sum_{k=1}^{\tau}\left(\Psi_k - \tilde{\Psi}_k\right)^2} \qquad (2.9)$$

$$\chi_c^2 = \sum_{k=1}^{\tau}\frac{\left(\Psi_k - \ddot{\Psi}_k\right)^2}{\ddot{\Psi}_k} \qquad (2.10)$$

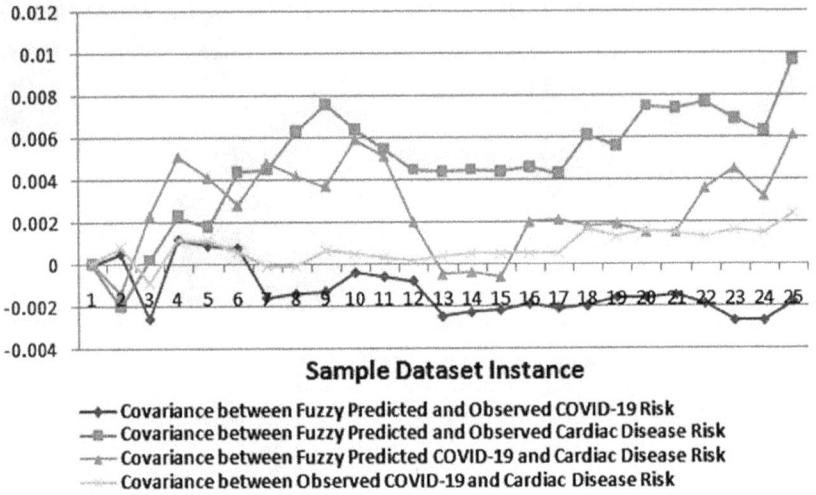

**Sample Dataset Instance**

—◆— Covariance between Fuzzy Predicted and Observed COVID-19 Risk
—■— Covariance between Fuzzy Predicted and Observed Cardiac Disease Risk
—▲— Covariance between Fuzzy Predicted COVID-19 and Cardiac Disease Risk
········· Covariance between Observed COVID-19 and Cardiac Disease Risk

*Figure 2.13* Evolution of the covariance metric between the proposed model estimation and the actual values of the two fuzzy outputs as a function of the sample data record instances.

$$\text{Pearson Correlation Coefficient} = \frac{\sum_{k=1}^{\tau}\left(\Psi_k - \tilde{\Psi}\right)\left(\ddot{\Psi}_k - \widetilde{\widetilde{\Psi}}\right)}{\sqrt{\sum_{k=1}^{\tau}\left(\Psi_k - \tilde{\Psi}\right)^2}\sqrt{\sum_{k=1}^{\tau}\left(\ddot{\Psi}_k - \widetilde{\widetilde{\Psi}}\right)^2}} \qquad (2.11)$$

The advancement of the covariance metric function with the sample data instances for the two investigated fuzzy outputs is shown in Figure 2.13. This covariance between the fuzzy optimized parameters and the associated analytical output values is numerically formulated as shown below in Equation (2.12). The maximum covariance of 0.0048 is conformed between the fuzzy assessed and the analogous theoretical values of the cardiovascular disease risk level. In contrast, the minimal covariance with mean of -0.001284 is exhibited by the COVID-19 illness risk output for the data from the fuzzy predicted and the corresponding actual samples varying together. The covariance between the two fuzzy outputs of COVID-19 and cardiac disease risk factors is alleviated by a factor of 1.85 as against maximal achieved covariance. In the same way, the two actual outputs of COVID-19 and heart risk levels exhibit the reduced covariance by a proportion of 6.168 contrasted with the peak covariance assessment.

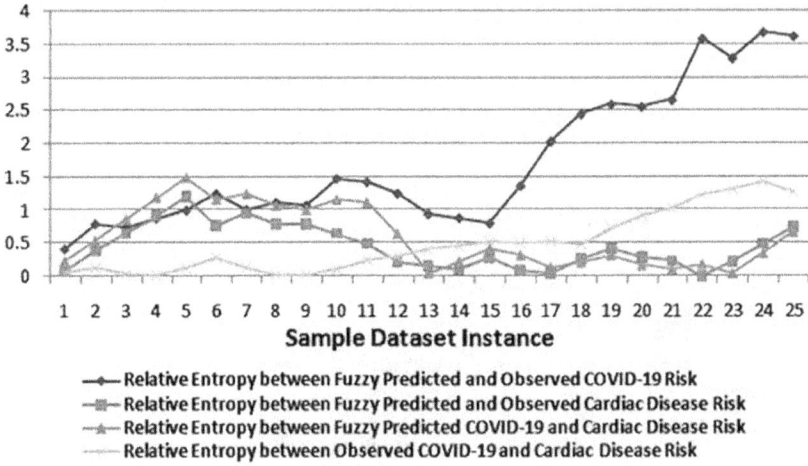

- ◆— Relative Entropy between Fuzzy Predicted and Observed COVID-19 Risk
- ▦— Relative Entropy between Fuzzy Predicted and Observed Cardiac Disease Risk
- ▲— Relative Entropy between Fuzzy Predicted COVID-19 and Cardiac Disease Risk
- ⋯⋯ Relative Entropy between Observed COVID-19 and Cardiac Disease Risk

*Figure 2.14* Evolution of the relative entropy between the proposed model estimated and the actual values of the two fuzzy outputs as a function of the sample data record instances.

$$\rho\left(\Psi, \ddot{\Psi}\right) = \sum_{k=1}^{\tau} \frac{\left(\Psi_k - \tilde{\Psi}\right)\left(\ddot{\Psi}_k - \widetilde{\ddot{\Psi}}\right)}{\tau - 1} \tag{2.12}$$

The evolution of the relative entropy measure as a function of the sample dataset instances is plotted in Figure 2.14. This metric is evaluated as the distance between the two distributions linked with the fuzzy estimation and the actual output vector of risk probability values. The relative entropy or Kullback-Leibler distance between the actual distribution $\Psi$ and the fuzzy-approximated distribution $\ddot{\Psi}$ is consistently nonnegative and is represented as given in Equation (2.13). Utmost relative entropy with an average value of 1.7086 is attained between the heuristic prediction and standard analysis of the COVID-19 risk output. This is reduced by around 73.47, 65.28, and 71.59% in accordance with the relative entropy between the fuzzy predicted and observed cardiac failure risk, relative entropy between fuzzy prediction COVID-19 and cardiovascular disease risk, and relative entropy between the theoretically observed COVID-19 and cardiac disease risk.

$$\delta(\Psi \| \ddot{\Psi}) = \sum_{k=1}^{\tau} \Psi_k \log \frac{\Psi_k}{\ddot{\Psi}_k} \tag{2.13}$$

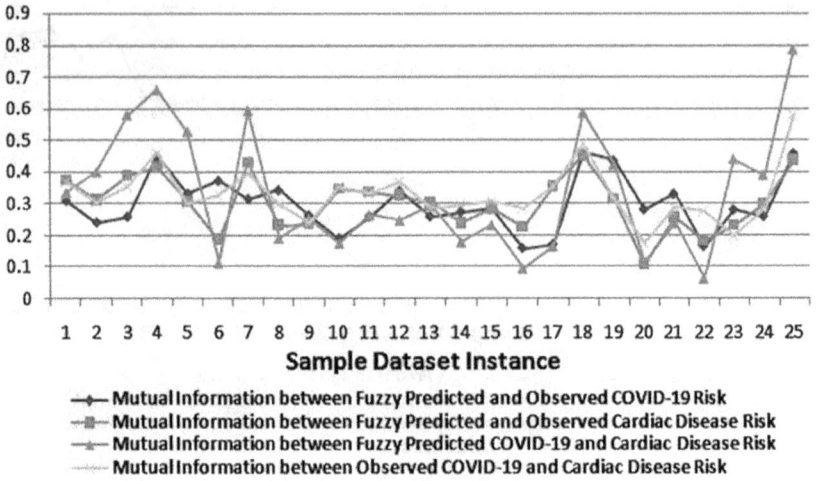

*Figure 2.15* Evolution of the mutual information metric between the proposed model estimated and the actual values of the two fuzzy outputs plotted against the increasing sample record instances.

Finally, the variation of the mutual information performance metric for the employed sample dataset is depicted in Figure 2.15. Perceived as the statistical dependence measure of the reduction in uncertainty within the context of Shannon entropy in network information theory, it can be alternately considered as the relative entropy between the joint distribution and the individual product marginal distributions. The mutual information $\Gamma$ between the actual distribution $\Psi$ and the fuzzy heuristic distribution $\ddot{\Psi}$ is computed as the difference between the entropy associated with the estimated distribution and its conditional entropy for the given actual distribution. This expression in Equation (2.14) can be further elaborated in Equation (2.15) in terms of the individual probability of the output attributes. As can be comprehended, the highest mutual information is obtained between the fuzzy predicted COVID-19 and cardiac disease risk probabilities that are sampled simultaneously with the mean value of 0.334. The average mutual information is mitigated by substantially 10.48% for the presented optimization system execution to compute the COVID-19 pandemic risk level.

$$\Gamma\left(\Psi;\ddot{\Psi}\right) = \mathcal{H}\left(\ddot{\Psi}\right) - \mathcal{H}\left(\ddot{\Psi} \mid \Psi\right) \tag{2.14}$$

$$\Gamma\left(\Psi;\ddot{\Psi}\right) = -\ddot{\Psi}_k \log \ddot{\Psi}_k - \left(-\Psi_k\left(\ddot{\Psi}_k \log \ddot{\Psi}_k + \left(1 - \ddot{\Psi}_k\right)\log\left(1 - \ddot{\Psi}_k\right)\right)\right) \tag{2.15}$$

## 2.5 CONCLUSION AND FUTURE WORK

In this work, we have designed and assessed a fuzzy logic-based healthcare monitoring model using the optimization of multiple physiological attributes. This method has been applied to retrieve a more reliable and accurate estimation of the risk factors [42] associated with the prevailing health conditions of cardiovascular disease and COVID-19 patients. The sample real-time medical dataset is employed to give the training reliability to the developed health system with enhanced precision performance. The experimental results acquired through the simulative evaluation demonstrate that the presented smart healthcare management system supported by the data analytical framework accomplishes higher accuracy by validating through the information-theoretical and the corresponding error prediction metrics. The proposed fuzzy-integrated cardiac and COVID-19 model exhibits lower risk associated with the development of COVID-19 infectious disease and higher risk of heart failure when implemented with the considered sample patients' data record. The progression of various entropy-related attributes such as mutual information, relative entropy, Pearson correlation, and covariance are plotted for the fuzzy estimation and actual dual disease output values. In addition, median absolute deviation, mean gamma deviance, R-squared, and Chi-square metrics are demonstrated for the employed dataset comprising of the cardiovascular patients suffering simultaneously from the ongoing worldwide pandemic. These diverse parameters plotted for the developed healthcare intelligence system are used to verify the correctness of the presented smart home health design and adaptive monitoring model.

In the next focus of study, the proposed model contemplated with the employed laboratory dataset can be extended in large-scale scenarios with more number of patient health data observations to incorporate the effects of the improved statistical efficiency and greater system accuracy. The performance of different artificial intelligence techniques can be explored in the subsequent research for autonomous rule generation and optimization for smart cardiac patient healthcare systems in the advancing pandemic situation of COVID-19 [43]. Furthermore, we will investigate the impact of applying dynamic heuristic strategies such as multiple-objective genetic algorithm, ant colony algorithm, and deep learning neural network to accomplish the generic control operation in the proposed remote patient health monitoring architecture. This can be substantiated through the execution of the developed multivariate system model with the additional specific features of human physiological characteristics to implement the enhanced decision-making process.

## REFERENCES

[1] Malik, S., Singh, N., & Anand, R. (2012). Compression artifact removal using SAWS technique based on fuzzy logic. *International Journal of Electronics and Electrical Engineering*, 2(9), 11–20.

[2] Malik, S., Saroha, R., & Anand, R. (2012). A simple algorithm for reduction of blocking artifacts using SAWS technique based on fuzzy logic. *International Journal of Computational Engineering Research*, 2, 1097–1101.

[3] Zadeh, L. A. (1965). Fuzzy sets. *Information and Control*, 8, 338–353.

[4] Kirubasri, G., Sankar, S., Pandey, D., Pandey, B. K., Singh, H., & Anand, R. (2021, September). A Recent Survey on 6G Vehicular Technology, Applications and Challenges. In *2021 9th International Conference on Reliability, Infocom Technologies and Optimization (Trends and Future Directions)(ICRITO)* (pp. 1–5). IEEE.

[5] Anand, R., & Chawla, P. (2020). Optimization of inscribed hexagonal fractal slotted microstrip antenna using modified lightning attachment procedure optimization. *International Journal of Microwave and Wireless Technologies*, 12(6), 519–530.

[6] Singh, L., Saini, M. K., Tripathi, S., & Sindhwani, N. (2008). An Intelligent Control System for Real-Time Traffic Signal Using Genetic Algorithm. In *AICTE Sponsored National Seminar on Emerging Trends in Software Engineering* (Vol. 50).

[7] Kakria, P., Tripathi, N. K., & Kitipawang, P. (2015). A real-time health monitoring system for remote cardiac patients using smartphone and wearable sensors. *International Journal of Telemedicine and Applications*, 2015, 1–11. http://dx.doi.org/10.1155/2015/373474.

[8] Bakshi, G., Shukla, R., Yadav, V., Dahiya, A., Anand, R., Sindhwani, N., & Singh, H. (2021). an optimized approach for feature extraction in multi-relational statistical learning. *Journal of Scientific & Industrial Research*, 80, 537–542.

[9] Rayan, Z., Alfonse, M., & Salem, A. B. M. (2019). Machine learning approaches in smart health. *Procedia Computer Science*, 154, 361–368.

[10] Nishiga, M., Wang, D. W., Han, Y., Lewis, D. B., & Wu, J. C. (2020). COVID-19 and cardiovascular disease: From basic mechanisms to clinical perspectives. *Nature Reviews Cardiology*, 17(9), 543–558.

[11] Abdullah, D. A., Akpınar, M. H., & Şengür, A. (2020). Local feature descriptors based ECG beat classification. *Health Information Science and Systems*, 8(1), 1–10. DOI: 10.1007/s13755-020-00110-y.

[12] Otoom, M., Otoum, N., Alzubaidi, M. A., Etoom, Y., & Banihani, R. (2020). An IoT-based framework for early identification and monitoring of COVID-19 cases. *Biomedical Signal Processing and Control*, 62, 102149. DOI: 10.1016/j.bspc.2020.102149.

[13] Swayamsiddha, S., & Mohanty, C. (2020). Application of cognitive internet of medical things for COVID-19 pandemic. *Diabetes & Metabolic Syndrome: Clinical Research & Reviews*, 14(5), 911–915.

[14] Javaid, M., Haleem, A., Vaishya, R., Bahl, S., Suman, R., & Vaish, A. (2020). Industry 4.0 technologies and their applications in fighting COVID-19 pandemic. *Diabetes & Metabolic Syndrome: Clinical Research & Reviews*, 14(4), 419–422. DOI: 10.1016/j.dsx.2020.04.032.

[15] Taiwo, O., & Ezugwu, A. E. (2020). Smart healthcare support for remote patient monitoring during covid-19 quarantine. *Informatics in Medicine Unlocked*, 20, 100428. DOI: 10.1016/j.imu.2020.100428.

[16] Hashem, I.A.T., Ezugwu, A.E., Mohammed A. Al-Garadi, M.A., Abdullahi, I.N., Otegbeye, O., Ahman, Q.O., Mbah, G.C.E., Amit K. Shukla, A.K., & Chiroma, H. (2020). A machine learning solution framework for combatting COVID-19 in smart cities from multiple dimensions. medRxiv 2020.05.18.20105577. DOI: 10.1101/2020.05.18.20105577.

[17] Chatterjee, P., Tesis, A., Cymberknop, L. J., & Armentano, R. L. (2020). Internet of things and artificial intelligence in healthcare during COVID-19 pandemic—A South American perspective. *Frontiers in Public Health*, *8*. DOI: 10.3389/fpubh.2020.600213.

[18] Vedaei, S. S., Fotovvat, A., Mohebbian, M. R., Rahman, G. M., Wahid, K. A., Babyn, P., ... & Sami, R. (2020). COVID-SAFE: An IoT-based system for automated health monitoring and surveillance in post-pandemic life. *IEEE Access*, *8*, 188538–188551.

[19] Tersalvi, G., Winterton, D, Cioffi, G.M., Ghidini, S., Roberto, M., Biasco, L., Pedrazzini, G., Dauw, J., Ameri, P., & Vicenzi, M. (2020). Telemedicine in heart failure during COVID-19: A step into the future. *Frontiers in Cardiovascular Medicine*, *7*, 313. DOI: 10.3389/fcvm.2020.612818.

[20] Rincon, J. A., Guerra-Ojeda, S., Carrascosa, C., & Julian, V. (2020). An IoT and Fog computing-based monitoring system for cardiovascular patients with automatic ECG classification using deep neural networks. *Sensors*, *20*(24), 7353. DOI: 10.3390/s20247353.

[21] El-Rashidy, N., El-Sappagh, S., Islam, S. M., El-Bakry, H. M., & Abdelrazek, S. (2020). End-to-end deep learning framework for coronavirus (COVID-19) detection and monitoring. *Electronics*, *9*(9), 1439. DOI: 10.3390/electronics 9091439.

[22] Seshadri, D. R., Davies, E. V., Harlow, E. R., Hsu, J. J., Knighton, S. C., Walker, T. A., ... & Drummond, C. K. (2020). Wearable sensors for COVID-19: A call to action to harness our digital infrastructure for remote patient monitoring and virtual assessments. *Frontiers in Digital Health*, *2*, 8. DOI: 10.3389/ fdgth.2020.00008.

[23] Rajesh Kumar, N.V., Arun, M., Baraneetharan, E., Stanly Jaya Prakash, J., Kanchana, A., & Prabu, S. (2020). Detection and monitoring of the asymptotic COVID-19 patients using IoT devices and sensors. *International Journal of Pervasive Computing and Communications*. DOI: 10.1108/IJPCC-08-2020-0107.

[24] Valsalan, P., Baomar, T. A. B., & Baabood, A. H. O. (2020). IoT based health monitoring system. *Journal of critical reviews*, *7*(4), 739–743.

[25] Conway, R., Kelly, D. M., Mullane, P., Bhuachalla, C. N., O'Connor, L., Buckley, C., ... & Doyle, S. (2021). Epidemiology of COVID-19 and public health restrictions during the first wave of the pandemic in Ireland in 2020. *Journal of Public Health (Oxford, England)*. DOI: 10.1093/pubmed/fdab049.

[26] Haleem, A., Javaid, M., Singh, R. P., & Suman, R. (2021). Applications of artificial intelligence (AI) for cardiology during COVID-19 pandemic. *Sustainable Operations and Computers*, *2*, 71–78. DOI: 10.1016/j.susoc.2021.04.003.

[27] Krittanawong, C., Rogers, A. J., Johnson, K. W., Wang, Z., Turakhia, M. P., Halperin, J. L., & Narayan, S. M. (2021). Integration of novel monitoring devices with machine learning technology for scalable cardiovascular management. *Nature Reviews Cardiology*, *18*(2), 75–91.

[28] Bayoumy, K., Gaber, M., Elshafeey, A., Mhaimeed, O., Dineen, E. H., Marvel, F. A., ... & Elshazly, M. B. (2021). Smart wearable devices in cardiovascular care: Where we are and how to move forward. *Nature Reviews Cardiology*, 1–19. DOI: 10.1038/s41569-021-00522-7.

[29] Miller, J. C., Skoll, D., & Saxon, L. A. (2021). Home monitoring of cardiac devices in the era of COVID-19. *Current Cardiology Reports*, 23(1), 1–9. DOI: 10.1007/s11886-020-01431-w.

[30] Juneja, S., Juneja, A., & Anand, R. (2020). Healthcare 4.0-digitizing healthcare using big data for performance improvisation. *Journal of Computational and Theoretical Nanoscience*, 17(9–10), 4408–4410.

[31] Rana, K., Tripathi, S. & Raw, R. S. "Fuzzy Logic-Based Directional Location Routing in Vehicular Ad-hoc Network", Proceedings of the National Academy of Sciences, India Section A: Physical Sciences Springer, (SCI, SCOPUS, DBLP) (IF = 1.544, Q-3R), ISSN: 0369-8203 (print version)/ISSN: 2250-1762 (electronic version), 2019.

[32] Zimmermann, H. J. (2011). *Fuzzy set theory—and its applications*. Springer Science & Business Media.

[33] Kohli, L., Saurabh, M., Bhatia, I., Shekhawat, U. S., Vijh, M., & Sindhwani, N. (2021). Design and Development of Modular and Multifunctional UAV with Amphibious Landing Module. In *Data Driven Approach Towards Disruptive Technologies: Proceedings of MIDAS 2020* (pp. 405–421). Springer Singapore.

[34] Kohli, L., Saurabh, M., Bhatia, I., Sindhwani, N., & Vijh, M. (2021). Design and Development of Modular and Multifunctional UAV with Amphibious Landing, Processing and Surround Sense Module. *Unmanned Aerial Vehicles for Internet of Things (IoT): Concepts, Techniques, and Applications*, eds. V. Mohindru, Y. Singh, R. Bhatt and A.K. Gupta, (pp. 207–230). Wiley.

[35] Anand, R., & Chawla, P. (2016, March). A Review on the Optimization Techniques for Bio-Inspired Antenna Design. In *2016 3rd International Conference on Computing for Sustainable Global Development (INDIACom)* (pp. 2228–2233). IEEE.

[36] Sindhwani, N., & Bhamrah, M. S. (2017). An optimal scheduling and routing under adaptive spectrum-matching framework for MIMO systems. *International Journal of Electronics*, 104(7), 1238–1253.

[37] Chawla, P., & Anand, R. (2017). Micro-switch design and its optimization using pattern search algorithm for applications in reconfigurable antenna. *Modern Antenna Systems*, 10, 189–210.

[38] Sindhwani, N. (2017). Performance analysis of optimal scheduling based firefly algorithm in MIMO system. *Optimization*, 2(12), 19–26.

[39] Sindhwani, N., & Singh, M. (2014). Comparison of adaptive mutation genetic algorithm and genetic algorithm for transmit antenna subset selection in MIMO-OFDM. *International Journal of Computer Applications*, 97(22), 22–28.

[40] http://www.mathworks.com/products/matlab.html.

[41] Anand, R., Shrivastava, G., Gupta, S., Peng, S. L., & Sindhwani, N. (2018). Audio Watermarking with Reduced Number of Random Samples. In *Handbook of Research on Network Forensics and Analysis Techniques*, eds. G. Shrivastava, P. Kumar, B.B. Gupta, S. Bala, N. Dey (pp. 372–394). IGI Global.

[42] Juneja, S., Juneja, A., & Anand, R. (2019, April). Reliability Modeling for Embedded System Environment Compared to Available Software Reliability Growth Models. In *2019 International Conference on Automation, Computational and Technology Management (ICACTM)* (pp. 379–382). IEEE.

[43] Anand, R., Sindhwani, N., & Saini, A. (2021). Emerging Technologies for COVID-19. In *Enabling Healthcare 4.0 for Pandemics: A Roadmap Using AI, Machine Learning, IoT and Cognitive Technologies*, eds. A. Juneja, V. Bali, S. Juneja, V. Jain and P. Tyagi (pp. 163–188).

# Chapter 3

# Internet of things implementation and challenges during COVID-19 in healthcare industries

*P. M. Manohar*

Raghu Engineering College (Autonomous), Visakhapatnam, India

## CONTENTS

DOI: 10.1201/9781003239888-3

## 3.1 INTRODUCTION

Kevin Ashton initially created the phrase "Internet of Things" (IoT) in a presentation concerning Procter & Gamble's implementation of radio-frequency identification (RFID) for supply chain management [1, 2]. IoT [3–5] is an advanced technology that can connect all the smart things in a network without requiring any human input [6]. An IoT device is anything that can be linked to the internet to track or send data [7, 8]. IoT has gained traction as a novel research area in a wide range of academic and industry domains in recent years, particularly in healthcare. Modern healthcare systems are being reshaped by the IoT revolution, which has technical, economic, and societal implications. It is converting old healthcare systems into more individualized ones, making it simpler to diagnose, treat, and monitor patients.

IoT is becoming increasingly prevalent in healthcare systems, where it has the potential to reduce costs, enhance service quality, and enable sophisticated user experiences [9–12]. IoT in healthcare is anticipated to grow at an exponential pace from USD 72 billion in 2020 to USD 188 billion in 2025 [7, 13] due to its complete capabilities, such as monitoring, identification and authentication, and data collection.

All the nations, including India, are combating COVID-19 in the present pandemic crisis and are still seeking a feasible and cost-effective strategy to cope with the issues that have developed in several ways. Physical scientists and engineers are creating new theories to address these difficulties, describing new research issues, developing user-centered explanations, and educating the public and ourselves. This brief overview sought to raise the awareness of this cutting-edge technology and its potential use in the COVID-19 outbreak.

To combat the pandemic, the healthcare industry has invested a lot of work toward COVID-19 diagnosis, screening, and treatment of affected people. Governments and international organizations are working to provide adequate healthcare to minimize the virus effects. Consequently, several treatment strategies and medications are used as needed to combat this condition. Authorities, on the other hand, are taking several steps to prevent the pandemic from spreading further, such as social isolation, area closure, and adequate sanitization. As a result, all the social institutions, most importantly, the community, must work together to prevent the illness from spreading. Furthermore, the extensive integration of future technology with excellent healthcare management and robust governance would strengthen the society's ability to defend itself from COVID-19 illness [14].

From a global perspective, advanced artificial intelligence (AI) approaches, machine learning (ML), IoT, and big data have all emanated as intelligent technologies in this era of information, promising massive applications in a wide range of sectors, particularly in addressing COVID-19 pandemic's healthcare and social sector problems. Sharing and disseminating research ideas, as well as gaining knowledge from analytics and simulations, are crucial for accelerating the pandemic response [15]. IoT can be quite useful in these situations. In terms of intelligent decision-making, AI combined with IoT is more powerful and can help in the fight against this epidemic.

Before the IoT, patients' correspondence with doctors was restricted to visits, teleconferences, and text messaging. There was no means for doctors or hospitals to monitor the patient's health frequently and offer suitable recommendations. We should be thankful to IoT-enabled products due to which remote tracking in the healthcare business is now possible, allowing physicians to give better treatment while keeping patients safe and healthy. As the interactions with doctors have grown easier and more efficient, patients' involvement and pleasure have also grown. IoT has a substantial influence on healthcare cost reduction and treatment results.

Various medical devices and apparatus such as oxygen concentrators, cylinders, nebulizers, scales, wheelchairs, and other devices are utilized for checking, tracking, and controlling the patient's condition during the medication of COVID-19 patients using IoT-enabled devices with real-time location service. The smart hospital offers all the information through system's total digitalization, minimizing the patient's waiting time. It provides a record analysis for the process of improving COVID-19 patient care.

The correct information like their location, time identification, and database is sent to the healthcare workers. IoT can allow the patients in remote locations distant from hospitals to communicate with the physicians through smart mobile phone applications. IoT analyzes the distance and accesses the patient information before arriving at the hospital in an emergency. It aids in the contact-tracing process.

In IoT, technologies like healthcare, eHealth, mHealth, and wireless body sensor networks (WBSN) are significant for tracking the patients. WBSN is made up of sensors that are placed all over the body. These sensors collect some crucial information such as the patient's body temperature, blood pressure, heartbeat rate, respiration rate, electrocardiogram (ECG), and blood glucose [16]. Over the last few years, actuators have been used to raise the warnings and change the ambient factors as needed. Because IoT-based systems generate massive amounts of data, they are unable to store it. Many cloud-based platforms for data storage, such as ThingWorx, OpenIoT, Google Cloud, Amazon, Nimbits, GENI [16], are available to circumvent this constraint. These solutions help in data management and storage. ML-based classification techniques for predicting ML-based diseases, ML-based prediction system for detection of fatal diseases, ML-based data aggregation, and ML-based living assistance are the techniques based on ML for big data analysis in IoT healthcare. IoT-based solutions are supporting elderly people by providing care and preventive steps. Medical super sensors (MSS) are new types of sensors that have additional memory, processing, and communication capabilities than standard sensor nodes [16].

The process of collecting and analyzing enormous amounts of data is known as big data. It can save all of a patient's medical records to assess risk. It is used to store people's travel histories to assess risk. It aids in the detection of those who are in close contact with a COVID-19 patient. With the necessary data, it aids in the identification of suspicious symptoms (e.g., black fungus). It aids in the early detection of viruses as well as the identification and analysis of fast-moving diseases. During the lockdown, this technology captures information on the virus [16].

We may conclude from the preceding discussion that organizations and researchers from many nations are working hard to establish resilience against the epidemic. This work focuses on examining the extent of these novel technologies and current advancements in designing countermeasures against the COVID-19 pandemic, because AI, ML, and IoT have all been shown to be important in a variety of applications.

The purpose of this research is to examine the current state-of-the-art COVID-19 control designs, implementations, platforms, applications, and IoT-based solutions, as well as to assess the significance of IoT-based technologies in COVID-19 monitoring and controlling.

The rest of the chapter is laid out as follows. Section 3.2 discusses the significance of IoT-based healthcare architecture. Section 3.3 highlights IoT technologies for the healthcare during COVID-19 pandemic. Section 3.4 covers processes involved in IoT during COVID-19. Section 3.5 presents IoT stakeholders. Section 3.6 reviews the application of advanced technologies in the medical field. Section 3.7 covers IoT applications during COVID-19. Section 3.8 discusses the potential risks of IoT. Section 3.9 describes the major advantages of IoT in healthcare. Section 3.10 highlights the challenges of IoT in healthcare. Finally, we discuss conclusions and outline future work.

## 3.2 IOT-BASED HEALTHCARE ARCHITECTURE

The architecture of an IoT-based healthcare system is fairly similar to that of traditional IoT architecture. Sensors are specifically developed to assess and quantify distinct physiological conditions of users/patients in IoT-based healthcare services. Figure 3.1 depicts a typical IoT healthcare architecture. The architecture is divided into four layers. The following is a full description of these layers:

  **Layer 1 - Devices:** The main drivers of IoT infrastructure deployment include networked devices such as sensors, actuators, monitors, detectors, and video systems. Different physiological systems are deployed on the human body at Layer 1. These sensors collect the values of various physiological parameters. To extract useful information, the physiological data is examined. These devices are the ones that collect the data.

  **Layer 2 - Data Aggregation and Preprocessing:** The data obtained from Layer 1 during the data aggregation and preprocessing phase is typically in an analog format which must be converted to digital format for subsequent operations.

  **Layer 3 - Data Storage:** The preprocessed, standardized data are transferred to a data center or the cloud once it has been digitized and aggregated.

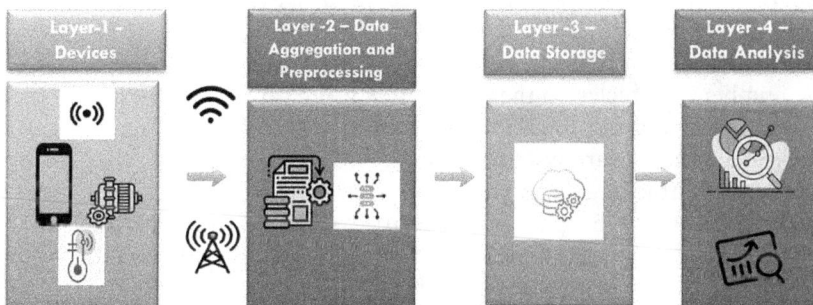

*Figure 3.1* The IoT healthcare four-layer architecture.

Layer 4 - **Data Analysis:** At the final phase, data is handled, examined, and analyzed. When applied to this data, advanced analytics generates actionable business insights for enhanced decision-making [17].

Good healthcare, improved treatment results, and lower rates for patients are all advantages of the IoT, as it leads to better processes that lead to improved performance and a patient satisfaction experience for healthcare professionals [18].

## 3.3 IOT TECHNOLOGIES FOR THE HEALTHCARE DURING COVID-19 PANDEMIC

### 3.3.1 Implementation technologies for IoT

Sensor networks are a critical component in gathering the data that smart environments require. Because of its ease of installation and maintenance, a sensor network is required. Running wires is not a viable option in these situations. RFID and wireless sensor networks (WSN) technology are the crucial drivers for IoT concept. RFID is an automated technology that uses radio waves to identify items and is considered a necessity for IoT applications. It may be employed in a variety of sectors, including logistics, engineering, chemical manufacture, retail construction, and many more. Better security, more productivity, more revenues, enhanced quality, cheaper cost, and time savings are all advantages of employing this technology.

WSNs are made up of tiny nodes that can detect, calculate, and communicate wirelessly. It's often used for low-power and low-data-connection-rate sensors. WSNs have the capability to handle many sensor nodes, have a sufficient battery life, and have the ability to cover a broad region. Indoor and outdoor applications are the examples of WSN environmental monitoring.

Hospitals, pharmacies, and long-term care communities can benefit from RFID by enhancing patient safety, increasing asset utilization with real-time tracking, increasing income with automated invoicing, and reducing the occurrence of medical errors with track-and-match applications. To keep track of who is on the road, e-Passes can be generated using RFID tags that can be placed on a vehicle. This type of enforcement can also help to reduce the number of vehicles on the road at any given time.

WSNs play a critical role in IoT healthcare applications. WSNs improve medical and healthcare systems by providing valuable applications like real-time patient tracking, drug administration, diagnostic assistance, patient tracking inside the hospital, and so on. Doctors can benefit from remote monitoring of a patient's status if the patient is not in the hospital.

AmbuSens is a system developed by Smart Wireless Applications and Networking (SWAN) laboratory of Indian Institute of Technology Kharagpur. The Ministry of Human Resource and Development (MHRD) of the Indian government provided the majority of the funding for the system. This product system is an important part of the IoT healthcare system. The AmbuSens system's key goals are healthcare data digitization and standardization and real-time monitoring of patients. Also, multiple doctors can view a patient's health data at the same time because of accessibility. Confidentiality of patient health data in the cloud is also guaranteed [17].

Researchers at Penn State University have developed a wearable sensor device that can be put directly to a person's skin to assess the parameters such as body temperature, heartbeat rate, and blood oxygen levels.

Body area sensors, advanced healthcare systems, wearable sensors, cloud-based platforms for wireless transfer, storage, and display of clinical data, and other IoT-related technologies are all of interest.

### 3.3.2 IoT technologies for healthcare during the COVID-19 outbreak

The IoT integrates medical instruments and equipment to develop the intelligent information systems tailored to the needs of individual COVID-19 patients. To improve production, quality, and information about impending illnesses, a distinct multidisciplinary strategy is required [19, 20]. Changes in essential patient data are detected by IoT technology, which allows important information to be determined. IoT technologies have a significant influence on elevated medical equipment, allowing for a more tailored response during the COVID-19 outbreak. It can digitally capture, store, and analyze data. All the healthcare records are kept digitally, and patient data and information may be readily transferred in emergencies, allowing clinicians to work more effectively [21]. Using smart sensors, we can track and control [22–24] all of the major needs of body temperature, sugar level, oxygen level, blood pressure, and COVID-19 patient health information [25–27]. For most effective communication and monitoring, the software is essential. All the records are kept in strict confidence to provide the best possible care in the future. AI improves the performance of doctors and surgeons to improve treatment accuracy, efficiency, and consistency. This technology can help patients feel better by reducing discomfort and identifying abnormalities so that appropriate treatment may be given. Various actuators are used to introduce physical object motion and control [28, 29]. Virtual reality is the most successful IoT solution for improving the quality of organizing real-time data.

Various IoT technologies to be used in healthcare during the COVID-19 pandemic are:

1. Big data: Currently, big data seems to be the ideal strategy for capturing, storing, and analyzing the COVID-19 patient's data. Data is historically saved in hard form in the medical field, which adds to the expense. Big data has a great deal of digital data storage capabilities. Big data keeps track of all patient's information, the billing system,

and the clinical record. Data is organized in such a way that the optimum option for healthcare may be found rapidly [30].

2. Cloud computing: It uses computer system resources and the Internet to save on-demand data storage and describe data. In emergencies, it swiftly communicates COVID-19 patient's information. There has been shared confidential data resources that assist doctors and surgeons in doing their duties more efficiently and successfully. It improves data quality while lowering data storage costs [30].

3. Smart sensors: Smart sensors have a great ability to communicate via digital network and provide accurate and dependable findings in the medical industry. They keep track of and regulate all the aspects of the patient's health. The blood pressure, temperature, oxygen level, sugar level, and so on of the COVID-19 patient may all be easily monitored. Obtaining information about one's health, a defective area, and the biological tissue around it is advantageous [30].

4. Software: There is a specialized software available for the medical industry that enhances patient care, stores patient records, prescribes therapy, runs tests, and makes diagnoses. It aids in the improvement of patient–doctor communication. The COVID-19 patient's medical history, sensitive information, and sickness are all readily detected and maintained by software [30].

5. AI: In a predetermined environment, AI aids in the performance, evaluation, validation, prediction, and analysis of data to provide strong viral infection prediction and control capabilities. Doctors and surgeons benefit from greater efficiency, precision, and efficacy because of this technology. It assesses the COVID-19 patient's pain in response to drug changes [30].

6. Actuators: An actuator is a mechanism that introduces action and regulates the system to act upon in a certain setting. Medical actuators are mostly used to maintain precision and regulate needed parameters. It aids in the development of a hospital bed that can be elevated or lowered to accommodate COVID-19 patients' demands [30].

7. Virtual reality/augmented reality: It is the most effective technique to merge human and technological technologies to give real-time data. Virtual reality aids in improving the quality of COVID-19 patient treatment planning, patient safety, and efficiency. To enhance surgery planning quality, necessary information to COVID-19 patients and clinicians is provided. In addition, augmented reality gives digital life information in the form of digital pictures and sound [30].

### 3.3.3 COVID-19 IoT processes

IoT is a cutting-edge technical framework for combating the COVID-19 pandemic that may meet considerable hurdles during a lockdown. Figure 3.2 depicts the key procedures employed by IoT for COVID-19.

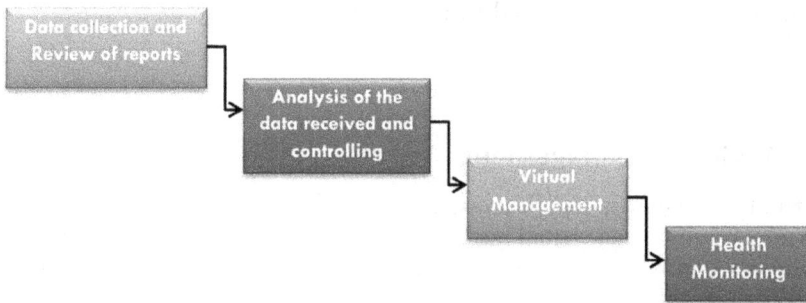

*Figure 3.2* Process flow for using IoT in the fight against the COVID-19 pandemic.

This technique is useful for capturing real-time data as well as other important information about an infected patient [31–33]. IoT is used in the initial step to gather health record from infected patients' various locations and manage it using a virtual management system [34, 35, 36, 37, 38]. This technology assists with data management and post-report follow-up.

### 3.3.4 Data collection and review of reports

This technology aims to use a set of wearable sensors to capture real-time symptom data from the user's body. Based on an actual COVID-19 patient dataset, we determined the most significant COVID-19 symptoms in a previous study. Symptoms to be noted include fever, cough, fatigue, sore throat, and shortness of breath [39].

These symptoms can be detected using a variety of biosensors. Temperature-based sensors are used to detect fever. Coughs can be detected and classified using audio-based sensors. Motion-based and heart-rate sensors can both identify fatigue. A sore throat can be detected using image-based categorization. Oxygen-based sensors can also detect shortness of breath [39].

Other vital information, such as travel and contact history over the past three to four weeks, can be acquired on the fly utilizing mobile applications. Finally, experts review the information gathered. Expert doctors can use this information to detect and diagnose COVID-19 disease [39].

### 3.3.5 Analysis of the data received and controlling

Experts use data analysis and ML techniques [40] to analyze the reviewed data. These algorithms are utilized to create a COVID-19 model as well as a real-time summary of the processed data. The algorithm can therefore be used to swiftly detect or predict potential COVID-19 incidents based on available data gathered and posted by users. The model can also anticipate how the patient will respond to treatment. The disease models generated with this data will eventually disclose important details about the disease's nature [39].

### 3.3.6 Virtual management

Virtual management applications allow the patients to consult with their doctors remotely via virtual meetings, resulting in fewer hospital visits. This approach can be used at any time during the COVID-19 pandemic [39].

## 3.4 HEALTH MONITORING

Physicians will keep an eye on suspected patients for whom our proposed ML-based detection/prediction model predicts an infection based on actual symptom data. Physicians will be able to swiftly respond to these reported instances by conducting any extra clinical investigations necessary to check the condition. As a result, verifiable cases can be isolated and properly dealt with [39].

## 3.5 IOT STAKEHOLDERS

*IoT for Patients* – Wearable devices such as fitness bands and other wirelessly connected equipment such as blood pressure and heart rate monitoring cuffs, glucometers, and other devices provide patients with the individualized attention. These devices may be configured to remind you of things like calorie counts, exercise, appointments, blood pressure fluctuations, and a variety of other things.

People's lives have been changed by the IoT, particularly the lives of elderly patients, who can now track their health concerns in real time. This has a big impact on single parents and their families. If a person's typical behaviors are disturbed or modified, an alert system sends signals to concerned family members and healthcare providers [18].

*IoT for Physicians* – Wearables and other IoT-enabled home monitoring devices can help physicians keep a better eye on their patients' health. They can monitor whether or not patients are adhering to their treatment plans and whether or not they require emergency medical care. Healthcare practitioners can be more watchful and proactive in their contact with patients thanks to the IoT. Data from IoT devices can assist physicians in determining the optimal treatment method for their patients and achieving the desired outcomes [18].

*IoT for Hospitals* - Hospitals may profit from IoT devices in a variety of ways in addition to monitoring patients' health. Wheelchairs, defibrillators, nebulizers, oxygen pumps, and other monitoring devices are all tracked in real-time utilizing IoT devices with sensors. The deployment of medical workers in various locations may also be monitored in real time.

Infection spread is a major issue among hospital patients. Hygiene monitoring devices with IoT capabilities help in the prevention of infection in patients. Asset management, such as pharmaceutical inventory control and environmental monitoring, like checking refrigerator temperatures and managing humidity and temperature, can also benefit from IoT devices [18].

*IoT for Health Insurance Companies* – Health insurers have a lot of opportunities with IoT-connected intelligent equipment. Insurance companies can utilize the data acquired by health-tracking devices for underwriting and claims processing. Using this data, they will be able to detect fraud claims and determine underwriting opportunities [18].

## 3.6 APPLICATIONS OF ADVANCED TECHNOLOGIES IN THE MEDICAL FIELD

In the medical field, AI and ML have a wide range of applications, including statistical data estimation and categorization. BlueDot Toronto, in particular, produced the first risk-based approach for identifying the SARS-COV-2 virus epidemic [41], which was created by scientists to study creative strategies for minimizing the virus. This approach detected anomalous numbers of pneumonia cases with unknown causes in Wuhan (China) and cautioned of the disease's presence far earlier than when COVID-19 was legally acknowledged [14]. As a result, these modern technologies can predict epidemics and raise public awareness about the need to take the necessary precautions in the event of an outbreak.

In the medical field, AI applications for identifying infectious illnesses are incredibly beneficial and have the potential to revolutionize healthcare procedures. Within the healthcare industry, incorporating AI into imaging operations has got a lot of interest. Machine-learning prototypes can examine medical photos to detect illness early on. These prototypes use big data [42] and deep learning [43] techniques to achieve the task. Pathology, ophthalmology, radiography, and dermatology are some of the potential fields where image-based learning might be used [14]. The prevention of illnesses like COVID-19 is heavily reliant on people being screened by pathogenic testing, which is a lengthy process and hence accuracy is essential. The author of the research employed deep learning to construct a COVID-19 medical identification technique based on radiographic changes in computed tomography (CT) images in the verification and validation stage with an accuracy of 85.2% [14].

Medical practitioners may benefit from ML by evaluating and organizing vast amounts of patient data housed in digital medical records. Furthermore,

ML is used in a variety of medical applications, such as detecting patients in critical condition, early detection of illness signs, analyzing chest X-rays to understand the patient's breathing condition, and so on. As a result, AI and ML increase the performance of the identification and prediction processes and result in determining how the administrative choices are made in the medical field [14].

### 3.6.1 Medical imaging for COVID-19 patients

CT scans and X-rays are commonly utilized in medical imaging for diagnosis and therapy. CT scans and X-ray imaging played a critical role in the discovery of the SARS-COV-2 virus during the COVID-19 pandemic. Latest technologies such as AI and ML can help with this by enhancing image analysis [44–47] with intelligent identification and categorization of anomalies.

The RT-PCR (reverse transcription-polymerase chain reaction) test is commonly used to determine the quantity of any form of RNA. The COVID-19 infection is diagnosed with this RT-PCR [48]. However, there are several drawbacks to the RT-PCR test. The newest AI-powered technologies and methodologies must contribute greatly to creating resistance against the COVID-19 outbreak to tackle the aforementioned problem of false-positive diagnosis.

Meng [49] offers a method for detecting COVID-19 in X-ray pictures of a patient's chest using deep transfer learning and a generative adversarial network (GAN). Another research [50] describes the identification of COVID-19 early on CT images in the abdomen using ML algorithms.

### 3.6.2 Using clinical data to track a patient's condition

The patient's condition can be observed remotely using remote monitoring technology [51], which collects the patient's status or clinical data. These devices use WiFi, Bluetooth, or a cellular connection to connect to the networks wirelessly. A similar concept may be applied to infectious disease surveillance, such as COVID-19. People who have been infected to COVID-19, as well as close family members and friends of the affected person, may be screened using this approach of remote surveillance. These technologies can also be used to protect medical practitioners from being exposed to high-risk patient groups. The same technical arrangements that are now utilized by remote monitoring programs might theoretically be utilized to include a temperature measurement gadget, such as a smart thermometer, for patient tracking thought of having COVID-19 [51]. AI and ML may greatly assist in improving monitoring and detecting aberrant patterns or behaviors. Advanced data analytics and signal processing based on ML and AI can assist in filtering data and identifying trends.

### 3.6.3 Drug development, selection, and delivery

Alwashmi [52] employed a drug–target prototype termed molecule trans-former–drug target interaction (MT-DTI) that react with SARS-COV-2 viral proteins using a deep learning methodology. Beck et al. [53] developed a model that uses ML technology to predict the possible inhibitory synthetic antibodies for the SARS-COV-2 virus. The accessible data can forecast the complicated biological scenarios to examine the viral protein structure and possible antibodies using ML approaches. A ML approach may be employed to construct relationships between the viral entity and its likely antibody responses using adequate and appropriate training data. A pretrained ML program can identify the probable antibodies for a particular viral protein sequence quicker than the human immune system, which can be extremely beneficial in the fight against pandemics like COVID-19 that can potentially save many lives.

### 3.6.4 Modeling and prediction of virus propagation

The rapid spread of the COVID-19 illness might be due to several factors. One aspect was lack of openness in the early stages of the pandemic. It is vital to share contagion information completely and correctly for society's anti-epidemic response. The early stages of the epidemic may have been prevented if information exchange had been more transparent. Another factor is the lack of comprehensive systemic diagnostic criteria for this virus. The rapid creation of checking procedures for a new virus is quite difficult. Finally, owing to the lack of an effective epidemic indication and forecast system, we missed the opportunity to stop the illness from spreading in its early stages.

The epidemiological investigation is critical in the current SARS-COV-2 transmission scenario for avoiding transmission by following infectious trails and finding the link chains that contribute to the rapid spread. The COVID-19 epidemic, on the other hand, was aided by the increased mobility of people during China's most important traditional carnival, which enhanced the virus's transmission while also considerably amplifying the epidemiological investigation's obstacles [54]. While making decisions on how to deal with a health crisis, it's critical to keep an eye on and forecast the progression of the epidemic. In this perspective, the mathematical propagation model has got increasing attention and consideration in epidemiological studies. One of these mathematical propagation models presented earlier is susceptible–infected–removed (SIR) model. Some important parameters inducing epidemic transmission have been integrated into the traditional SIR model termed as SEIRS (susceptible–exposed–infectious–recovered–susceptible) model.

### 3.6.5 COVID-19 syndromes early prediction or detection

By collecting and analyzing all the past data linked to this epidemic, AI plays a crucial function in recognizing the accumulation of incidents and predicting the region where this infection will spread in the future. Based on the information obtained from social media and other media platforms, such as the propensity for contagion and the nature of its spread, this technology may detect sickness symptoms and predict its type. It may also anticipate the number of infected cases and fatalities in any particular place according to associated facts and information [55].

In Ref. [55], the authors reported ML investigation of the COVID-19 outbreak using data from the early phases of infection dynamics. The purpose is to gather the information that will help us understand public health better. These include the likelihood of disease spread, the rate at which a mild sickness progresses to a major illness, asymptomatic contagion estimates, and forecasts of new infections over time.

### 3.6.6 Protecting healthcare workers

The significance of healthcare professionals cannot be overstated. They are not only assisting in the collection of COVID data, but they are also assisting vulnerable patients personally, risking their lives in danger. AI and ML may assist in identifying risks and automating a variety of functions. The AI technology can help safeguard the healthcare professionals in the context of the current epidemic's fast-expanding concern over medical staff infection [55]. Researchers and manufacturers are also aiming to employ the AI-enabled medical equipment to prevent direct contact during SARS-COV-2 infection detection and treatment.

## 3.7 IOT APPLICATIONS DURING COVID-19

As technology advances, the healthcare application developers are interested in IoT-based approaches. Without a doubt, IoT technologies appear to be a highly realistic choice for managing the COVID-19 epidemic. IoT technology might be used to track COVID-19's spread, diagnose affected patients, provide telemedicine, and link these apps with smart gadgets. The subsections below explore several IoT applications for COVID-19 illness management.

### 3.7.1 Current contact-tracing mechanisms

IoT-based contact-tracing tools have been shown to be a useful tool for controlling COVID-19 across nations and regions [55]. As a part of the contact monitoring system, citizens having COVID-19 must unveil their contact list to a trustworthy party, such as public health authorities. Other people who have been in the same place or had contact with the COVID-19-infected person are then requested to participate in the activities such as self-quarantine or testing depending on the tested citizen's location [55]. Contact tracking using IoT technology can increase the efficiency in terms of automated analysis, rapid response, and, most crucially, the secrecy of the individual impacted [55]. Several IoT-based contact-tracking tools have been devised for the COVID-19 pandemic, which are outlined below.

*Aarogya Setu*: Aarogya Setu is a contact-tracing tool that people can download on their smartphones to help in promoting the viral awareness and combating it. Aarogya Setu was created to improve the communication between citizens and healthcare providers. The user will be asked about any experience with COVID-19 indications due to their international travel in the recent times in the application. By analyzing the input data from users as well as their tracking information, Aarogya Setu can detect if the user has had contact with someone who is already or will become a proven case [1].

*Trace Together*: The Singapore government published this software for mobile apps in March 2020. To interact with the central server and distribute randomly produced time-varying tokens among neighboring mobiles, the program uses Bluetooth technology [55]. If someone tests positive for COVID-19, the government will demand that they give information about tokens obtained by their phones, which the government will decode and link to contact numbers and names [55].

*Decentralized Privacy-Preserving Proximity Tracing (DP3T)*: The Pan-European Privacy-Preserving Proximity Tracing project team [55] proposes a decentralized method. The individual users must produce new keys every day and broadcast ephemeral identifiers in a random sequence. All IDs, as well as their proximity, are stored in the device database by the users. If a user is confirmed to be COVID-positive, the central health department will request the user's secret key for the first day of infection and distribute it to other users. As a consequence, other users will be able to check if they were in the same area as the COVID-19 individual [55].

*Contact Categorization*: To identify illness transmission, the approach uses contact categories rather than locations. Based on the received Bluetooth communications, the user devices save a list of contacts. The built program compares this list to the list of virus-infected persons acquired from the health authorities. When a match is detected, the program classifies the contact depending on how long the noninfected user was in communication with the COVID-19-infected user. When the amount of illness dissemination is particularly high, the classification aids the health authorities in prioritizing testing. Signal strength may be used to assess the closeness of infected and nonaffected users, much as the prior methods [55].

*Privacy-Sensitive Protocols and Mechanisms for Mobile Contact Tracing (PACT)*: When the amount of illness dissemination is particularly high, the classification aids the health authorities in prioritizing testing. Similar to the previous ways, the closeness of infected and noninfected persons may be determined based on signal strength [55]. The solution involves a time delay before the ID and the inclusion of timestamps to the public list to prevent replay attacks. Furthermore, it employs a specified seed update schedule for a pseudorandom generator [55].

### 3.7.2  COVID-19 diagnosis using IoT

IoT technology has the potential to speed up, increase accuracy, and streamline the COVID-19 diagnostic and treatment process [55]. A COVID-19 Intelligent Diagnosis and Treatment Assistant Program has been incorporated into a cloud-based application by the Abir et al. [56]. For automatic diagnosis, the software makes use of electronic medical information and ML algorithms. By gathering the data from the patient, maintaining coordination, and allowing patients to self-diagnose, the health authority can be assisted. The application is built on fifth-generation (5G) technologies, which make use of such networks' increased capacity and communication efficiency. It provides a collaborative environment for doctors, medical scientists, and health professionals [55] and allows improved coordination between diagnosis and treatment using WeChat.

### 3.7.3  During COVID-19 IoT telemedicine services

To avoid the disease from spreading, people infected with COVID-19 must get proper healthcare remotely [55]. Many health authorities are concentrating on building chatbots to automate disease screening and follow-up appointments. Robotic telemedicine carts (such as Vici InTouch) can be utilized to monitor patients under quarantine without the need for health staff to be there. A handful of hospitals in the United States utilize bidirectional audio and video connections to monitor patients in intensive care units [55].

### 3.7.4  COVID-19 prediction using IoT-enabled wearable technologies

The development of IoT-enabled smart devices has spawned a slew of smartphone apps for tracking physiological data, including heart rate, temperature, and sleep cycles [55]. The stages of COVID-19 can be predicted using these devices in combination with ML technologies. Temperature and blood oxygen levels can be monitored automatically, which can trigger the alerts that require immediate care from medical staff. Several studies have linked heart rate and activity patterns reported by COVID-19 patients with those recorded by Fitbit or Apple Watch users [55].

### 3.7.5 Drone and unmanned aerial vehicle to fight the pandemic

COVID-19's infectious nature will force the majority of health-monitoring tasks to be done online, putting a strain on current WiFi connections. Different communication technologies such as the long range wide area network (LoRaWAN) have sparked a lot of interest as a result. Unmanned aerial vehicles (UAVs), for example, have been suggested as a means of improving data interchange reliability [57] between infected individuals' long-range (LoRA) devices and the base station. The technique uses a distributed topology control algorithm to change the UAV topology based on the mobility of LoRA end devices at the base station, enhancing packet reception rates [55].

Drones and robots, likewise, can be extremely valuable in addressing a variety of technological difficulties originating from the pandemic [55].

### 3.7.6 Significant applications of IoT for COVID-19 pandemic

The IoT employs a huge number of networked devices to build a smart network for effective healthcare. To protect the patient's safety, it identifies and monitors any type of disease. Without the requirement for human interaction, it digitally records the patient's record. This data can also help you make well-informed decisions [30].

#### 3.7.6.1 Treatment of COVID-19 patient

For the optimum handling of COVID-19 patients, IoT with actual location provision was deployed. In the context of IoT, various medical gadgets and gear such as nebulizers, scales, wheelchairs, and other equipment are utilized for tracking. Also, we have to keep an eye on, monitor, and manage the environment, such as temperature, humidity, and so on.

#### 3.7.6.2 Smart hospital

IoT provides a smart hospital by connecting specialized networks and automating processes. The software delivers accurate information on the patient's continuous problems. With comprehensive digitization of the system, the smart hospital offers all information, minimizing the patient's waiting time. It does a record analysis for both the process and the patient. Data analysis aids everyday operations in improving COVID-19 patient care.

#### 3.7.6.3 COVID-19 patient data storage

COVID-19 patient data may be sent, effectively stored, and analyzed via IoT devices, allowing for improved treatment in the future to raise the alertness about the virus's origins. Checking and analyzing the patient's retrieved data is beneficial.

### 3.7.6.4 Acquire information from various sources and devices

IoT in healthcare gives a variety of sources and devices that may be automatically analyzed. COVID-19 patients' data is automatically collected, reported, and stored via an IoT device. It aids in the decision-making process in difficult instances, reducing surgical and medical errors as a result.

### 3.7.6.5 Accurate decision-making

Due to the several forms of communication required for effective operation, this technology saves data and produces precise and quality judgment. It was particularly useful in getting correct COVID-19 patient records, which doctors had previously struggled to get.

### 3.7.6.6 Focus on COVID-19 patient's condition

It forecasts the COVID-19 patient's arrival and keeps track of the state of support facilities. It aids in the monitoring of infection and hygiene in the hospital and support sectors. The COVID-19 patient's information, as well as other data, is obtained and kept.

### 3.7.6.7 Warning about the COVID-19 disease

This technology informs the human of COVID-19 illness and allows real-time tracking in life-threatening situations. It alerts users via connected devices on time. It reports on the state of human health and appropriately expresses an opinion. It provides more accurate real-time alerts, on-time treatment, and tracking.

### 3.7.6.8 Details for the healthcare professional

The details include the right information to give to a healthcare worker, including their location, time stamp, and database. Proper lighting is achieved by personal management and an intimate understanding of the patient's requirements. It is the most effective approach for doctors to interact with patients and their families.

### 3.7.6.9 Proper medication

It keeps track of the COVID-19 patient's medicine, as well as his or her protein and food consumption. It examines and tracks the patient's progress in daily life.

### 3.7.6.10 Proper facilities

During the COVID-19 pandemic, IoT can simply automate the patient process to offer suitable healthcare services. It shares data to improve the efficiency of healthcare services. It appears to be an effective method for using high-quality resources and improving complex surgical planning in a better way.

### 3.7.6.11 Assess level of glucose

It refers to examining the glucose level and flow concerning the patient's requirements. The insulin dosage is automatically adjusted to keep it within a healthy range.

### 3.7.6.12 Assist in remote areas

IoT can allow patients in far-flung places to communicate with the doctors using smart mobile phone apps. It aids in the examination of a COVID-19 patient and the determination of the infection's etiology. It enhances patient safety and enhances hospital digitalization.

### 3.7.6.13 Assessment of an asthma attack

It detects asthma symptoms early in the course of an attack. The attack is reported and guidance on how to avoid it is given.

### 3.7.6.14 Reminder about medication time

This technology's primary use is to remind patients to take their medications. When there are missed doses, it alerts the patient to take them as soon as possible.

### 3.7.6.15 Emergency case

Before approaching a facility/hospital in an emergency, IoT analyses the proximity and accesses the patient information. As a result, emergency care has improved and related losses have decreased.

### 3.7.6.16 Smart bed

IoT applications are attempting to develop a smart bed that can adjust its elevation to suit COVID-19 patients' needs.

## 3.8 POTENTIAL RISKS OF IOT

Existing IoT apps undoubtedly have certain privacy and security shortcomings. The contact-tracing technologies now in use by the various governments offer substantial security threats. Because government officials may be able to discover the sensitive data from those infected with COVID-19, the process utilized in TraceTogether, for example, necessitates a high level of confidence in them. As a result, while the TraceTogether software can keep the information private from third parties in general, it cannot provide the privacy-preserving solutions for the affected group [30]. Backend impersonation, false report, replay attack, and relay assault are some examples of new forms of privacy threats that can be introduced by the decentralized approach in DP3T [30]. Data breaches in healthcare systems may have a significant influence on the treatment process and patient well-being, and they've become a severe concern in modern healthcare systems as hacking assaults have become more common [30]. Because they rely on data retrieved from linked networks, IoT-based apps can exacerbate this vulnerability.

### 3.8.1 Enhancing the privacy and security of AI and IoT techniques

Due to the sensitivity of the data exposed and the potential consequences, it's vital to provide appropriate privacy and security to the approaches in AI and IoT applications, given the fundamental issues of AI and IoT methodologies. In COVID-19 contact-tracing apps, polling is used to protect the privacy of COVID-19-infected users from nonaffected users. Private messaging systems [30] and confidential set intersection protocols can be used to keep information from the health authority private.

Using cutting-edge technology to safeguard information exchange during a pandemic like COVID-19 can be extremely successful. In this context, for smooth integration in healthcare systems, adequate standardized procedures for new communication and network protocols are necessary [30]. Because IoT applications provide extensive exposure to system tracking data, new data-driven security strategies for building predictive ML models to identify IoT threats may be created [30]. Blockchain and other distributed ledger technologies can ensure data integrity without the need for a third party, allowing for secure information transmission among several parties in the healthcare sector, thus resulting in the privacy-preserving solutions for smart healthcare systems [30].

## 3.9 SIGNIFICANT ADVANTAGES OF IOT IN HEALTHCARE

The significant benefits of IoT in healthcare include:

- **Reduction of Cost:** IoT enables significant patient monitoring, minimizing the number of needless doctor appointments, hospitalization, and re-admissions.
- **Effective Treatment:** It allows doctors to make the educated judgments based on facts and ensures complete openness.

- **Quicker Disease Diagnosis:** Real-time data and continuous patient monitoring help in the early detection of diseases, even before symptoms manifest.
- **Proactive Treatment:** The ability to provide proactive medical therapy is enabled through continuous health monitoring.
- **Management of Drugs and Equipment:** In the healthcare industry, managing drugs and medical equipment is a huge concern. Linked devices efficiently manage and utilize them, resulting in cheaper costs.
- **Error Reduction:** Not only can IoT data aid in better decision-making, but it also ensures that healthcare operations run smoothly with minimum errors, waste, and system expenses.

## 3.10 CHALLENGES OF IOT IN HEALTHCARE

Security, privacy, interoperability, storage management, server technology, and data center networking are among the hurdles of IoT development, according to the authors in Ref. [58–60]. Ultralow-power design and real-time restrictions are two issues in the medical and healthcare fields [61]. Data confidentiality is a security issue that is engaged with IoT. According to Shahid and Aneja [62], secrecy refers to preventing unauthorized parties from accessing information. It is critical to guarantee that data is safe and accessible only to authorized individuals. Only those who are authorized have access to sensitive information. A loss of confidentiality happens when someone gains access to data that they shouldn't have.

According to Mahmoud et al. [63], users of IoT have to be familiar with management policies and processes to ensure data security [64, 65]. Privacy and trust are two further issues that IoT presents. For example, giving information confidence in a shared medium, ensuring safe data sharing, and implementing protective procedures etc. Interoperability is another issue that has to be addressed. Interoperability has always been the foundational value for ensuring device communication. Different industries now utilize several standards to deal with a wide range of different data and devices. As a result, the IoT system must maintain a high level of compatibility.

## 3.11 CONCLUSION

In this work, the importance of IoT in the medical sector using advanced technologies has been elaborated. The IoT architecture for healthcare is outlined. The different optimized [66–68] technologies used for IoT implementation are discussed. Furthermore, the latest advances in IoT for tracking and analyzing COVID-19-infected patients, as well as the future uses of IoT, were discussed. Furthermore, modern technologies such as AI and ML applications [69] for anticipating illness patterns and generating social awareness campaigns have been detailed. The potential risks, major advantages, and challenges of IoT in healthcare are discussed. Future research will be conducted to expand on the findings to build some new algorithms for COVID-19 health-tracking applications using IoT.

## REFERENCES

[1] Nasajpour, M., Pouriyeh, S., Parizi, R. M., Dorodchi, M., Valero, M., & Arabnia, H. R. (2020). Internet of things for current COVID-19 and future pandemics: An exploratory study. *Journal of Healthcare Informatics Research*, 1–40.

[2] Andrea, I., Chrysostomou, C., & Hadjichristofi, G. (2015, July). Internet of Things: Security vulnerabilities and challenges. In *2015 IEEE Symposium on Computers and Communication (ISCC)* (pp. 180–187). IEEE.

[3] Gupta, A., Srivastava, A., Anand, R., & Tomažič, T. (2020). Business Application Analytics and the Internet of Things: The Connecting Link. In *New Age Analytics*, eds. G. Shrivastava, S.L. Peng, H. Bansal, K. Sharma, M. Sharma (pp. 249–273). Apple Academic Press.

[4] Anand, R., Sinha, A., Bhardwaj, A., & Sreeraj, A. (2018). Flawed Security of Social Network of Things. In *Handbook of Research on Network Forensics and Analysis Techniques*, eds. G. Shrivastava, P. Kumar, B.B. Gupta, S. Bala, N. Dey (pp. 65–86). IGI Global.

[5] Gupta, R., Shrivastava, G., Anand, R., & Tomažič, T. (2018). IoT-Based Privacy Control System through Android. In *Handbook of E-business Security*, eds. J.M.R.S. Tavares, B.K. Mishra, R. Kumar, N. Zaman, M. Khari (pp. 341–363). Auerbach Publications.

[6] Ali, Z. H., Ali, H. A., & Badawy, M. M. (2015). Internet of Things (IoT): definitions, challenges and recent research directions. *International Journal of Computer Applications*, *128*(1), 37–47.

[7] HaddadPajouh, H., Dehghantanha, A., Parizi, R. M., Aledhari, M., & Karimipour, H. (2019). A survey on internet of things security: Requirements, challenges, and solutions. *Internet of Things*, 100129.

[8] Kumar, A., Tripathi, S., & Raw, R. S. (2016). Bringing Healthcare to Doorstep using VANETs. In *3rd IEEE International Conference as INDIACom-2016*, ISSN (0973-7529), 16–18 March, Delhi, pp. 4747–4750.

[9] Da Costa, C. A., Pasluosta, C. F., Eskofier, B., Da Silva, D. B., & da Rosa Righi, R. (2018). Internet of health things: Toward intelligent vital signs monitoring in hospital wards. *Artificial Intelligence in Medicine*, *89*, 61–69.

[10] Islam, S. R., Kwak, D., Kabir, M. H., Hossain, M., & Kwak, K. S. (2015). The internet of things for health care: A comprehensive survey. *IEEE Access*, *3*, 678–708.

[11] Hu, F., Xie, D., & Shen, S. (2013, August). On the application of the internet of things in the field of medical and health care. In *2013 IEEE International Conference on Green Computing and Communications and IEEE Internet of Things and IEEE Cyber, Physical and Social Computing* (pp. 2053–2058).

[12] Yang, P., Qi, J., Min, G., & Xu, L. (2017). Advanced internet of things for personalised healthcare system: A survey. *Pervasive and Mobile Computing*, *41*, 132–149.

[13] Kishor, A., & Chakraborty, C. (2021). Artificial intelligence and internet of things based healthcare 4.0 monitoring system. *Wireless Personal Communications*, 1–17.

[14] Elavarasan, R. M., & Pugazhendhi, R. (2020). Restructured society and environment: A review on potential technological strategies to control the COVID-19 pandemic. *Science of the Total Environment*, *725*, 138858.

[15] Bullock, J., Luccioni, A., Pham, K. H., Lam, C. S. N., & Luengo-Oroz, M. (2020). Mapping the landscape of artificial intelligence applications against COVID-19. *Journal of Artificial Intelligence Research*, *69*, 807–845.

[16] Li, W., Chai, Y., Khan, F., Jan, S. R. U., Verma, S., Menon, V. G., & Li, X. (2021). A comprehensive survey on machine learning-based big data analytics for IoT-enabled smart healthcare system. *Mobile Networks and Applications*, *26*(1), 1–19.

[17] Misra, S., Mukherjee, A., & Roy, A. (2021). *Introduction to IoT*. Cambridge University Press.

[18] Besher, K. M., Subah, Z., & Ali, M. Z. (2020). IoT sensor initiated healthcare data security. *IEEE Sensors Journal*, *21*(10), 11977–11982.

[19] Končar, J., Grubor, A., Marić, R., Vučenović, S., & Vukmirović, G. (2020). Setbacks to IoT implementation in the function of FMCG supply chain sustainability during COVID-19 pandemic. *Sustainability*, *12*(18), 7391.

[20] Al-Turjman, F., & Deebak, B. D. (2020). Privacy-aware energy-efficient framework using the internet of medical things for COVID-19. *IEEE Internet of Things Magazine*, *3*(3), 64–68.

[21] Sun, G., Trung, N. V., Hiep, P. T., Ishibashi, K., & Matsui, T. (2020). Visualisation of epidemiological map using an internet of things infectious disease surveillance platform. *Critical Care*, *24*(1), 1–2.

[22] Kohli, L., Saurabh, M., Bhatia, I., Shekhawat, U. S., Vijh, M., & Sindhwani, N. (2021). Design and Development of Modular and Multifunctional UAV with Amphibious Landing Module. In *Data Driven Approach towards Disruptive Technologies: Proceedings of MIDAS 2020*, eds. T.P. Singh, R. Tomar, T. Choudhury, T. Perumal, H.F. Mahdi (pp. 405–421). Singapore: Springer.

[23] Srivastava, A., Gupta, A., & Anand, R. (2021). Optimized smart system for transportation using RFID technology. *Mathematics in Engineering, Science and Aerospace (MESA)*, *12*(4).

[24] Kohli, L., Saurabh, M., Bhatia, I., Sindhwani, N., & Vijh, M. (2021). Design and Development of Modular and Multifunctional UAV with Amphibious Landing, Processing and Surround Sense Module. In *Unmanned Aerial Vehicles for Internet of Things (IoT): Concepts, Techniques, and Applications*, eds. V. Mohindru, Y. Singh, R. Bhatt and A.K. Gupta (p. 207). Wiley.

[25] Li, C. T., Wu, T. Y., Chen, C. L., Lee, C. C., & Chen, C. M. (2017). An efficient user authentication and user anonymity scheme with provably security for IoT-based medical care system. *Sensors*, *17*(7), 1482.

[26] Lai, Y. L., Chou, Y. H., & Chang, L. C. (2018). An intelligent IoT emergency vehicle warning system using RFID and Wi-Fi technologies for emergency medical services. *Technology and Health Care*, *26*(1), 43–55.

[27] Vafea, M. T., Atalla, E., Georgakas, J., Shehadeh, F., Mylona, E. K., Kalligeros, M., & Mylonakis, E. (2020). Emerging technologies for use in the study, diagnosis, and treatment of patients with COVID-19. *Cellular and Molecular Bioengineering*, *13*(4), 249–257.

[28] Bamidis, P. D. (2017). Internet of things in health trends through bibliometrics and text mining. *Informatics for Health: Connected Citizen-Led Wellness and Population Health, 235*, 73.

[29] Dai, H. N., Imran, M., & Haider, N. (2020). Blockchain-enabled internet of medical things to combat COVID-19. *IEEE Internet of Things Magazine, 3*(3), 52–57.

[30] Javaid, M., & Khan, I. H. (2021). Internet of Things (IoT) enabled healthcare helps to take the challenges of COVID-19 Pandemic. *Journal of Oral Biology and Craniofacial Research, 11*(2), 209–214.

[31] Javaid, M., Haleem, A., Vaishya, R., Bahl, S., Suman, R., & Vaish, A. (2020). Industry 4.0 technologies and their applications in fighting COVID-19 pandemic. *Diabetes & Metabolic Syndrome: Clinical Research & Reviews, 14*(4), 419–422.

[32] Allam, Z., & Jones, D. S. (2020, March). On the Coronavirus (COVID-19) Outbreak and the Smart City Network: Universal Data Sharing Standards Coupled with Artificial Intelligence (AI) to Benefit Urban Health Monitoring and Management. In *Healthcare* (Vol. 8, No. 1, p. 46). Multidisciplinary Digital Publishing Institute. DOI:10.3390/healthcare8010046.

[33] Dewey, C., Hingle, S., Goelz, E., & Linzer, M. (2020). Supporting clinicians during the COVID-19 pandemic. *Annals of Internal Medicine, 172*(11), 752–753. DOI:10.7326/M20-1033.

[34] Stoessl, A. J., Bhatia, K. P., & Merello, M. (2020). Movement disorders in the world of COVID-19. *Movement Disorders Clinical Practice, 7*(4), 355.

[35] Gupta, M., Abdelsalam, M., & Mittal, S. (2020). Enabling and enforcing social distancing measures using smart city and its infrastructures: A COVID-19 Use case. *arXiv preprint arXiv:2004.09246.*

[36] Singh, P., Raw, R. S., Khan, S. A., Mohammed, M. A., Aly, A. A., & Le, D. -N. (2021). W-GeoR: Weighted geographical routing for VANET's Health monitoring applications in urban traffic networks. *IEEE Access.* DOI: 10.1109/ACCESS.2021.3092426.

[37] Singh, P., Raw, R. S., & Khan, S. A. (2021). Link risk degree aided routing protocol based on weight gradient for health monitoring applications in vehicular ad-hoc networks. *Journal of Ambient Intelligence Humanized Computing.* https://doi.org/10.1007/s12652-021-03264-z

[38] Kumar, S., & Raw, R. S. (2020). Health Monitoring Planning for On-Board Ships through Flying Ad Hoc Network. In *Advanced Computing and Intelligent Engineering*, eds. B. Pati, C.R. Panigrahi, R. Buyya, K.C. Li (pp. 391–402) Springer, ISBN: 978-981-15-1483-8.

[39] Otoom, M., Otoum, N., Alzubaidi, M. A., Etoom, Y., & Banihani, R. (2020). An IoT-based framework for early identification and monitoring of COVID-19 cases. *Biomedical Signal Processing and Control, 62*, 102149.

[40] Jain, S., Kumar, M., Sindhwani, N., & Singh, P. (2021). SARS-Cov-2 detection using Deep Learning Techniques on the basis of Clinical Reports. In *2021 9th International Conference on Reliability, Infocom Technologies and Optimization (Trends and Future Directions) (ICRITO)*, pp. 1–5, DOI: 10.1109/ICRITO51393.2021.9596455. (Scopus Indexed).

[41] Singh, H., Rehman, T. B., Gangadhar, C., Anand, R., Sindhwani, N., & Babu, M. (2021). Accuracy detection of coronary artery disease using machine learning algorithms. *Applied Nanoscience*, 1–7.

[42] Bogoch, I. I., Watts, A., Thomas-Bachli, A., Huber, C., Kraemer, M. U., & Khan, K. (2020). Pneumonia of unknown aetiology in Wuhan, China: Potential for international spread via commercial air travel. *Journal of Travel Medicine*, 27(2), taaa008.

[43] Sansanwal, K., Shrivastava, G., Anand, R., & Sharma, K. (2019). Big Data Analysis and Compression for Indoor Air Quality. In *Handbook of IoT and Big Data*, eds. V.K. Solanki, V.C. Diaz, J.P. Davim (pp. 1–21). CRC Press.

[44] Sindhwani, N., Verma, S., Bajaj, T., & Anand, R. (2021). Comparative analysis of intelligent driving and safety assistance systems using YOLO and SSD model of deep learning. *International Journal of Information System Modeling and Design (IJISMD)*, 12(1), 131–146.

[45] Vyas, G., Anand, R., & Holê, K. E. (2011). Implementation of advanced image compression using wavelet transform and SPHIT algorithm. *International Journal of Electronic and Electrical Engineering*, 4(3), 249–254. ISSN: 0974-2174.

[46] Kumar, R., Anand, R., & Kaushik, G. (2011). Image compression using wavelet method & SPIHT algorithm. *Digital Image Processing*, 3(2), 75–79.

[47] Choudhary, P., & Anand, M. R. (2015). Determination of rate of degradation of iron plates due to rust using image processing. *International Journal of Engineering Research*, 4(2), 76–84.

[48] Saini, P., & Anand, M. R. (2014). Identification of defects in plastic gears using image processing and computer vision: A review. *International Journal of Engineering Research*, 3(2), 94–99.

[49] Meng, L. (2020). Review: Chest CT features and their role in COVID-19. *Radiology of Infectious Diseases*. Available online: www.sciencedirect.com (accessed on 30 March 2020).

[50] Loey, M., Smarandache, F., & Khalifa, N. E. M. (2020). Within the lack of chest COVID-19 X-ray dataset: a novel detection model based on GAN and deep transfer learning. *Symmetry*, 12(4), 651.

[51] Öztürk, Ş., Özkaya, U., & Barstuğan, M. (2021). Classification of coronavirus (COVID-19) from X-ray and CT images using shrunken features. *International Journal of Imaging Systems and Technology*, 31(1), 5–15.

[52] Alwashmi, M. F. (2020). The use of digital health in the detection and management of COVID-19. *International Journal of Environmental Research and Public Health*, 17(8), 2906.

[53] Beck, B. R., Shin, B., Choi, Y., Park, S., & Kang, K. (2020). Predicting commercially available antiviral drugs that may act on the novel coronavirus (SARS-CoV-2) through a drug-target interaction deep learning model. *Computational and Structural Biotechnology Journal*, 18, 784–790.

[54] Magar, R., Yadav, P., & Farimani, A. B. (2021). Potential neutralizing antibodies discovered for novel corona virus using machine learning. *Scientific Reports*, 11(1), 1–11.

[55] Zhong, L., Mu, L., Li, J., Wang, J., Yin, Z., & Liu, D. (2020). Early prediction of the 2019 novel coronavirus outbreak in the mainland China based on simple mathematical model. *IEEE Access*, 8, 51761–51769.

[56] Abir, S. M., Islam, S. N., Anwar, A., Mahmood, A. N., & Oo, A. M. T. (2020). Building resilience against COVID-19 pandemic using artificial intelligence, machine learning, and IoT: A survey of recent progress. *IoT*, 1(2), 506–528.

[57] Juneja, S., Juneja, A., & Anand, R. (2019, April). Reliability Modeling for Embedded System Environment compared to available Software Reliability Growth Models. In *2019 International Conference on Automation, Computational and Technology Management (ICACTM)* (pp. 379–382). IEEE.

[58] Bai, L., Yang, D., Wang, X., Tong, L., Zhu, X., Zhong, N.,... & Tan, F. (2020). Chinese experts' consensus on the Internet of Things-aided diagnosis and treatment of coronavirus disease 2019 (COVID-19). *Clinical eHealth, 3*, 7–15.

[59] ILee, I., & Lee, K. (2015). The Internet of Things (IoT): Applications, investments, and challenges for enterprises. *Business Horizons, 58*(4), 431–440.

[60] Hassanalieragh, M., Page, A., Soyata, T., Sharma, G., Aktas, M., Mateos, G.,... & Andreescu, S. (2015, June). Health monitoring and management using Internet-of-Things (IoT) sensing with cloud-based processing: Opportunities and challenges. In *2015 IEEE International Conference on Services Computing* (pp. 285–292). IEEE.

[61] Chiang, M., & Zhang, T. (2016). Fog and IoT: An overview of research opportunities. *IEEE Internet of Things Journal, 3*(6), 854–864.

[62] Shahid, N., & Aneja, S. (2017, February). Internet of Things: Vision, application areas and research challenges. In *2017 International Conference on I-SMAC (IoT in Social, Mobile, Analytics and Cloud)(I-SMAC)* (pp. 583–587). IEEE.

[63] Mahmoud, R., Yousuf, T., Aloul, F., & Zualkernan, I. (2015, December). Internet of things (IoT) security: Current status, challenges and prospective measures. In *2015 10th International Conference for Internet Technology and Secured Transactions (ICITST)* (pp. 336–341). IEEE.

[64] Samie, F., Bauer, L., & Henkel, J. (2016, October). IoT Technologies for Embedded Computing: A Survey. In *2016 International Conference on Hardware/Software Codesign and System Synthesis (CODES+ ISSS)* (pp. 1–10). IEEE.

[65] Anand, R., Shrivastava, G., Gupta, S., Peng, S. L., & Sindhwani, N. (2018). Audio Watermarking With Reduced Number of Random Samples. In *Handbook of Research on Network Forensics and Analysis Techniques*, eds. G. Shrivastava, P. Kumar, B.B. Gupta, S. Bala, N. Dey (pp. 372–394). IGI Global.

[66] Sindhwani, N., Bhamrah, M. S., Garg, A., & Kumar, D. (2017, July). Performance Analysis of Particle Swarm Optimization and Genetic Algorithm in MIMO Systems. In *2017 8th International Conference on Computing, Communication and Networking Technologies (ICCCNT)* (pp. 1–6). IEEE.

[67] Sindhwani, N., & Singh, M. (2020). A joint optimization based sub-band expediency scheduling technique for MIMO communication system. *Wireless Personal Communications, 115*(3), 2437–2455.

[68] Sindhwani, N., & Singh, M. (2017, March). Performance Analysis of ant Colony based Optimization Algorithm in MIMO Systems. In *2017 International Conference on Wireless Communications, Signal Processing and Networking (WiSPNET)* (pp. 1587–1593). IEEE.

[69] Anand, R., Sindhwani, N., & Saini, A. (2021). Emerging technologies for COVID-19. Enabling healthcare 4.0 for pandemics: A roadmap using AI, *Machine Learning, IoT and Cognitive Technologies*, 163–188.

Chapter 4

# Internet of medical things

## Reduced energy consumption and data storage

*Mohammed Moutaib*
EST My Ismail University, Morocco

*Tarik Ahajjam*
LSTI-IDMS My Ismail University Faculty of Sciences and Technics, Morocco

*Mohammed Fattah*
EST My Ismail University, Morocco

*Youssef Farhaoui*
LSTI-IDMS My Ismail University Faculty of Sciences and Technics, Morocco

*Badraddine Aghoutane*
FS My Ismail University, Morocco

## CONTENTS

DOI: 10.1201/9781003239888-4

## 4.1 INTRODUCTION

Internet of things (IoT) is a concept that embodies the vision of ubiquitous computing: as Mark Weiser [1] imagined in 1991, technology gradually fades into the user's environment and blends naturally into everyday objects. This revolution cannot be represented by a single object, for instance a personal computer, but in the form of a simple to use and a powerful device capable of communicating on several types of networks.

This phenomenon [2, 3] and cloud computing [4–6] take advantage of the ubiquity of devices equipped with sensors to collect data at low cost [7–9], guaranteeing a new concept for high demand detection [10, 11]. Maintaining high data energy efficiency is essential. Therefore, IoTs have become more creative in several areas, for example, healthcare technology.

With the power of the IoT, several problems can be found, such as the integration of many types of expensive sensors that allow different people to benefit from medical health services, storage or bandwidth, and power consumption, etc. It must be adopted for a specific purpose, and it has a particular type of intelligence, a capacity using onboard sensors that allow data to be received and transmitted [12, 13]. The connected object has value when connected to other objects and software. A connected watch only has meaning within an oriented ecosystem, which goes far beyond the hour's knowledge.

Indeed, IoT [14–16] has currently reflected an increase in the connected objects, devices with their own identities and increasingly complex calculation and communication capacities, telephones, watches, household. IoT is also a way to communicate with the other objects and software, such as a watch. These objects increasingly carry either sensors or actuators [17, 18], which measure and act in an environment, thus establishing a connection between virtual and physical environments.

IoT poses specific challenges due to its large scale, as well as its dynamic nature and the heterogeneity of information and its constituent systems such as powerful devices with low power consumption or fixed devices or mobile phones as well as batteries. These functionalities require some suitable methods and tools to implement powerful applications to extract helpful information from many available data sources in order to store them in a heterogeneous database so that it can communicate with the environment via the actuators (rather than via the user) [19].

Some researchers speak of "hyper objects" [20] as those capable of pooling their resources. To accomplish the tasks, they are linked by links in the same environment. In this case, some researchers like Mavrommati and Kameas [21] have imagined today's computing where the deepest technologies are those which have become invisible. Those, when tied together, form the fabric of our daily life to the point of becoming inseparable from it.

In this work, we have proposed a new application solution based on IoT health that begins with a definition of connected objects, followed by a discussion on the connected object technologies used in the different fields. Then, a discussion of other solutions, which can target this subject, is done. Finally, our chapter ends with the solution of our study.

The rest of the chapter is organized like this. Section 4.2 presents the history and application of the IoT in healthcare. We list some IoT technologies in section 4.3. In section 4.4, we present the solution of our study. This solution is detailed and divided into two parts: design and implementation. Finally, section 4.5 concludes our chapter.

## 4.2 IOT ENERGY CONSUMPTION

IoT is an avant-garde technology, where traditionally unconnected objects around us (such as lamps, machines, clothes), whether physical or virtual, can communicate with each other in real time. This network of objects allows them to share their data via cloud interface without any intervention. Due to the reduction of human–machine interaction and the increase of data flow, these connected objects can define the individual's needs to provide with unique goods or services. IoT enables the reduction in energy consumption. With IoT, mobile devices can communicate via wireless networks. So, these processes are increasingly automated by reporting the types of information used for optimization [22, 23]. In addition, there is a real-time aspect that allows supply to adapt better to demand. Thus, to process large quantities, the producer can deduct from the future demand. All these elements have a significant impact: energy consumption, security, and data storage.

Minimizing the energy consumption of the connected objects requires optimized design [24, 25] and more efficient electronic components. European developers have developed very low-power technologies, and this is a discriminating factor with the manufacturers.

A connected object must communicate, and this consumes energy. Transmitting data via networks such as 3G or 4G and lately 5G is very energy consuming. Thus, specific networks such as Sigfox or Lora have emerged, allowing devices to communicate with lower energy consumption.

### 4.2.1 History of the IoT

Nikola Tesla said in 1926: "When the absence of loss is perfectly applied, the whole world becomes one huge brain, all things are part of a real and rhythmic whole. We will be able to communicate with each other at any time, regardless of the distance. Not only that, but thanks to television and telephony, we will see and hear so perfectly, as if we were standing face to face, despite the distance of thousands of kilometers, and whose tools with which we could do it, they will look like today's phones. Human will be able to carry such a device in a pocket" [26]. Figure 4.1 represents the History of

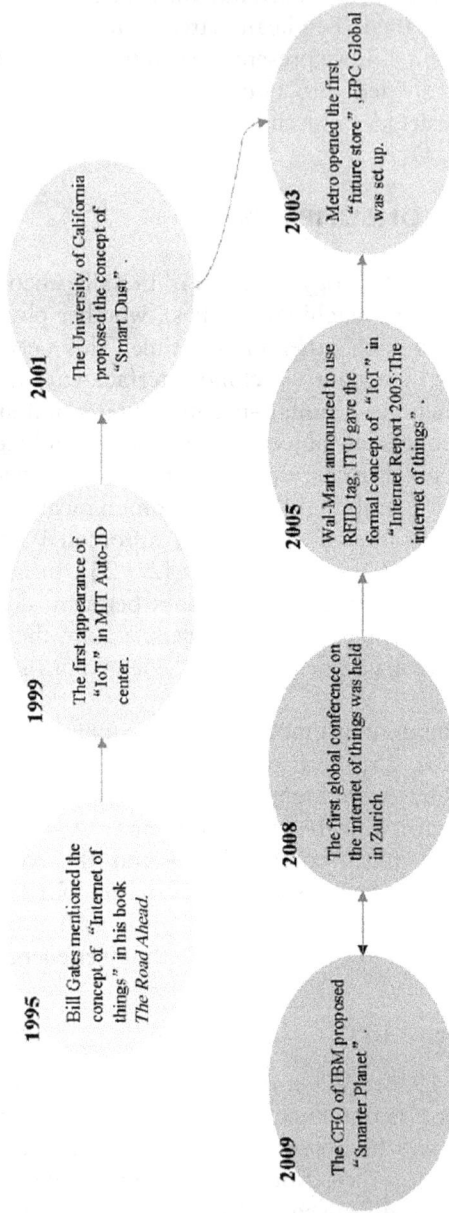

Figure 4.1  History of IoT.

IoT. In 1989, Tim Berners designed the Lee World Wide Web (WWW) and, later in 1990, launched the world's first web server [27]. An example of the Internet was probably made by one of the founders of the TCP/IP protocols, John Romkey, in 1990 when he plugged in his toaster [28]. The idea of a network of smart devices was first proposed in modern times and popularized by Kevin Ashton in 1999, who came up with the term "Internet of Things."

The emergence of the IoT as such dates back to 2008 and 2009, when CISCO estimated the number of devices linked to the network exceeds the amount of worldwide [29]. The great media coverage of the IoTs took place in 2014. In 2015, 4.9 billion devices were reportedly connected to the Internet. The analysts at Gartner predicted a daily increase of about 5.5 million new devices. In 2020, they estimated the number of connected devices at 20.8 billion. ABIR estimates that by 2020 the number of devices will reach 40.9B [30]. CISCO even predicts up to 50 billion connected devices [31]. Estimates vary from company to company due to the uncertainty of which devices are IoT devices [32]. One of these companies, which on its website states that their statistics do not include smartphones, tablets, or computers, in particular, Gartner confirms this fact [30].

## 4.2.2 Application

The potential granted by the IoT allows the growth of a massive number of applications. Currently, the company provides only a small number of applications, and we can find many areas that can change the quality of life: at home, when traveling at work, and in case of illness [33].

These environments are now equipped with objects of intelligence, which guarantee primitivity. Giving them the ability to create data perceived from the environment involves differences between them. Figure 4.2 shows the application domains of IoT. They can be applied in several fields such as the medical domain, transport, and logistics domain. Among the applications that can be distinguished, we can find those that are applicable or closer to our current lifestyles, such as health.

For example, in the medical field:

Remote patient monitoring: IoT has given us the ability to monitor patients remotely through medical devices.

Medical operations: With the IoT, it has become possible to perform operations easily and to detect the abnormality in our body.

## 4.3 IOT TECHNOLOGY

From a technical standpoint, the term IoT holds a considerable promise for the future. However, IoT technology is still in its infancy, with massive expansions expected in years soon. We can already encounter this

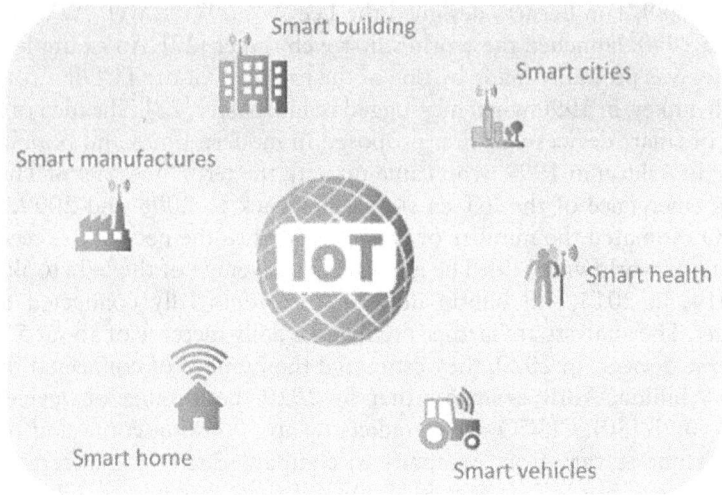

*Figure 4.2* Application domains of the IoT.

technology daily in everyday life, and we will encounter it more and more often; we will depend on it more and more, and we will demand more of it. The essence of IoT is the connection of the physical world, such as the sensor, with the virtual world, such as the cloud. The connection of these two worlds brings new possibilities.

Objects within the IoT can make decisions and execute based on the data collection activities in a completely autonomous way [34]. From reading many professional articles and reports on the IoT, we are convinced that there is no single and commonly used definition of the term. Different companies use different definitions to describe or disseminate a particular vision of what IoT represents and what its basic characteristics are.

The major technologies for IoT are:

## 4.3.1 RFID

RFID stands for radio frequency identification or radio identification [35] or "RFID Tags." These beacons, which can be linked or incorporated into products, react to the radio waves to send the information at a distance. This evolution could eventually renew the bar codes. However, its formidable efficiency poses ethical and confidentiality problems.

This technology has been used, even if it is at the beginning, in confidentially, for military applications since the Second World War. However, it was not until the 2000s that it became popular. In the logistics sector, it participates in the traceability of products from the warehouse to the store. Then, it is transformed into an anti-theft system and a means of identifying products at the checkout. In libraries, RFID helps to identify the books. Moreover, it is found on passports, public transport access cards, and even in the chips used to identify our dogs and cats. More recently, it has made it possible to imagine the marketing of communicating objects.

- How RFID technology works:
  At the heart of RFID technology, there are, first of all, RFID readers. They emit radio frequencies intended to activate RFID chips located approximately a few centimeters to several hundred meters for the most efficient way, thus exchanging information. Higher frequencies are used to exchange more information at a higher rate. Lower frequencies help to penetrate the matter better.

  RFID tags may or may not be rewritable, consisting of an antenna [36], a thin silicon chip, and an encapsulation. Some are said to be passive when they rely on the energy of the RFID reader to function. Others are said to be active. They are also equipped with a battery, which allows them to transmit information to a reader located at a distance. RFID tags can encrypt the information they receive.

## 4.3.2 WSN

WSN [37–39] is composed of independent decentralized devices equipped with sensors. It aims to monitor the physical or environmental environment and can be used in conjunction with RFID systems to track the conditions such as temperature or location or movements [40, 41].

WSN allows communication with different network topologies and multihops. The latest technological advancements in low-power circuits and wireless interaction have made it possible to use miniature devices with high performance, low cost, and optimized power consumption for WSN use.

WSN is mainly used in the logistics cold chain, which uses temperature-sensitive transport methods for hot packaging and refrigerated products [42].

- How WSN technology works:
  The data processed by the nodes is routed via a multihop routing, considered as a "collection point," "called a receiving node."

  This latter can be connected to the network user or other systems. The user can transmit requests to other nodes in the network, specifying the data required and collecting the environmental data captured via the receiving node.

  The joint advancement of microelectronics as well as the revolution in other technologies such as microtechnology and wireless transmission technology and software applications have produced large volume microsensors that can operate in the network at an acceptable cost. They integrate a capture unit (responsible for capturing physical "heat, humidity, vibrations, radiation, etc." and transforming them into digital) with wireless transmission module. These microsensors are accurate onboard systems. Several of these deploy to transmit and collect data at one or more assembly points, in an autonomous manner to form a wireless sensor network called WSN.

### 4.3.3 Cloud computing

Cloud computing (CC) is an infrastructure where servers manage computing power and storage, and it is a provider of computing resources over the Internet such as servers, databases, storage, platforms, infrastructure, etc. CC is provided on a pay-per-use basis. CC refers to the storage and access to data through the intermediary of the IT infrastructure, that is, hardware and software can be stored online.

To access these servers, which host either the applications or the data, one needs an Internet connection.

CC services can be available with different methods, and this new creation has become the first choice for companies because of their power and security [43].

Several types of CC meets the need of all users:

- Types of CC
  There are three CC models that users can access:
  - *Public*:
    It is an infrastructure of the computing resources. These resources change depending on the cloud provider but can include many capabilities such as storage capacity, applications, or virtual machines. These kinds of clouds can achieve scalability and resource sharing that a single organization cannot achieve.
  - *Private*:
    This is an infrastructure that hosts only one company. In some features, it is similar to the other cloud. ACP hosts the resources of a single client, which makes it different from the public one and gives it stability. It is hosted on the company's internal servers using some virtualization technologies, and it also offers better protection.
  - *Hybrid*:
    It's a mix of private and public clouds that generally offer the best capabilities of both categories. In it, one can host the confidential data, while other resources are hosted in public to manage excessive traffic. A company can also return to the C. public.

### 4.3.4 Middleware

In the context of distributed computing, middleware is used for communication that allows the multiple processes to run on one or more machines through interact via a network. We can express middleware as the layer between O.system and application [44].

The role of middleware is to ensure communication and sharing services. The resources are transparent, that is, the application will use the advanced features provided by the middleware without worrying about how to process and transmit its data. In object-oriented language, this mechanism is particularly suited to the realization of middleware to characterize their packaging.

## 4.4 NETWORK ARCHITECTURE

### 4.4.1 Consumption

Several solutions exist to optimize [45, 46] the energy consumption of connected objects in the medical field. In a desire for hyper-connectivity, the choice of a data transfer in continuous flow already exists. So, in many cases, a device only needs to connect episodically, as is the case for all the devices operating in automation [47–49].

The connected objects are structured around two large families:

*Nodes*: They are usually equipped with a low-powered processor, a wireless communication interface, and limited memory. They carry out the measurements in the field with obligation to the sensors they carry on board.

*Basics*: These are much more powerful devices, but they don't have sensors. They are generally limited in number in the network. They are used as centralized collection points receiving the measurements acquired by the nodes, as intermediaries between two networks of sensors, or with another network (Internet, in particular), or as points of interaction with users.

After analyzing the existing models [50–52], we propose a fully distributed trust model. We did not apply the rules of a direct link to the base, but we introduced a new rule according to which nodes exchange data: "Nodes A and B send to C, then C and D and E also send F to go immediately."

A single bit sent can sometimes consume as much power as the execution of a thousand instructions by the processor. To reduce this power consumption, there are several solutions to choose from:

*Time slots*: In this solution, nodes are only allowed to communicate regularly, whereas the network interface is disabled rest of the time, which is useful in some cases, but not available in most cases (sensitive data).

*Mono-jump*: Each device only exchanges information with devices that are close enough to communicate. However, in order to minimize power consumption, the range of these links has been markedly reduced.

*Multihop*: Each node can serve as an intermediary (routing role) for other nodes. Self-organizing is done to build a route through which messages pass.

Scenarios often use a centralized approach (Figure 4.3), where the node sends all information to the base. The nodes typically store this information in a database and allow users to retrieve and process this information. In our solution, we want to create a distributed scenario (Figure 4.4), where each node communicates with another node and sends data to the base node. This solution aims to distribute the tasks of the base between the different nodes.

We have implemented our two previous architectures in the medical field. In these architectures, several sensors have been distributed homogeneously on the human body to look for the signs of health. Each of these sensors collects a set of information and transfers it to the database, sending these data depending on the method used.

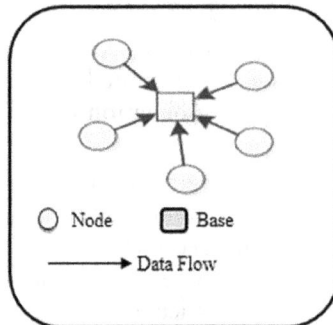

*Figure 4.3* Centralized collection.

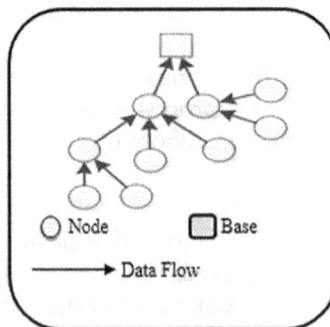

*Figure 4.4* Distributed collection.

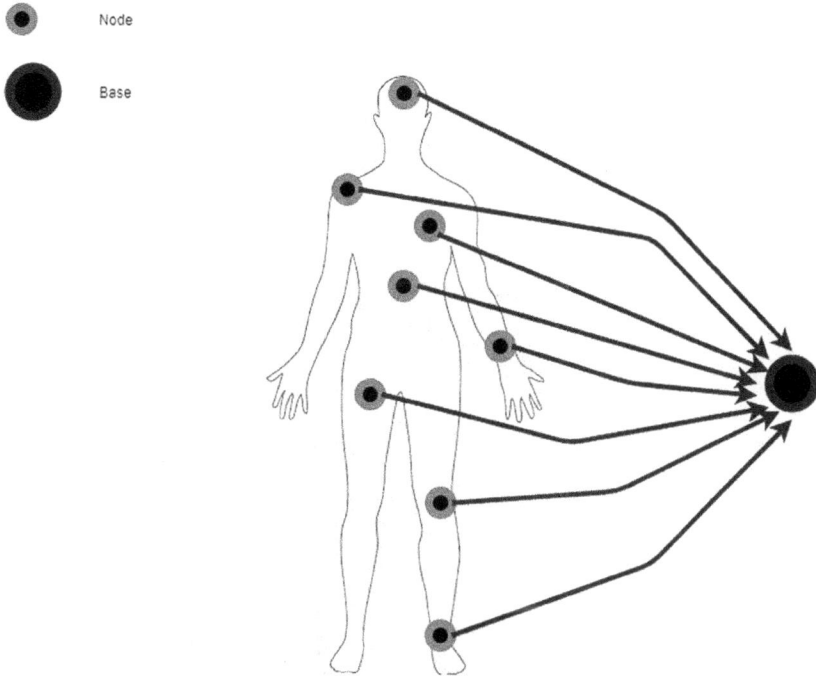

*Figure 4.5* Centralized collection of nodes in the human body.

The first traditional network architecture is illustrated in Figure 4.5. This topology validates the direct link between the base and the nodes, that is, when a sensor receives a signal in a human organ, this node sends these data to the base to be stored, analyzed, and reported. In Figure 4.6, a new network architecture is designed. Each node in this solution has the role of node and base at the same time. We aim not to disrupt the base with a vast number of information submissions. We choose to make a direct connection between the nodes.

As an example, in our case, the first node will send this data to the node closest to it, the latter will send the first node's data, and this data is collected to the base. In this way, we are able to make a single connection with as much information as possible.

## 4.4.2 Storage

A cloud database is a set of data that can be structured or unstructured according to our need that occupies a platform of private or public CC infrastructure or hybrid, as we already quote.

The CC databases are divided into two main models. A database runs on IT department's infrastructure via a virtual machine in a traditional CC. The enterprise IT team is responsible for monitoring and administering the database.

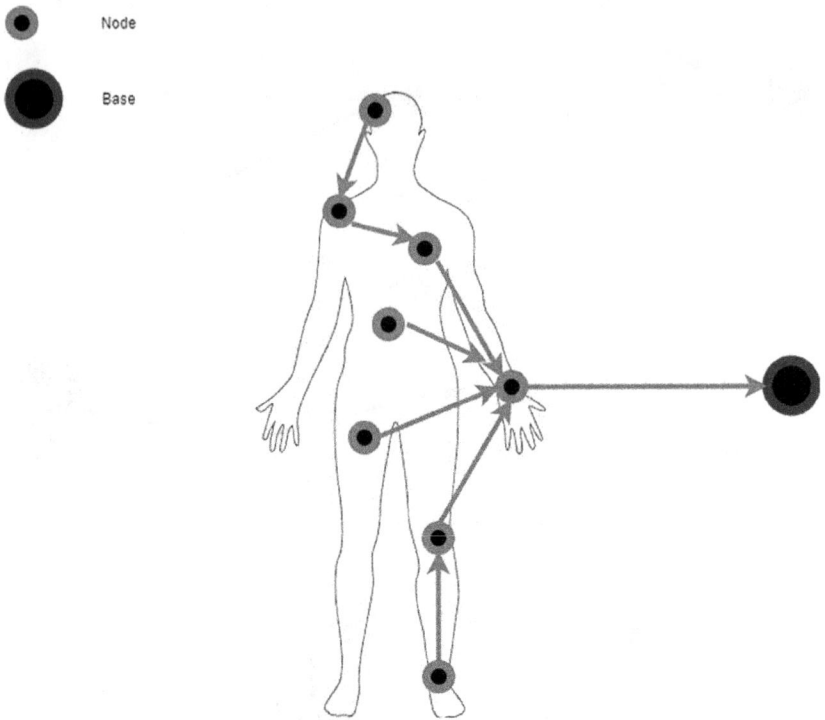

*Figure 4.6* Distributed collection of nodes in the human body.

The advantages of our approach are:

- Increased access to data
- An automatic switchover
- Fast and automated recovery in case of failure
- Minimal investment and maintenance of internal equipment
- Better performance

Consequently, our goal is to structure and minimize the EC and storage charges. That is why this technology will offer us several advantages and benefits. The first three benefits are self-service, flexibility, and pay-as-you-go. Self-service configuration allows us to access any IT resource. Flexibility offers the ability to increase or decrease the resource usage. Finally, pay-per-use allows the users to pay only for what they use, making this technology efficient compared to traditional databases.

For our use of CC databases for our solution, we based our solution on the fact that our data streams, which transmit information, must be stored in order to be processed. This case hinders the traditional databases. We could schematize our solution to link our first design with the cloud in the following way.

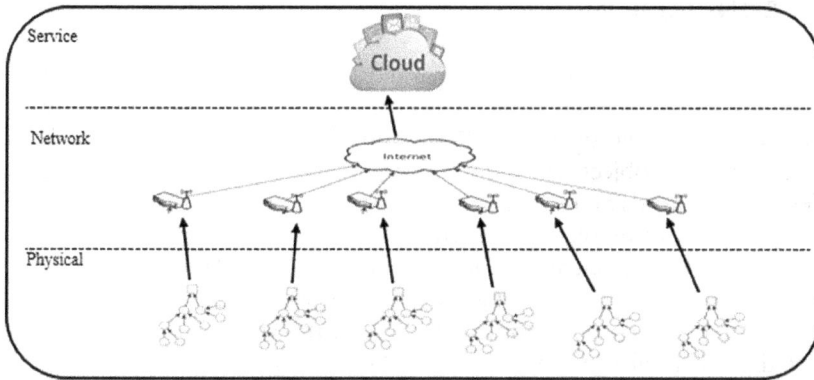

*Figure 4.7* Data storage.

As shown in Figure 4.7, after collecting data on the different bases of the physical layer, it will be transmitted via the Internet network. Then, all this data will be sent to the cloud platform. For this reason, the cloud can be considered as the best way to store and process the data. In this way, when we use different methods to process data, we will have a considerable amount of data.

### 4.4.3 Contribution of our solution

Compared with the use of a standard database, with a physical server and a storage platform, a database in CC has significant advantages compared with our solution:

*Elimination of physical infrastructure*: In a cloud-based database, providers of servers and data storage and other types of infrastructure are in charge of their maintenance and availability.
*Savings*: This physical structure can neither be owned nor used by the IT department; much money can be saved as capital expenses, personnel, operating costs (electricity, ventilation, and air-conditioning), and physical space requirements are reduced.
*Instant scalability*: If the database capacity needs to be increased for any reason, we can apply via our infrastructure to increase capacity, throughput, and bandwidth for a database implemented in an infrastructure.

The cloud naturally adapts to the increase in load.
Several packaged solutions are available today. These solutions host a volume of data at the affordable prices. Dumped onto the platform, this data can be stored in different ways: raw or contextualized.

## 4.5 CONCLUSION

The new technologies market is marked by a new discipline: "connected objects." These technological concentrates are the objects that use the Internet to improve their functioning, often the technical evolution of an already existing object. During the first part of this article, we were able to identify these fields and explain the progress they were undergoing. The IoT and its users can be receivers or transmitters of data. The IoT has opened up new concepts to science in the fields of health [53]. The new digital technologies analyze connected objects to meet several user needs. The role of our chapter is to provide some solutions to the various problems of connected objects linked to medical fields, linked to the consumption and volume of data and the heterogeneity of objects. However, the solution aims to give benefit to these connected objects. Indeed, after the study and the research, our solution will be implemented to be applicable. Our work is a step toward a medical internet of objects answering all the problems we evoked in this chapter's introduction.

## GLOSSARY

| Term | Designation |
| --- | --- |
| CC | Cloud computing |
| WSN | Wireless sensor network |
| IoT | Internet of things |
| RFID | Radio frequency identification |
| EC | Energy consumption |

## REFERENCES

[1] Weiser, M. (1999). The computer for the 21st century. *ACM SIGMOBILE Mobile Computing and Communications Review*, *3*(3), 3–11.

[2] Liu, X., Zhao, S., Liu, A., Xiong, N., & Vasilakos, A. V. (2019). Knowledge-aware proactive nodes selection approach for energy management in Internet of Things. *Future Generation Computer Systems*, *92*, 1142–1156.

[3] Boumaiz, M., El Ghazi, M., Mazer, S., Fattah, M., Bouayad, A., El Bekkali, M., & Balboul, Y. (2019). Energy harvesting based WBANs: EH optimization methods. *Procedia Computer Science*, *151*, 1040–1045.

[4] Wang, J., Liu, A., Yan, T., & Zeng, Z. (2018). A resource allocation model based on double-sided combinational auctions for transparent computing. *Peer-to-Peer Networking and Applications*, *11*(4), 679–696.

[5] Sakkila, L., Elhillali, Y., Rivenq, A., Tatkeu, C., & Rouvaen, J. M. (2007, June). Short range automotive radar based on UWB pseudo-random coding. In *2007 7th International Conference on ITS Telecommunications* (pp. 1–6). IEEE.

[6] Ahmed, A., Abdul Hanan, A., Omprakash, K., Lobiyal, D. K., & Raw, R. S. (2017). Cloud Computing in VANETs: Architecture, Taxonomy and Challenges. *IETE Technical Review* (Vol. 35, pp. 523–547). India & USA: Taylor & Francis.

[7] Kumar, S., & Raw, R. S. (2020). "Health Monitoring Planning for On-Board Ships Through Flying Ad Hoc Network," *Advanced Computing and Intelligent Engineering*, eds. B. Pati, C.R. Panigrahi, R. Buyya, K.C. Li (pp. 391–402). Singapore: Springer, ISBN: 978-981-15-1483-8.

[8] Singh, P. (2020). "Vehicle Monitoring and Surveillance through Vehicular Sensor Network" IGI book series "Cloud-Based Big Data Analytics in Vehicular Ad-Hoc Networks" by the publisher, IGI Global.

[9] Singh, P., Pareek, V., & Ahlawat, A. K. (2017). Designing an energy efficient network using integration of KSOM, ANN and data fusion techniques. *International Journal of Communication Networks and Information Security (IJCNIS)*, 9 (3), 466–474.

[10] Mahmood, K., Chaudhry, S. A., Naqvi, H., Kumari, S., Li, X., & Sangaiah, A. K. (2018). An elliptic curve cryptography based lightweight authentication scheme for smart grid communication. *Future Generation Computer Systems*, 81, 557–565.

[11] Buford, J. F., & Yu, H. (2010). Peer-to-peer networking and applications: Synopsis and research directions. In *Handbook of peer-to-peer networking*, eds. X. Shen, H. Yu, J. Buford, M. Akon (pp. 3–45). Boston, MA: Springer.

[12] Liu, X., Liu, A., Li, Z., Tian, S., Choi, Y. J., Sekiya, H., & Li, J. (2017). Distributed cooperative communication nodes control and optimization reliability for resource-constrained WSNs. *Neurocomputing*, 270, 122–136.

[13] Parveen, K., Ali, A., & Asadullah, G. (2018). Survey on Operating Systems for the Applications of the Internet of Things. *Journal of Information Communication Technologies and Robotic Applications*, 7(1), 9–16.

[14] Anand, R., Sinha, A., Bhardwaj, A., & Sreeraj, A. (2018). "Flawed Security of Social Network of Things. In *Handbook of Research on Network Forensics and Analysis Techniques*, eds. G. Shrivastava, P. Kumar, B.B. Gupta, S. Bala, N. Dey, (pp. 65–86). Hershey, PA: IGI Global.

[15] Gupta, A., Srivastava, A., Anand, R., & Tomažič, T. Business Application Analytics and the Internet of Things: The Connecting Link. In *New Age Analytics: Transforming the Internet through Machine Learning, IoT, and Trust Modeling*, eds. G. Shrivastava, S.L. Peng, H. Bansal, K. Sharma, M. Sharma, (pp. 249–273). Boca Raton, FL: CRC Press.

[16] Gupta, R., Shrivastava, G., Anand, R., & Tomažič, T. (2018). IoT-based privacy control system through android. In *Handbook of E-business Security*, eds. J.M.R.S. Tavares, B.K. Mishra, R. Kumar, N. Zaman, M. Khari (pp. 341–363). Boca Raton, FL: Auerbach Publications.

[17] Kohli, L., Saurabh, M., Bhatia, I., Shekhawat, U. S., Vijh, M., & Sindhwani, N. (2021). Design and Development of Modular and Multifunctional UAV with Amphibious Landing Module. In *Data Driven Approach towards Disruptive Technologies: Proceedings of MIDAS 2020* (pp. 405–421). Singapore: Springer.

[18] Kohli, L., Saurabh, M., Bhatia, I., Sindhwani, N., & Vijh, M. (2021). Design and Development of Modular and Multifunctional UAV with Amphibious Landing, Processing and Surround Sense Module. In *Unmanned Aerial Vehicles for Internet of Things (IoT): Concepts, Techniques, and Applications*, eds. V. Mohindru, Y. Singh, R. Bhatt, R.K. Gupta, (pp. 207–230).

[19] Moutaib, M., Fattah, M., & Farhaoui, Y. (2020). Internet of things: Energy Consumption and Data Storage. *Procedia Computer Science*, *175*, 609–614.

[20] Roxin, I., & Bouchereau, A. (2017). Ecosystème de l'Internet des Objets. https://hal.archives-ouvertes.fr/hal-02178723

[21] Mavrommati, I., & Kameas, A. (2003). The evolution of objects into hyper-objects: will it be mostly harmless?. *Personal and Ubiquitous Computing*, *7*(3), 176–181.

[22] Sindhwani, N., & Bhamrah, M. S. (2017). An optimal scheduling and routing under adaptive spectrum-matching framework for MIMO systems. *International Journal of Electronics*, *104*(7), 1238–1253.

[23] Sindhwani, N., Bhamrah, M. S., Garg, A., & Kumar, D. (2017, July). Performance analysis of particle swarm optimization and genetic algorithm in MIMO systems. In *2017 8th International Conference on Computing, Communication and Networking Technologies (ICCCNT)* (pp. 1–6). IEEE.

[24] Sindhwani, N., & Singh, M. (2020). A Joint Optimization Based Sub-band Expediency Scheduling Technique for MIMO Communication System. *Wireless Personal Communications*, *115*(3), 2437–2455.

[25] Sindhwani, N. (2017). Performance Analysis of Optimal Scheduling Based Firefly algorithm in MIMO system. *Optimization*, *2*(12), 19–26.

[26] Novak, M. Nikola Tesla's Incredible Predictions For Our Connected World [online].[cit. 2. 8. 2017]. Dostupné z: http://paleofuture.gizmodo.com/nikola-teslas-incrediblepredictions-for-our-connected-1661107313.

[27] Omarov, A. (2017). *Využití internetu věcí (IoT) ve skladování* (Bachelor's thesis, České vysoké učení technické v Praze. Vypočetní a informační centrum.).

[28] Deoras, S. First ever IoT device- "The internet Toaster" [online].[cit. 2. 8. 2017]. Dostupné z: http://iotindiamag.com/2016/08/first-ever-iot-device-the-internet-toaster.

[29] Boumaiz, M., El Ghazi, M., Bouayad, A., Fattah, M., El Bekkali, M., & Mazer, S. (2019, December). The impact of transmission power on the performance of a WBAN prone to mutual interference. In *2019 International Conference on Systems of Collaboration Big Data, Internet of Things & Security (SysCoBIoTS)* (pp. 1–4). IEEE.

[30] Says, G. (2015). 6.4 billion connected "Things" will be in use in 2016, up 30 percent from 2015. URL: http://www.gartner.com/newsroom/id/3165317

[31] Maroua, A., & Mohammed, F. (2019, October). Characterization of Ultra Wide Band indoor propagation. In *2019 7th Mediterranean Congress of Telecommunications (CMT)* (pp. 1–4). IEEE.

[32] Smetanová, L. (2016). *Internet věcí a možnosti jeho využití pro komerční účely* (Bachelor's thesis, České vysoké učení technické v Praze. Vypočetní a informační centrum.).

[33] Deepak, K. S., & Babu, A. V. (2016). Energy consumption analysis of modulation schemes in IEEE 802.15. 6-based wireless body area networks. *EURASIP Journal on Wireless Communications and Networking*, *2016*(1), 1–14.

[34] Bubílek, A. (2018). Využití technologic IoT.

[35] Fattah, M., Abdellaoui, M., Daghouj, D., Mazer, S., El Ghazi, M., El Bekkali, M.,. & Bouayad, A. (2019). Multi band OFDM alliance power line communication system. *Procedia Computer Science*, *151*, 1034–1039.

[36] Dahiya, A., Anand, R., Sindhwani, N., & Deshwal, D. (2021). Design and Construction of a Low Loss Substrate Integrated Waveguide (SIW) for S Band and C Band Applications. *MAPAN*, 1–9.

[37] Anisi, M. H., Abdullah, A. H., & Abd Razak, S. (2011). Energy-efficient data collection in wireless sensor networks. *Wireless Sensor Network*, 3(10), 329.

[38] Meelu, R., & Anand, R. (2010, November). Energy Efficiency of Cluster-based Routing Protocols used in Wireless Sensor Networks. In *AIP Conference Proceedings* (Vol. 1324, No. 1, pp. 109–113). American Institute of Physics.

[39] Paliwal, K. K., Israna, P. R. A., & Garg, P. Energy efficient data collection in Wireless sensor network-a survey. In *International Conference on Advanced Computing, Communication and Networks' II*.

[40] Atzori, L., Iera, A., & Morabito, G. (2010). The internet of things: A survey. *Computer networks*, 54(15), 2787–2805.

[41] Gubbi, J., Buyya, R., Marusic, S., & Palaniswami, M. (2013). Internet of Things (IoT): A vision, architectural elements, and future directions. *Future generation computer systems*, 29(7), 1645–1660.

[42] Tarik, A., & Farhaoui, Y. (2019, April). Recommender System for Orientation Student. In *International Conference on Big Data and Networks Technologies* (pp. 367–370). Springer, Cham.

[43] Anand, R., Shrivastava, G., Gupta, S., Peng, S. L., & Sindhwani, N. (2018). Audio Watermarking With Reduced Number of Random Samples. In *Handbook of Research on Network Forensics and Analysis Techniques*, eds. G. Shrivastava, P. Kumar, B.B. Gupta, S. Bala, N. Dey (pp. 372–394). Hershey, PA: IGI Global.

[44] Ando, N., Suehiro, T., Kitagaki, K., Kotoku, T., & Yoon, W. K. (2005, August). RT-middleware: Distributed component middleware for RT (robot technology). In *2005 IEEE/RSJ International Conference on Intelligent Robots and Systems* (pp. 3933–3938). IEEE.

[45] Anand, R., & Chawla, P. (2016, March). A review on the optimization techniques for bio-inspired antenna design. In *2016 3rd International Conference on Computing for Sustainable Global Development (INDIACom)* (pp. 2228–2233). IEEE.

[46] Chibber, A., Anand, R., & Arora, S. (2021, September). A Staircase Microstrip Patch Antenna for UWB Applications. In *2021 9th International Conference on Reliability, Infocom Technologies and Optimization (Trends and Future Directions) (ICRITO)* (pp. 1–5). IEEE.

[47] Boumaiz, M., Bekkali, M. E., Bouayad, A., & Fattah, M. (2019, October). The Impact of Distance between Neighboring WBANs on IEEE 802.15. 6 Performances. In *2019 7th Mediterranean Congress of Telecommunications (CMT)* (pp. 1–4). IEEE.

[48] Boumaiz, M., El Ghazi, M., Mazer, S., El Bekkali, M., Bouayad, A., & Fattah, M. (2018, November). Performance analysis of DQPSK and DBPSK modulation schemes for a scheduled access phase based Wireless Body Area Network. In *2018 9th International Symposium on Signal, Image, Video and Communications (ISIVC)* (pp. 163–167). IEEE.

[49] Boumaiz, M., Bekkali, M. E., Bouayad, A., & Fattah, M. (2019, October). The Impact of Distance between Neighboring WBANs on IEEE 802.15. 6 Performances. In *2019 7th Mediterranean Congress of Telecommunications (CMT)* (pp. 1–4). IEEE.

[50] Omar, M., Challal, Y., & Bouabdallah, A. (2012). Certification-based trust models in mobile ad hoc networks: A survey and taxonomy. *Journal of Network and Computer Applications*, 35(1), 268–286.

[51] Omar, M., Challal, Y., & Bouabdallah, A. (2009). Reliable and fully distributed trust model for mobile ad hoc networks. *Computers & Security*, *28*(3–4), 199–214.

[52] Boumaiz, M., El Ghazi, M., Mazer, S., Fattah, M., Bouayad, A., El Bekkali, M., & Balboul, Y. (2019). Energy harvesting based WBANs: EH optimization methods. *Procedia Computer Science*, *151*, 1040–1045.

[53] Anand, R., Sindhwani, N., & Saini, A. (2021). Emerging Technologies for COVID 19. *Enabling Healthcare 4.0 for Pandemics: A Roadmap Using AI, Machine Learning, IoT and Cognitive Technologies* (pp. 163–188).

Chapter 5

# Communication and detection of sanitation solutions during epidemics

*Shiela David, G Saranya, and C Ashwini*

SRM Institute of Science and Technology, Ramapuram, India

## CONTENTS

DOI: 10.1201/9781003239888-5

## 5.1 INTRODUCTION

In low- and middle-income nations, a lack of access to proper and sufficient sanitation and hygiene can be a persistent public health problem that contributes to disease transmission. During natural crises and public health crises, this condition will get even worse. To deter disease transmission during floods and crises, open defecation prevention and waste containment are important. Though long-term waste disposal is essential, urgent sanitation solutions are also required to prevent disease spread during crises. These solutions may include sanitation services, hand-washing stations with soap and water, service and maintenance regimes, operator training, and community education. During all infectious disease outbreaks, including the coronavirus illness of 2019, clean drinking water, sanitation, waste control, and sanitary conditions are crucial for protecting and maintaining human health. Preventing human-to-human transmission of pathogens such as some virus that causes COVID-19 would require evidence-based and routinely practiced wash and waste management procedures in neighborhoods, households, workplaces, marketplaces, and healthcare facilities [1]. Sanitation applies to public health issues such as safe drinking water and proper care and recycling of industrial waste and sewage. Hygiene includes avoiding human contact with urine and washing hands with soap. Sanitation systems are designed to protect human health by providing a clean environment that prevents disease transmission, especially through the fecal–oral route. For example, proper sanitation may minimize diarrhea, which is a leading cause of malnutrition and stunted growth in infants. Many other diseases, such as ascariasis (a form of intestinal worm infection or helminthiasis), cholera, hepatitis, polio, schistosomiasis, and trachoma, are easily spread in populations with poor sanitation, to name a few. There are a variety of sanitation technology and methods available. Complete sanitation directed by the crowd, container-based sanitation

(CBS), urban sanitation, emergency sanitation, natural sanitation, onsite sanitation, and integrated sanitation are some examples. Human excreta and wastewater are captured, stored, transported, treated, and disposed of or reused in a sewage system. The nutrients, water, electricity, and organic matter found in excreta and wastewater can be the target of reuse practices within the sanitation system. The "sanitation value chain" or "sanitation economy" refers to this. Sanitation workers are those who are in charge of washing, maintaining, running, or emptying sanitation technology at any point along the sanitation chain. To compare the sanitation service standards inside and across countries, many sanitation "levels" are used. The sanitation ladder developed by the Joint Monitoring Program (JMP) in 2016 begins with open defecation and progresses upward using the words "improved," "restricted," and "basic," with "safely controlled" as the highest category. This is particularly true in developed countries The World Health Organization (WHO) defines the term "sanitation" as follows: "The provision of facilities and services for the safe disposal of human urine and faeces is referred to as sanitation." The term 'sanitation' also refers to the upkeep of sanitary conditions through rubbish collection and wastewater disposal services.

Sanitation encompasses all these technological and nontechnical schemes: excreta management systems, wastewater management systems (which incorporate wastewater treatment plants), solid waste management systems, and rainwater runoff (also known as storm water drainage). Many in the WASH market, on the other hand, only include excreta control when defining sanitation. Another example of what sanitation entails can be seen in Sphere's "Humanitarian Charter and Minimum Standards in Humanitarian Response" handbook, which outlines minimum standards in four "primary response fields" in humanitarian situations. "Water Supply, Sanitation, and Hygiene Promotion" (WASH) is one of them, and it covers the following topics: promotion of hygiene and water supply. Many people consider hygiene promotion to be an essential aspect of sanitation. "The collection, transport, storage, disposal or reuse of human excreta, household wastewater, and solid waste, are related to hygiene promotion," according to the Water Supply and Sanitation Collaborative Council. Despite the fact that sanitation requires wastewater treatment, the words "sanitation and wastewater disposal" are still used interchangeably.

Personal sanitation and public hygiene are examples of sanitation. Handling menstrual waste, washing domestic toilets, and controlling household garbage are all examples of personal sanitation function. Garbage collection, transport, and disposal (municipal solid waste management), sweeping drains, parks, classrooms, trains, public areas, communal toilets and public toilets, sewers, and running sewage treatment plants are all examples of public sanitation work. Sanitation staffs are individuals who offer these resources to others.

## 5.2 TYPES AND CONCEPTS

In alphabetical order, the term sanitation is associated with several descriptors or adjectives to denote different types of sanitation systems (which may deal solely with human excreta management or with the full sanitation system, including greywater, stormwater, and solid waste management).

### 5.2.1 Basic sanitation

JMP coined the phrase "basic sanitation service" in 2017. This is defined as using better sanitary facilities that are not shared with other homes. "Limited sanitation service" is a new term for a lesser level of service that refers to the use of improved sanitation facilities shared by two or more homes [2].

### 5.2.2 Container-based sanitation

CBS is a sanitation technique in which human excreta is collected in sealable, detachable containers (also known as cartridges) and transferred to treatment facilities [3]. This method of sanitation entails the use of a commercial service that offers specific sorts of portable toilets and distributes empty containers when full ones are picked up. The expense of excreta collection is often paid by the users. CBS may be utilized to offer low-income urban areas with safe collection, transportation, and treatment of feces at a lesser cost than establishing and maintaining sewers with the right development, support, and collaborations [4]. CBS is based on the usage of urine-diverting dry toilets (UDDTs) in the majority of situations.

### 5.2.3 Sanitation guided by the community

CLTS (community-led total sanitation) is a method of improving sanitation and hygiene practices in a community that is mostly employed in poor nations. The method aims to modify behavior in mostly rural populations through a "triggering" process that results in spontaneous and long-term renunciation of open defecation habits. It focuses on an entire spontaneous and long-term behavioral transformation. The CLTS method revolves around the phrase "triggering": it refers to methods for stimulating community enthusiasm in stopping open defecation, mainly through the construction of rudimentary toilets like pit latrines. CLTS entails taking steps that promote one's self-esteem and pride in one's community [5]. It also includes feelings of humiliation and disgust about one's own open defecation habits [5]. CLTS provides a unique approach to rural health care.

### 5.2.4 Sanitation in the absence of water

The term "sanitation without water" isn't properly defined and isn't often used. It generally refers to a system that transports excreta using a form of dry toilet rather than sewers. When people talk about "dry sanitation," they are usually referring to a sanitation system that employs a UDDTs [6–8].

### 5.2.5 Ecological sanitation

Ecological sanitation, often known as ecosan (sometimes written eco-san or EcoSan), is a sanitation system that tries to properly reuse excreta in agriculture [9]. It is a concept, not a technology or a device, that is defined by a goal to "complete the loop" between sanitation and agriculture in a safe manner, primarily for nutrients and organic matter. One of the goals is to utilize nonrenewable resources as little as possible. Ecosan systems, when correctly built and run, provide a hygienically safe mechanism for converting human excreta into nutrients and water that may be returned to the ground. Resource-oriented sanitation is another name for Ecosan.

### 5.2.6 Sanitation in an emergency

The administrative and technical techniques necessary to provide sanitation in an emergency are known as emergency sanitation as shown in Figure 5.1.

During humanitarian, assistance activities for refugees, victims of natural catastrophes, and internally displaced individuals, emergency sanitation is essential [10]. Emergency response is divided into three phases: immediate, short term, and long term [10]. The immediate focus is on controlling open defecation, with toilet technologies such as extremely rudimentary latrines, pit latrines, bucket toilets, container-based toilets, and chemical toilets being used. In the medium run, technology such as UDDTs, septic tanks, and decentralized wastewater systems may be used.

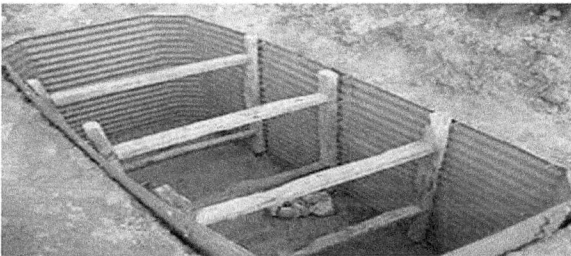

Figure 5.1 Emergency pit.

### 5.2.7 Environmental sanitation

The regulation of environmental conditions linked to disease transmission is referred to as environmental sanitation. Solid waste management, water and wastewater treatment, industrial waste treatment, and noise pollution control are all subcategories of this category.

### 5.2.8 Sanitation, both improved and unimproved

Improved sanitation (not to be confused with "safely managed sanitation service") is a term used to describe different forms of sanitation for monitoring. The management of human excrement at the home level is referred to as this. The phrase was established in 2002 by United Nations International Children's Emergency Fund (UNICEF) and WHO's JMP for Water Supply and Sanitation to track progress toward Goal #7 of the Millennium Development Goals. In the JMP definitions, "unimproved sanitation" is the polar opposite of "improved sanitation." From 2015 onward, the same words are used to track progress toward Sustainable Development Goal 6 [11] that are a part of the definition of "safely managed sanitation service" in this case.

### 5.2.9 Lack of sanitation

The absence of sanitation is referred to as lack of sanitation. In practice, this frequently translates to a shortage of bathrooms or sanitary toilets that anyone would want to use voluntarily. Open defecation (and open urination, though this is less of a worry) is a common effect of poor sanitation, with major public health consequences [12]. As of 2015, it was projected that 2.4 billion people required adequate sanitation, with 660 million people lacking access to safe drinking water [13, 14].

### 5.2.10 Onsite sanitation

It is a sanitation system in which excreta and wastewater are collected, stored, or treated on the plot where they are created, according to the definition of onsite sanitation (or on-site sanitation). The level of therapy might range from nonexistent to advanced. Pit latrines (without treatment) and septic tanks are two examples (primary treatment of wastewater). On-site sanitation systems are frequently linked to off-site fecal sludge management (FSM) systems, which treat fecal sludge generated on-site only when a piped water supply is present within or close to a building does wastewater (sewage) occur. A decentralized wastewater system, which refers to the wastewater component of on-site sewage treatment, is a similar phrase.

## 5.2.11 Safely managed sanitation

The Sustainable Development Goal Number 6 envisions the greatest degree of household sanitation: safely managed sanitation [15]. It is quantified as the "Proportion of population using securely managed sanitation services, including a hand-washing facility with soap and water" under Sustainable Development Goal 6.2 [16]. According to JMP's 2017 baseline estimate, 4.5 billion people do not have access to properly managed sanitation.

Following is the operation definition: the percentage of the population who uses a better sanitation facility that is not shared with other homes and where the excreta generated is either recycled or composted.

## 5.2.12 Sustainable sanitation

A sanitation system that is intended to satisfy specific standards and perform well over time is known as sustainable sanitation.

From the user's experience through excreta and wastewater collection technologies, waste transportation or conveyance, treatment, and reuse or disposal, sustainable sanitation systems examine the full "sanitation value chain" [17]. The Sustainable Sanitation Alliance (SuSanA) defines "sustainable sanitation" as having five characteristics (or criteria): systems must be economically and socially acceptable, as well as technically and institutionally sound and environmentally friendly [18].

## 5.3 ENVIRONMENTAL CONSIDERATIONS

## 5.3.1 Indicator organisms

Various types of indicator organisms are employed to screen for fecal contamination in environmental samples when they are analyzed. The bacteria *Escherichia coli* (abbreviated as *E. coli*) and nonspecific fecal coliforms are often employed as indicators for bacteriological water analysis. Helminth eggs are a common indication in soil, sewage sludge, biosolids, and feces from dry toilets. Eggs are retrieved from the sample and a viability test is performed to distinguish between viable and nonviable eggs in helminth egg analysis. The number of viable helminth eggs in the sample is next determined.

## 5.3.2 Climate change

Climate change may have a severe influence on current sanitation systems in a number of ways, including flood damage and service loss, as well as lower carrying capacity of wastewater-receiving rivers [19]. "Weather and climate-related factors such as variability, seasonality, and extreme weather occurrences" already have an impact on the sanitation industry in a variety of ways [20]. Climate change is increasing the frequency and intensity of extreme weather events like floods and droughts. Water supply, storm drainage and sewerage systems, and wastewater treatment facilities are all affected [21]. A WHO paper outlines how adaptation programs should account for the hazards posed by extreme weather occurrences. [20]. Water and sanitation services contribute to the emission of greenhouse gases. Sanitation services are predicted to contribute 2–6% of worldwide man-made methane, which is one of the greenhouse gases [22]. Anaerobic treatment methods such as septic tanks, pit latrines, anaerobic lagoons, and anaerobic digesters generate methane, which may or may not be collected (typically not in the case of septic tanks). By creating renewable energy in the form of biogas, heat recovery, or directly from excreta, sustainable sanitation systems can help to reduce greenhouse gas emissions [23]. "Nearly all National Adaptation Plans issued by the UN Framework Convention on Climate Change list improving sanitation and hygiene as a priority," according to researchers at the International Institute for Sustainable Development (IISD) in 2017 [24].

## 5.4 WHAT IS EPIDEMICS AND HOW TO REACT DURING EPIDEMICS?

The rapid spread of disease to a large number of people in a certain community in a short period of time is known as an epidemic (from Greek epi "upon or above" and o demos "people"). In meningococcal infections, for example, an attack rate of more than 15 cases per 100,000 persons for two weeks is termed an epidemic [25, 26]. In most cases, an epidemic begins when host immunity to an established disease or a newly developing novel disease is rapidly decreased below that observed in the endemic equilibrium, and the transmission threshold is crossed [4].

An infectious agent can undergo a number of alterations that can lead to an epidemic. These are some of them:

- Virulence has increased.
- Introduction to a new environment
- Changes in the infectious agent's susceptibility in the host

## 5.5 TYPES OF EPIDEMICS

### 5.5.1 Common source outbreak

Affected people were exposed to a common agent in a common source outbreak epidemic. A point source epidemic occurs when a single exposure occurs and all of the afflicted individuals get the illness during the course of a single exposure and incubation period. A continuous epidemic or an intermittent epidemic occurs depending on whether the exposure was continuous or varied.

## 5.5.2 Propagated outbreak

The afflicted people were exposed to a common agent in a common source outbreak pandemic. A point source epidemic occurs when a single exposure occurs and all of the afflicted individuals get the illness throughout the course of one exposure and incubation period. A continuous epidemic or an intermittent epidemic depends on whether the exposure is constant or fluctuating.

## 5.5.3 Transmission

- Airborne transmission
- Arthropod transmission
- Biological transmission
- Contact transmission
- Developmental transmission
- Fecal–oral transmission
- Horizontal transmission
- Propagative transmission
- Vertical transmission

## 5.5.4 Potential sanitation solutions during an emergency response

In low- and middle-income nations, a lack of access to adequate and sufficient sanitation and hygiene can be a chronic public health concern that contributes to disease transmission. During environmental disasters and public health emergencies, this scenario might become even worse. To avoid disease transmission during catastrophes and emergencies, open defecation avoidance and waste containment are crucial. While long-term waste management is important, emergency sanitation solutions are often required to prevent disease transmission during catastrophes. These solutions should include sanitation facilities, hand-washing stations with soap and water, operation and maintenance regimens, operator training, and community education. The possibilities for sanitation are explored further down.

## 5.6 SANITATION SOLUTIONS

### 5.6.1 Packet latrines

These are individual, single-use biodegradable bags that are buried or appropriately disposed of for point-of-use sanitation. For example, bags typically inside reusable buckets, brand names like Peepoople, Wagbag

*Advantages*: There is no need for infrastructure. They are transportable and lightweight. They can be employed in regions where space is at a premium or in flood-prone locations.

*Constraints*: A functioning supply chain is required to offer around one bag per person every day. Some types of bags have exorbitant prices. There is a requirement for a dumping facility and potentially collection services. Bags may be abandoned in open spaces or in situations where others may be at danger. Social acceptability varies, and the target population's acceptability would need to be determined. It requires a comprehensive hygiene effort to educate the public about proper handling and disposal.

### 5.6.2 Bucket latrines or elevated toilets

It is a temporary construction that is elevated above a big container or tank and it can be lined with a big, replaceable plastic bag.

*Advantages*: Some of the advantages are:

- Large containers are usually easy to get by.
- It's ideal for locations where digging latrines isn't practicable or practical.
- It's ideal for places with a high water table or flooding.
- A larger tank needs fewer emptying.

*Constraints*: Some of the constraints are:

- Tanks and a superstructure are required.
- Trucks and employees must be dislodged.
- Vehicle access is necessary to empty containers; hence, a sewage disposal facility is necessary.
- Social acceptability varies, and the target population's acceptability would need to be determined.
- To guarantee that bags are buried/disposed of and containers are sterilized, an intensive hygiene effort is required.
- Accessibility may be problematic for disabled, elderly, and young children.

### 5.6.3 Chemical toilets

They are portable prefabricated sanitation units with a chemical solution to promote digestion. They minimize odor and contain a water-tight excreta-holding tank.

*Advantages*: Some of the benefits are:

- Hygiene on the go.
- Reduces the amount of odor.
- Can be quickly mobilized.
- Flooding in the Dominican Republic in 2003 was a resounding success.
- It's ideal for places with a high water table or flooding.

*Constraints*: Some of the restrictions are:

- High priced.
- Transport is difficult.
- Desludging vehicles and workers, as well as disposal locations, are required.
- To service the toilets, you'll need access to a vehicle.
- Because of the tiny size of the tank, it must be emptied often.
- A sewage disposal facility is required.

## 5.6.4 Trench latrines

They are narrow ditches with a makeshift privacy structure; waste is covered with dirt on a regular basis.

*Advantages*: The main advantages are:

- Implementation is quick (one worker may dig a 50-m [165 ft] trench per day).
- It is simple to hide feces with dirt.

*Constraints*: Some of the constraints are:

- Life expectancy is limited.
- During the wet season, trenches flood.
- Drainage is necessary to redirect surface water away from the trench.
- Limited privacy and unsuitable if water table is high.

## 5.6.5 Communal or family pit latrines with short-term structure

They are shallow holes with simple privacy construction, roughly 0.3 m x 0.5 m x 0.5 m (1ft x 1.6 ft x 1.6 ft) in depth; waste is covered with earth when latrine is nearly full.

*Advantages*: Some of the important benefits are:

- Increased personal privacy.
- Implementation is quick.
- Labor input is reduced.
- User engagement and ownership are at a higher degree.

*Constraints*: Some of the constraints are:

- Appropriate area is required for pit digging.
- Flooding of pits may occur during the rainy season.
- Where the water table is high, it is unsuitable.

- Pit latrines build up and must be capped in the long run.
- A large number of tools and equipment are needed.
- The community must be capable of and willing to build latrines.

## 5.6.6 Ecological sanitation (Eco-San) latrines

A raised structure that sits on top of a container or bin that holds organic waste for decomposition. Urine is diverted from organic waste in dehydrating toilets, which need bulk drying and pH additives. Nonurine diverting toilets collect all waste and require the addition of organics for decomposition. When referring to familiar people or agricultural communities, the term "agricultural community" is used.

*Advantages*: The common advantages are:

- Reduces the amount of odor.
- It's ideal for places with a high water table or flooding.
- In agriculture, decomposed organics can be used to supplement top soil and fertilizers.

*Constraints*: They have some restrictions like:

- Construction is more challenging.
- It is necessary to have a high level of user awareness.
- Management at the highest level is essential.
- Consumables (ash/lime and/or organics) are necessary.
- It is difficult to operate and maintain.
- To guarantee proper usage, an intensive cleanliness effort is required.

The sanitation solution in urban area and rural area is shown in Figures 5.2 and 5.3.

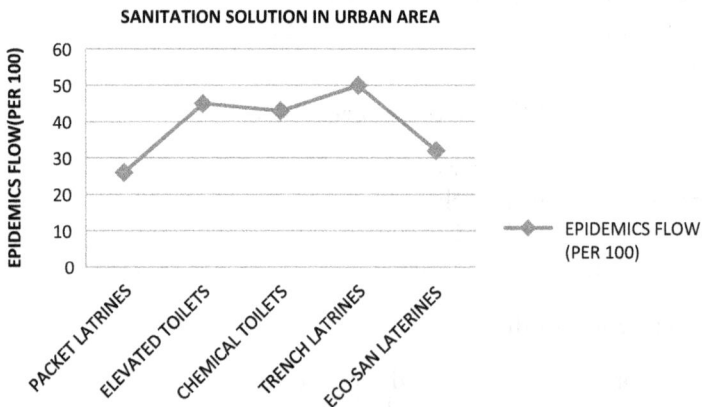

*Figure 5.2* Sanitation Solution in Urban Area.

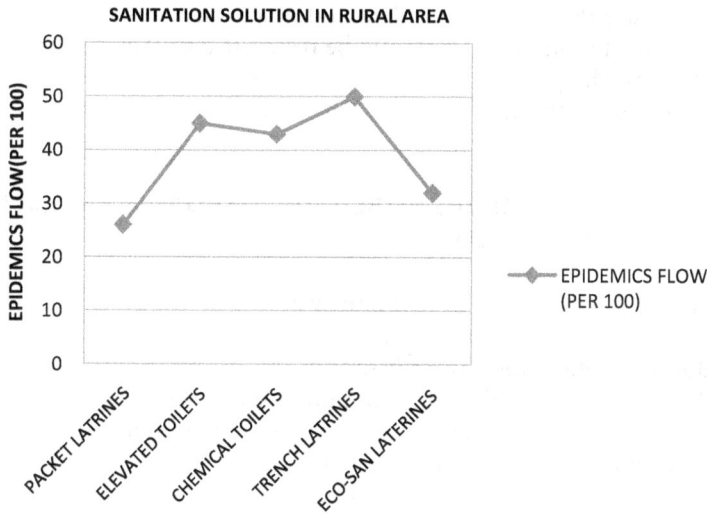

Figure 5.3 Sanitation Solution in Rural Area.

## 5.7 SANITATION RECOMMENDATIONS FOR CHOLERA-PRONE AREAS AND IMPROVISED SETTLEMENTS

- Chemical toilets should be utilized in the short term where they are available and when proper servicing is possible.
- If chemical toilets aren't an option, trench latrines or temporary pit latrines should be built as soon as possible where there aren't any.
- Elevated latrines should be considered in regions where digging is neither practicable nor appropriate, or in locations where the water table is high.
- For the time being, the Sphere emergency standard external icon of 50 people per latrine should be employed, with the goal of reducing to the Sphere minimum standard for excreta disposal of 20 people per latrine.
- Internally displaced persons (IDP) settlement residents should be included in selecting acceptable solutions.
- Existing habits should be studied further to uncover additional viable options (e.g., are people in temporary villages utilizing toilets in nearby less damaged buildings?)
- Further research into the viability and acceptability of packet and bucket latrines on a local level is needed.
- Information concerning latrine usage and care (in local languages) should be included in health communication materials, as should facilities for communicating with no literate communities.

- To reduce the spread of cholera and other infectious illnesses, longer-term sanitation methods should be researched further.
- Hand-washing stations should be placed at every sanitary facility, regardless of the kind of sanitation facility.

## 5.8 AWARENESS AMONG PUBLIC RELATED TO SANITATION AND HYGIENE ISSUES

There are four major ways to promote awareness as follows:

- Boosting total public awareness.
- Professional marketing of sanitation to those without access.
- Stimulating private sector interest in the sanitation market.
- Reaching decision makers in the public, commercial, and civil sectors.

## 5.9 ACTIONS TO TAKE DURING, BEFORE, AND AFTER A PANDEMIC

The following are the activities that national authorities and WHO should take.

1. planning and coordination.
2. situation monitoring and assessment.
3. reducing the spread of disease.
4. continuity of health care provision.
5. Communications.

The purpose of cross-sector planning and coordination is to offer leadership and coordination. Integrating pandemic preparation into national emergency preparation frameworks is a crucial part. The purpose of scenario monitoring and assessment is to gather, evaluate, and distribute information on the danger of a pandemic before it starts, as well as to track pandemic activity and characteristics after it has begun. It will be necessary to track the infectious agent, its ability to cause disease in people, and illness distribution patterns in order to determine if the danger of a pandemic is rising. It is critical to collect information on influenza viruses, their genetic mutations, and the resulting changes in biological properties, as well as to study and analyze epidemics quickly. It will be critical to assess the success of response measures after a pandemic influenza virus has begun to circulate. Increasing the "social distance" between people will play a big role in reducing disease spread. Individual/household-level, societal-level, and international travel-level measures, as well as the use of antivirals, other medications, and vaccinations, will be critical.

During a pandemic, healthcare systems will need to offer services while dealing with an inflow of influenza patients. The extent to which the present health system can grow to handle the extra patient load will be determined by planning for surge capacity in healthcare institutions. Health- care institutions will need to keep up with triage and infection control protocols.

Before and during a pandemic, the purpose of communications is to share and communicate essential information with the public, partners, and stakeholders, so that they may make well-informed decisions and take necessary steps to protect health and safety and respond, and it is a critical component of good risk management. The five principles established in WHO's outbreak should guide communications.

## 5.10 RISK COMMUNICATION – A LIFE-SAVING ACTION IN PUBLIC HEALTH EMERGENCIES

One of the most important aspects of outbreak management is risk coordination. It refers to the sharing of facts, recommendations, and opinions between health experts or officials and people who are facing a danger (hazard) to their survival, health, economic, or social well-being in real time. Its ultimate aim is for anyone who is at risk to be able to make educated decisions about how to deal with the consequences of a disease epidemic. Effective risk coordination not only saves lives and prevents sickness (by educating people about how to protect their health), but it also allows countries and cities to maintain social, economic, and political cohesion in the face of disasters. As a result, risk coordination is one of the key capabilities that all countries have agreed to establish in order to deter disease and other threats from spreading internationally, as mandated by the International Health Regulations (2005).

Risk coordination only happens where people who know (experts), those in control (authorities or response teams), and those that are concerned communicate in a way that is built on confidence (communities). People are less likely to take advice if they lack confidence. It's just as important to listen to and consider people's views, concerns, and perceptions as it is to provide them with information and advice.

## 5.11 TEN THINGS TO KNOW AND DO

*a. Build trust*
  • People must have faith in those in charge of handling the epidemic and disseminating knowledge about it. Compliance with prescribed control measures would be influenced by public belief that a government or organization is working first and foremost to protect their welfare, hastening disease containment.

- Accountability is crucial: communicators and epidemic administrators must show that they are responsible for what they claim, promise, and do.
- Danger communication strategies should, according to evidence, be linked to functioning and available program, straightforward, prompt, and easy-to-understand, identify ambiguity, target impacted communities, connect to self-efficacy, and be disseminated using various formats, processes, and networks to create trust.
- Being viewed as experts with integrity by offering expert guidance that is right and factual and by being compliant with other trustworthy institutions and entities.
- Being perceived as having a strong character by speaking the truth and not omitting vital information are some of the foundation blocks of confidence.
- Identifying with the afflicted community as bearing the same problems and fate.
- Demonstrating good will by understanding and care of messages and their distribution.

b. *Communicate uncertainty proactively*
- Officials' official communications should provide clear details about the uncertainty involved with threats, incidents, and interventions, as well as what is understood and what is unknown at any given moment.
- Publicize the event as soon as possible, even though the details aren't final. This will create you as the go-to person for communicating risk; it will build confidence in you and the response; it will allow improvements in procedure and action to get the outbreak under control; and it will reduce confusion and rumors.
- The following is a good guide for communicating uncertainty:
  - State what is known, what is unknown, and what you/your organization is doing to address the problem.
  - Communicate early, if possible, be the first to announce the case, communicate often, and communicate on a daily basis.
  - Provide information about the risk/danger, as well as some suggestions for how people can defend themselves.
  - Speak like a human being, with enough empathy.
  - Avoid being too reassuring.

c. *Engage communities*
- Identify individuals in the neighborhood that the group trusts, form relationships with them, and include them in decision-making to facilitate collaborative, context-appropriate strategies and community-owned contact.
- Community interaction is a good place to proceed when it comes to communicating risk and promoting behavioral and practice improvements.

d. *Message well*

Threat should not be explained in technical terms, according to the new research, since this is ineffective in encouraging risk avoidance behaviors. Early in the epidemic, consistent signals can appear from the various intelligence outlets. Messages should encourage people to take practical steps to protect their health that they will realistically take.

e. *Establish good feedback systems*

- Must listen to the public and impacted groups, use a variety of methods (surveys, focus group meetings, neighborhood walk-throughs, primary whistleblowers, input from frontline responders, feedback from allies and stakeholders, social media, etc.).
- Use them to learn about people's questions about the epidemic and the steps we're urging them to take.
- Use these systems to test messaging and materials developed to support risk communication.

f. *Correct usage of social media as appropriate*

- During an emergency, social media can be used to engage the public, promote peer-to-peer contact, build situational awareness, track and respond to rumors, public reactions, and complaints, and facilitate local level responses, among other things.
- To ensure integration with authenticated, factual information, social media and conventional media must be part of an interconnected strategy with other modes of communication.

g. *Risk communication operations requires resources*

- In epidemics, risk coordination is a major organizational undertaking that necessitates personnel, logistics, material, and funds.
- Diverse types of skills are expected in a variety of areas: stakeholder relations, communication related to travel and trade; media interactions, social media, spokespersons, social mobilization, wellness education, group participation, and behavioral improvement communication.

h. *Consider emergency risk communication to be a strategic responsibility rather than an afterthought.*

- In global and national emergency preparedness and response leadership teams, emergency risk coordination should be a designated strategic position.
- The International Health Regulations (2005) mandate that all Member States develop national risk communication capability in two areas: systems and people.
- The Global Health Security Agenda's Joint External Evaluation (JEE) framework assesses risk coordination capability in many areas:
  - National agendas
  - Programs
  - Plans
  - Coordination

- Cooperation with stakeholders
- Mass media approaches to public communication
- Communicating and interacting with communities
- Dynamic listening (to disinformation, worries, and concerns) and rumor control

i. *Create information and coordination systems*
   • Develop and expand agency and organizational networks across geographic, disciplinary, and national borders, as needed.
   • Tailor information and communication systems to users' needs and involve local stakeholders to ensure information flows across sectors.

j. *Build capacity for the next emergency*
   • Personnel preparation and training for emergency risk communication should be scheduled [27–29] on a regular basis, with a focus on cross-agency collaboration.
   • Emergency risk communication necessitates a well-defined and long-term budget, which should be included in emergency preparedness and response core budgeting.

## 5.12 CONCLUSION & DISCUSSION

The global vision that has enhanced travel and trade while increasing interdependence among countries also necessitates a global health vision. Infectious disease outbreaks, endemics, and epidemics are a constant threat to all nations. Around the same time, because many countries suffer from similar problems, there are prospects for mutual innovation and social intent. There is a need for a more comprehensive review of global health issues and concerns in this consensus report. This approach is applicable not only to global health security issues [30], but also to external factors that affect health security, such as the development of general capability in countries and the establishment of strong communities that promote peace, healthier lifestyles, and a healthy environment.

The global danger of infectious disease will continue to endanger the United States' health and security, unless key capabilities and robust health networks are established around the world. Aside from the pressing need to counter infectious disease challenges, it's also critical to comprehend the profound connection between health and economic development. Many countries are currently dealing with the dual challenge of a dramatic rise in noncommunicable diseases (NCDs) such as cardiovascular disease (CVD) and cancer, as well as the ongoing need to eradicate infectious diseases such as malaria and tuberculosis (TB), in addition to the priority of reducing the burden of HIV/AIDS. Based on the preliminary considerations established in this chapter, the sanitation systems defined as options cannot be considered entirely feasible in any coastal or waterfront location. Because sanitation programs are built on a project-by-project basis, special assessments and choice changes can be required based on the needs of a particular population. Before making a final decision and implementing the chosen alternative, community-specific economic, social, cultural, and structural needs should be considered during this tentative selection process.

When an illness breaks out and expands, it immediately attracts the attention of the majority of emergency responders and consumes the majority of the health system's human and financial capital, as well as prescription supplies and technology [31]. Furthermore, healthcare facilities, especially emergency rooms, may serve as transmission centers. If prevention and preventive mechanisms are not adequately applied, a large number of individuals may become sick. This is particularly true for new and unknown pathogens. A delay in recognizing the disease can result in a delay in implementing the appropriate protective steps. Because healthcare staff, family members, and other patients will not know how to defend themselves, infected patients will be able to spread the disease. Because healthcare facilities and emergency departments are often busy, a lack of adequate infection prevention and management, such as triage, isolation, and other measures, may have a major impact [32, 33]. The two things that play a significant role in a person's life are fitness and grooming. Human life expectancy is largely determined by an individual's fitness.

Access to education can raise awareness of the health benefits of improved sanitation technologies, whereas a household's ability to acquire specific facilities is influenced by income. Personal experience and demonstrations of alternative technologies can aid in persuading people that the investment's benefits will outweigh the costs. By highlighting factors valued locally, community groups and influential figures will help market the idea. This could involve the prestige that comes with owning a facility or its utility in terms of comfort. Similarly, factors such as rapid population growth, which reduces privacy, could increase the perceived need for sanitation developments. People are resistant to reform for a variety of causes. There may be indignation against outside "experts" who are unfamiliar with local traditions and are seen as benefiting more from the breakthrough than locals. Inside a society, leadership cannot be unified. Those of established authority who fear losing their influence and prestige, for example, may be opposed to creativity that is widely promoted by political or educated elite.

New innovations can be unattractive or incompatible with long-standing norms of personal and social conduct. Furthermore, households have a wide range of financial, labor, and time capital, as well as their own interests. When weighed against their need for food, the short-term risks of an ostensibly "low-cost" scheme can be too high for those with minimal capital. Furthermore, if latrines take a long time to clean, are cumbersome to use, or need dramatic improvements in social practices, they can be very expensive for households in terms of capital expenditure. Seasonal fluctuations in the supply of capital and labor are also possible. As a result, the pacing of a project's promotional facets in relation to, say, agricultural seasons could be crucial in determining its success.

Specific household demographics, economic characteristics, and attitudes toward sanitation shift over time. People's interest in latrines is likely to increase as they begin to upgrade their homes, according to experience. As a result, as part of the modernization process, some households will be encouraged to add a latrine. Households should be able to engage in on-site sanitation not only when they are inspired, but also when they have the financial means to do so. Indeed, it could be more fitting to implement a variety of on-site technology within a city, from which residents can choose based on their evolving preferences and interests. Identifying a need for better sanitation is preferable to initiating a supply of infrastructure that is considered beneficial to populations. The former is dependent on mutual collaboration between providers and recipients, which is achieved by dialog and knowledge sharing. Individual consumers are the final arbiters on whether emerging technology is accepted or rejected. They are the ones that decide a project's progress, because the investment's worth is determined not just by group interest, but also by the consensus of households and individual consumers. They must be persuaded that the gains of better sanitation, as well as the modern technology that comes with it, outweigh the costs. It is also the responsibility of providers to recognize the social context. They need to learn from communities about why better sanitation can evoke negative reactions, as well as the positive aspects of community values, beliefs, and practices that can be used to foster change.

Taking hygienic food at regular intervals helps to keep one's health in check. If a person eats only hygienic food and keeps his health in good shape, he will lower his morality score. This is due to the fact that certain foods can be used to treat such diseases. As a result, staying safe and eating hygienic food are important.

Vaccines, increased sanitation and hygiene, cleaner environments, expanded food and drug control, and preventive health programs helped to reduce deaths and increase public health throughout the twentieth century. A well-trained public health staff is essential for effective public health actions. Individuals from a variety of disciplines, including doctors, nurses, public health professionals, epidemiologists, and health educators, are among those that make up such a population. The emphasis of this study is on physicians' vital positions in supporting and improving the public health system, as well as what these physicians need to know in order to participate in successful public health intervention.

## REFERENCES

[1] Juneja, S., Juneja, A., & Anand, R. (2020). Healthcare 4.0-Digitizing Healthcare Using Big Data for Performance Improvisation. *Journal of Computational and Theoretical Nanoscience*, 17(9–10), 4408–4410.

[2] World Health Organization. (2017). Progress on drinking water, sanitation and hygiene: 2017 update and SDG baselines.

[3] Tilmans, S., Russel, K., Sklar, R., Page, L., Kramer, S., & Davis, J. (2015). Container-based sanitation: assessing costs and effectiveness of excreta management in Cap Haitien, Haiti. *Environment and urbanization*, 27(1), 89–104. doi:10.1177/0956247815572746.PMC4461065.PMID26097288.

[4] Mikhael, G., Shepard, J., & Stevens, C. (2017). The world can't wait for sewers: advancing container-based sanitation businesses as a viable answer to the global sanitation crisis. Available at. http://www.wsup.com/wp-content/uploads/2017/02/Clean-Team-whitepaper.pdf, p. 14.

[5] Venkataramanan, V., Crocker, J., Karon, A., & Bartram, J. (2018). Community-led total sanitation: a mixed-methods systematic review of evidence and its quality. *Environmental health perspectives*, 126(2), 026001. doi:10.1289/EHP1965. PMC6066338.PMID29398655.

[6] Akorede, S. N., Nofiu, O. D., Musa, C., & Olofu, E. E. (2019). Attitude towards water sanitation among senior boarding secondary schools student in Kaduna state, Nigeria. *Global Journal of Health Related Researches*, 1(1).

[7] Platzer, C., Hoffmann, H., & Ticona, E. (2008, November). Alternatives to waterborne sanitation–a comparative study–limits and potentials. In *Proceedings of the IRC Symposium: Sanitation for the Urban Poor, Delft, The Netherlands* (pp. 19–21).

[8] Flores, A. E. (2011). *Towards sustainable sanitation: evaluating the sustainability of resource-oriented sanitation* (Doctoral dissertation, University of Cambridge).

[9] Werner, C., Fall, P. A., Schlick, J., & Mang, H. P. (2003, April). Reasons for and principles of ecological sanitation. In *IWA 2nd international symposium on ecological sanitation* (pp. 23–30).

[10] Harvey, P. (2007). *Excreta disposal in emergencies: a field manual*. Water, Engineering and Development Centre (WEDC) Loughborough University of Technology.

[11] Who, U. (2017). Progress on drinking water, sanitation and hygiene: 2017 update and SDG baselines.

[12] Mara, D. (2017). The elimination of open defecation and its adverse health effects: a moral imperative for governments and development professionals. *Journal of Water, Sanitation and Hygiene for Development*, 7(1), 1–12.1

[13] MacArthur, J., Carrard, N., & Willetts, J. (2020). WASH and Gender: a critical review of the literature and implications for gender-transformative WASH research. *Journal of Water, Sanitation and Hygiene for Development*, 10(4), 818–827.

[14] World Health Organization, & UNICEF. (2013). *Progress on sanitation and drinking-water*. World Health Organization.

[15] Berendes, D. M., Sumner, T. A., & Brown, J. M. (2017). Safely managed sanitation for all means fecal sludge management for at least 1.8 billion people in low and middle income countries. *Environmental Science & Technology*, 51(5), 3074–3083.

[16] World Health Organization. (2021). Progress on household drinking water, sanitation and hygiene 2000–2020: five years into the SDGs.

[17] Mara, D., & Evans, B. (2018). The sanitation and hygiene targets of the sustainable development goals: scope and challenges. *Journal of Water, Sanitation and Hygiene for Development*, 8(1), 1–16.

[18] Tilley, E. (2014). *Compendium of sanitation systems and technologies*. Eawag.
[19] Alliance, S. S. Towards More Sustainable Sanitation Solutions—SuSanA Vision Document.
[20] Howard, G., Calow, R., Macdonald, A., & Bartram, J. (2016). Climate change and water and sanitation: likely impacts and emerging trends for action. *Annual Review of Environment and Resources, 41*, 253–276.
[21] Barbier, E. B., & Burgess, J. C. (2020). Sustainability and development after COVID-19. *World Development, 135*, 105082.
[22] World Health Organization. (2011). *Guidance on water supply and sanitation in extreme weather events*. World Health Organization. Regional Office for Europe.
[23] Gambrill, M., Gilsdorf, R. J., & Kotwal, N. (2020). Citywide inclusive sanitation—business as unusual: shifting the paradigm by shifting minds. *Frontiers in Environmental Science, 7*, 201.
[24] Action, P. U., & can Contribute, H. D. A. Welcome Letter from the Directors 2 Introduction to the UN Sustainable Development Group 3 Rules of Procedure 4 Improving Youth Engagement in Sustainable Development 5.
[25] Hepburn, J. (2020). *WTO agriculture talks: Prospects for progress on SDG 2*. International Institute for Sustainable Development.
[26] Lee, L. M., Thacker, S. B., & Louis, M. E. S. (2010). *Principles and practice of public health surveillance*. Oxford University Press, USA.
[27] Sindhwani, N. (2017). Performance analysis of optimal scheduling based firefly algorithm in MIMO system. *Optimization, 2*(12), 19–26.
[28] Sindhwani, N., & Bhamrah, M. S. (2017). An optimal scheduling and routing under adaptive spectrum-matching framework for MIMO systems. *International Journal of Electronics, 104*(7), 1238–1253.
[29] Sindhwani, N., & Singh, M. (2020). A joint optimization based sub-band expediency scheduling technique for MIMO communication system. *Wireless Personal Communications, 115*(3), 2437–2455.
[30] Anand, R., Shrivastava, G., Gupta, S., Peng, S. L., & Sindhwani, N. (2018). Audio Watermarking With Reduced Number of Random Samples. In *Handbook of Research on Network Forensics and Analysis Techniques* (pp. 372–394). IGI Global.
[31] Singh, P., et al.; "Voice Control Device using Raspberry Pi", SOUVENIR, IEEE Conference, Amity International Conference on Artificial Intelligence (AICAI'19), Amity University Dubai, Dubai International Academic City, IEEE, UAE Section. February 4-6, 2019.
[32] Kumar, S., & Raw, R. S. (2020). "Health Monitoring Planning for On-Board Ships Through Flying Ad Hoc Network," In *Advanced Computing and Intelligent Engineering* (pp. 391–402). Singapore: Springer. ISBN: 978-981-15-1483-8.
[33] Kumar, A , Tripathi, S., & Raw, R. S. (2016). "Bringing Healthcare to Doorstep using VANETs," 3rd IEEE International Conference as INDIACom-2016, ISSN (0973-7529), 16-18 March, Delhi, pp. 4747–4750.

Chapter 6

# Security and privacy on the internet of medical things

## Challenges and issues

*Yahya Rbah, Mohammed Mahfoudi, and Younes Balboul*
Sidi Mohamed Ben Abdellah University of FES, Morocco

*Mohammed Fattah*
University of Moulay Ismail of Meknes, Morocco

*Said Mazer, Moulhime Elbekkali, and Benaissa Bernoussi*
Sidi Mohamed Ben Abdellah University of FES, Morocco

## CONTENTS

## 6.1 INTRODUCTION

The recent advancement of 5G technology, artificial intelligence, big data, and cloud networking technology has transformed people's traditional lifestyles [1]. These advancements have greatly fueled healthcare innovation, particularly the internet of medical things' (IoMTs') emergency [2]. IoMT is a component of the IoT ecosystem wherein different implanted and wearable medical devices (e.g., pressure sensors, smart bands, pacemakers, and glucometers) exist. Clinical systems are connected and interact with one another through networking technologies to share critical medical information used by healthcare providers (e.g., doctors and nurses) to provide better care and medicine [3, 4]. This confidential information is transmitted to the appropriate end-user after being stored on different cloud platforms through the gateway.

The application of IoMT has changed the intelligent healthcare industry. It enables different application scenarios, including chronic diseases (i.e., COVID-19), remote health monitoring, fitness programs, medication management, faster response, lower costs, and excellent treatment quality [5]. While smart medical devices provide a variety of benefits, they also have numerous privacy and security problems, especially when dealing with highly confidential and critical medical information in healthcare systems [6]. Patients' sensitive medical data, such as names, addresses, and health conditions, are particularly sent to cloud servers through open wireless channels interconnected via the internet. Throughout this procedure, intruders could eavesdrop on and intercept incoming and outgoing confidential and critical data, resulting in severe patient information leakage [7, 8]. Attackers, adversaries, and hackers may use various cyber exploitation techniques and network-related assaults to exploit specific vulnerabilities in these devices [9]. Eavesdropping, message modification, false data injection, asset destruction, malware attacks, and denial of service are examples of such attacks. The destructive effects of these cyberattacks not only severely disrupt the healthcare system (i.e., ransomware attacks) but also have a significant impact, putting patients' lives in danger [10]. For instance, hacks on medical insulin pumps can result in insulin overdosage and, in extreme cases, death. Connected cardiac devices, such as a pacemaker, can be attacked, putting patients' lives in danger [5].

The widespread adoption and evolution of IoMT, particularly during pandemics, could create significant security issues, making it more challenging to protect the privacy of sensitive and critical medical information [11]. Furthermore, IoMT is constrained by limitations, including limited battery power, computational power, and memory. Such limitations have the most important impact on interoperability and security [12]. Consequently, the critical challenge in IoMT is to achieve a higher security level while protecting the patient's privacy. Furthermore, suitable security and privacy methods must include minimum computations that require limited resources [9].

## 6.2 RELATED WORK

The rapid development and emergence of IoMT have resulted in numerous changes in the medical and health sectors. As a consequence of medical information's confidential and critical nature, patients' privacy and security are essential in IoMT applications. Many researchers have indeed been attracted to this significant issue. Several studies were conducted to investigate security and privacy issues related to IoMT [12–16]. The authors in [10] identified possible security problems that impacted the IoMT system and mentioned a list of security measures to tackle these risks. In [17], the authors provided a review on security assessment, assaults, and security strategies for network-connected medical devices. In [12], the authors examined various security modules and discussed diverse security mechanisms, anonymity and identification algorithms, and data destruction for medical device reusability. In [18], the authors have identified additional security and privacy issues in the surveyed medical sensor. In a related survey [19], the authors analyzed the security and privacy concerns of wearable IoMT systems to provide vulnerable-proof healthcare. The paper [20] has highlighted the recent privacy and security concerns related to IoMT. Also, the authors have classified and compared the existing security mechanisms based on their computational complexity and resource requirements. Then, in [21], the authors reviewed and analyzed various security issues and challenges related to IoMTs and identified multiple risk factors of security threats on the IoMT system. Recently, the paper [11] addressed the IoMT privacy and security concerns in addition to the existing methods and measurements for securing IoMT systems in the medical field to tackle COVID-19.

## 6.3 IOMT SECURITY CHALLENGES

IoMT applications present a plethora of security challenges that are discussed in this section. In [10, 22, 23], the authors discussed the main IoMT challenges. Because traditional security techniques cannot ensure IoMT security requirements (e.g., integrity, confidentiality, availability, authorization, anonymity, and non-repudiation), novel security measures are required to address new issues confronting the IoMT.

The main root causes of security vulnerabilities are the constraints of medical devices in computing capabilities, memory size, and energy resources. Furthermore, the features of these devices in terms of mobility

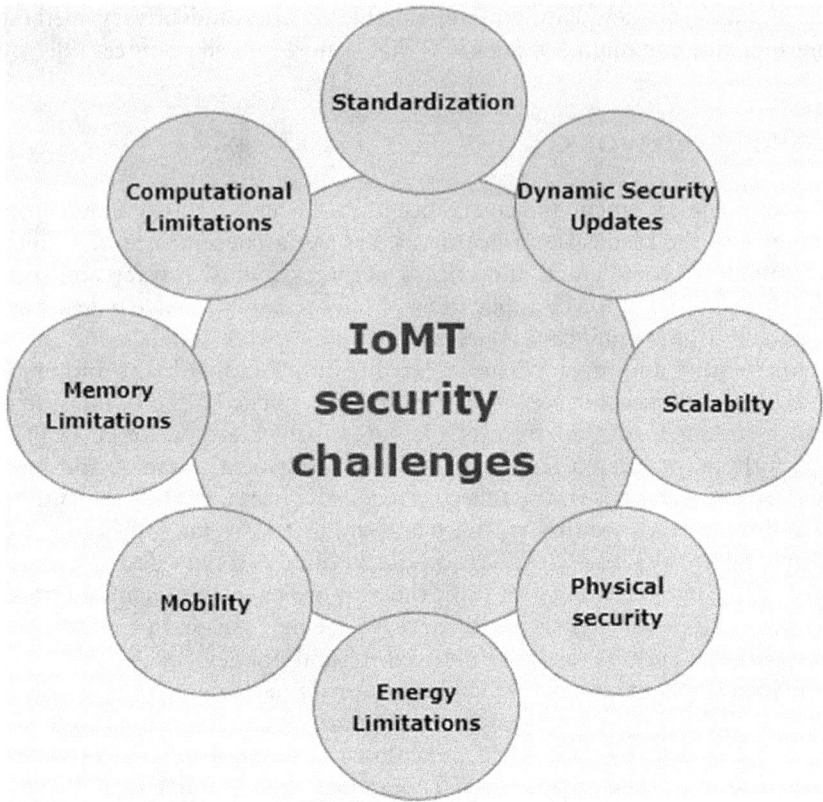

*Figure 6.1* IoMT security challenges.

and variety contribute to the complexity of designing feasible security methods [9]. Indeed, most of these challenges are primarily, but not exclusively, associated with different IoMT resource limitations (e.g., size and volume). The main challenges (Figure 6.1) for secure IoMT services are presented in this section.

- *Standardization*
  As soon as medical devices started to be integrated into IoT networks, IoMT challenges emerged. The heterogeneity is among the most significant challenges [20]. Due to the absence of standards, solution providers can develop their own proprietary security protocols. That is not always compatible with current norms and technologies, introducing dangers [10].
- *Computational limitations*
  IoMT devices and sensors [24, 25] are embedded with limited processing capabilities. In such devices, the central processing unit (CPU) is not particularly effective and efficient in terms of processing speed.

In addition, these devices are not designed to perform complex computational tasks [22]. In other words, they simply serve as actuators or sensors. Some security computations consume an important part of computing resources. Many wireless sensors [26–28] lack built-in encryption due to their limited capabilities (i.e., computation and power) [13].

- *Memory limitations*
Most IoMT devices have restricted on-device storage space. An application binary, a software system, and an embedded operating system are used to activate such devices [22]. Consequently, IoMT devices' memory is insufficient to handle complex security mechanisms because complex computing operations take much longer and cause significant delays in transmitting data, posing a risk to patients [9].

- *Mobility*
Medical devices, in general, are mobile rather than stationary. The mobility of such devices expands the scope of IoMT applicability. Furthermore, patients can keep moving from their homes to several other medical examinations without interfering with continuous medical monitoring, thanks to mobility. Medical devices could connect to or disconnect from the IoMT network at any time, resulting in dynamic changes in network topology as well as challenges with centralized control or private key distribution. Security configurations and settings differ between networks. Therefore, developing a mobile-compliant security algorithm is a significant challenge [9].

- *Energy limitations*
Medical devices that have limited battery power are common in the IoMT network (e.g., blood pressure sensors and body temperature). When no sensor readings are required, such devices focus on saving energy by activating the power-saving mode. Furthermore, when there is nothing significant to process, they operate at a slow speed. As a result of IoMT devices' energy constraints, finding an energy-aware security solution is difficult [22].

- *Physical security*
The majority of embedded system developers are unfamiliar with hardware security fundamentals. Furthermore, hardware security experts are not always able to design the overall system, and even if they were, the design costs would be much higher. As a result of these facts, several other manufacturers' medical devices have ignored security concerns that can have severe repercussions for the privacy, safety, or health of patients who entrust them [29, 30].

- *Scalability*
As the number of connected devices has grown, more medical devices are being integrated and linked to the internet. Therefore, developing a highly scalable protection mechanism while maintaining security procedures is now a complex process [22].

- *Dynamic security updates*
  Security protocols must be kept up to date to mitigate critical threats. Consequently, IoMT devices require security patches to be updated. Nevertheless, developing a process for the dynamic installation of security updates (patches) is challenging [22]. However, the appropriate security measures for medical devices are restricted by the computing capabilities, storage space, and energy power limitations of these devices. Therefore, the majority of current security mechanisms are inappropriate for regular operation under resource constraints. As a result, new security concerns about integrity, confidentiality, and availability emerge.

## 6.4 IOMT PRIVACY AND SECURITY ISSUES

In the case of IoMT, security issues could affect confidentiality, disrupt availability, and compromise integrity. Furthermore, medical information can be used to commit fraud or identity theft, as well as to discover health records [19]. An adversary who is not ill and does not need treatment can earn money by ordering expensive drugs through a medical cardholder to obtain resale medicines. For instance, attackers may also use extortion and blackmail against patients with common diseases that they do not want to disclose [31]. Access control and authorization are other security concerns. An assault, for instance, can rationally modify a drug dose that might kill or severely harm a specific patient [20]. The management of identities and users' authentication within the IoMT system are critical issues because integrity, confidentiality, and availability might be affected without them. For instance, if an attacker could authenticate as a valid user, he could access any given data, impacting integrity, confidentiality, and availability [32].

Furthermore, when terrorists hijack medical devices, they can use them for targeted assassination. Physical restrictions on connectivity and devices are another source of security concern. The limitations of IoMT devices (e.g., being integrated with low-power processors and small areas) limit their capability to process medical data at incredible speeds [33]. This has an impact on attempts to maintain IoMT systems' integrity and confidentiality. Several researchers discovered various security vulnerabilities in the IoMT [20, 21, 34]. In this section, we categorize privacy concerns related to IoMT systems. Our classification is based on the most critical security requirements, including data confidentiality, integrity, authenticity, and availability.

### 6.4.1 Confidentiality attacks

Patients are becoming more vulnerable to confidentiality threats due to the public and open access to IoMT communication networks. Eavesdropping, brute force, and traffic analysis attacks are the most common forms of confidentiality attacks.

- *Eavesdropping attacks*: (aka sniffing) These are mainly based on data collection. They exploit insecure transmission to gain access to the sensitive data being transmitted [35]. Such attacks could provide confidential data about the system being assaulted (e.g., usernames, passwords, node configuration, and identification) to the attacker when transmitted information is unencrypted. Adversaries could use and process this information to create their own custom-made assaults. Intruders, for example, could simply connect malicious devices to an IoMT system and exploit it if they could capture and extract the data needed to insert a new medical device into the group of authorized devices [36].
- *Data interception attacks*: These attacks take place as a consequence of the man-in-the-middle (MiTM) attack. This allows the attacker to intercept the medical data exchanged between a given transmitter and receiver and later re-transmit the intercepted medical information [37]. Such an assault is perilous when used to, for instance, prescribe the wrong drugs or inject a high dose of drugs into a patient, putting patients' lives in grave danger [20].
- *Packet sniffing attacks*: or packet attacks capturing, in which data packets are captured and critical medical data, including patients' passwords and medical conditions, can be extracted using sniffers (e.g., Wireshark) if the data packets are not encrypted while in transit [38].

## 6.4.2 Data integrity

Integrity attacks are based on modifying messages in transit to compromise the integrity of data or a system. To reach this objective, various attacks can be used, including interception and data injection attacks.

- *Message tampering alteration attacks*: In this case, the adversary attempts to compromise the integrity of the transmitted message. This occurs when an attacker alters received messages to achieve his objectives [39]. As a result, doctors will make wrong decisions that may compromise their patients' health.
- *Malicious data injection*: This attack effectively prevents legitimate messages from legitimate users from reaching the network rather than injecting falsified data into it. IoMT device software is updated over-the-air, allowing any perpetrator to inject malicious code that could cause unwanted activities and gain access to unauthorized health system levels [38]. False data injection represents a form of such assault that may result in false information being transmitted to a hospital data center [40] by sending a false message to the hospital data centers or doctors in order to manipulate the overall

result measurement or reading. This may have dangerous consequences in the medical system, and it can lead to serious accidents [41]. SQL injection is an alternative form of such attack that enables cybercriminals to obtain access to health databases by opening back doors [42].

- *Malicious script injection attacks*: These attacks initiate a falsified update script scheme, in which attackers can impersonate a legitimate medical server to back up the system. This allows the attackers to gain non-authorized access to a given medical device and possibly create a back door [42].
- *Spoofing attack*: The goal of these attacks is to obtain unauthorized access to the network. Attackers attempt to obtain information from a valid IP address or valid tag of authorized IoMT devices before sending malicious content with the obtained data to make the information appear valid [43]. IP spoofing, radio frequency identification (RFID) spoofing, and other spoofing attacks on IoMT systems are examples of spoofing attacks. Spoofing and cloning attacks could be integrated to create a more severe offense against an IoMT device or system [44]. Spoofing attacks take advantage of cloned information to obtain unauthorized access, whereas cloning attacks duplicate the spoofed data [45].
- *Buffer overflow*: A buffer overflow, according to the National Institute of Standards and Technology (NIST) definition, is a form of attack that enables an attacker to add more data into a buffer than the buffer's capacity limit permits. The intruder intends to overwrite the available data in the buffer with malicious code, which allows him to take full control of the system [46]. These attacks are intended to compromise the integrity and authenticity of systems, have a significant impact, and have a medium risk level. This threat is effectively countered by secure programming [47].

### 6.4.3 Availability attacks

To attack the availability of IoMT systems, various actions are being conducted to degrade the existing medical devices and systems' performance [48–50]. The attacker's purpose is to disrupt the data availability of the transmitted messages by dropping them. Consequently, crucial data such as patients' health conditions could be missing from the hospital's data centers or doctors [20]. The following are the various forms of system availability attacks.

- *Denial-of-service (DoS) attacks*: It consists of numerous network packets targeted directly at the smart medical device in the IoMT application, resulting in a real-time service interruption [51]. For example, an attacker may try to consume the medical devices' resources and affect the performance of the IoMT system, rendering their services unavailable. This form of attack occurs when an IoMT system seems unable to upload patients' health data onto the corresponding medical cloud center or when a healthcare professional fails to collect patient data via the IoMT system, making it difficult to make a good decision [52, 53]. Furthermore, these attacks keep IoMT devices turned on all the time, reducing battery life.

- *Distributed-denial-of-service (DDoS) attacks*: DDoS attacks medical devices from numerous sources in a distributed manner, using various IP addresses to generate multiple requests and maintain the server occupied. This makes differentiating between normal and attack traffic challenging [54]. DDoS attacks can be directed at a network or an application or be reflective and routed through a botnet. Spoofing attacks are commonly used in conjunction with flooding attacks to conceal the source of packets or to circumvent firewalls and filters [55].
- *SYN flooding attacks*: The main objective of such an assault is to crash a healthcare server by depleting its memory reserve, allowing insecure connections to be used for further attacks. Because they depend on Transmission Control Protocol (TCP) services to communicate, they are explicitly aimed at IoMT devices' high capacity [56].
- *ICMP flooding attacks*: These are ping flood or Internet Control Message Protocol (ICMP) attacks with DoS capability, which overwhelm a specific targeted IoMT device using ICMP echo/requests recognized as ping [57]. To carry out such attacks, attackers use manipulated medical devices (bots or zombies) that a bot master operates.
- *Wireless jamming*: It is a subcategory of denial-of-service attacks wherein the attacker attempts to disrupt the communication medium to severely interrupt and disrupt any wireless communication of the IoMT network that connects medical devices to healthcare professionals. Furthermore, by consuming more energy, memory, bandwidth, and so on, this attack affects the performance of IoMT devices and systems [58, 59].

## 6.4.4 Authentication attacks

Authentication attacks bypass passwords, which are considered to be the first and most important line of protection through gaining access to a particular system. When a password is too short, too weak, or static, then such attacks are often successful. Encryption cracking attacks, including dictionary, birthday, and brute force attacks, constitute the most frequent form of such attack [20]. Various forms of system authentication attacks are described as:

- *MiTM attacks*: In this instance, an intruder can monitor or intercept the communication between different IoMT devices and gain access to their confidential information. Therefore, this could easily disrupt communications by adding malicious and fake information to alter original data [54].

- *Brute-force attacks*: Such attacks are mainly driven by an exhaustive search, with different combinations that could break a given password [60]. An attack of this type attempts to obtain private and credentialed medical data of patients for fraud or theft purposes. Among the most commonly targeted devices are remote medical sensors and patient monitors [61].

- *Masquerading attacks*: These attacks occur when an IoMT device is exploited for malicious reasons by a specific attacker. These attacks can cause a constant stream of fake alarms about such medical emergencies and can interrupt healthcare services' availability [62]. Furthermore, such attacks may alter a patient's medical condition, resulting in the injection of improper medication or an overdose, which can lead to that patient's death.

- *Replay attacks*: These attacks attempt to modify control signals transferred to medical devices, this is particularly if the hacker gets access to the medical system with high privilege and the capacity to manage the system's control signals. This form of attack is usually carried out during the authentication process, resulting in leaking, disclosing, or stealing confidential data to have unauthorized entry and high privilege on a specific healthcare system [20].

- *Dictionary attacks*: These attacks attempt to guess the password using a massive set of alphanumeric passwords, enabling the attacker access. Actuality, such attacks are resource and time-intensive, anywhere between minutes to hours, or sometimes days. Such attacks typically occur when attempting to obtain access to a specific medical system, intending to attack a medical device with limited security mechanisms [63, 64].

- *Session hijacking attacks*: These attacks are carried out using a session sniffer, which is a packet sniffer with the ability to capture, read, and alter network traffic between different parties. This applies to both devices and users. These attacks are capable of capturing a valid Session ID (SID). As an extension of IP networks, session hijacking of TCP messages will also impact IoMT networks [20, 65].

### 6.4.5 Privacy attacks

Among the most challenging problems in IoMT is preserving patients' privacy, which is primarily concerned with mitigating the disclosure of their behaviors, true identities, and locations. Furthermore, the main privacy attacks discussed below are traffic analysis attacks and identity/location tracking attacks.

- *Traffic analysis attacks (TAA)*: The adversaries collect and analyze IoMT data packets to gather essential data, including traffic flow or the payload of unencrypted packets in medical device communication. TAA primarily affects patients' privacy as well as data confidentiality. This is because the medical devices' activity could potentially expose enough sensitive data for an attacker to provoke malicious damage to the IoMT devices [20, 47].

- *Identity and location tracking attacks*: To obtain the patient's identity and relate the patient to either a business or home address, the attacker spies on a medical device. Actuality, an adversary could be able to track the IoMT devices' movements. In addition to personal information, analyzing this trace might reveal the patient's real identity. Consequently, obtaining such confidential data of patients can compromise their privacy and potentially their life [20].

## 6.4.6 Implementation attacks

Hardware attacks are currently among the attack vectors for medical devices, posing a significant risk by limiting or even suspending their levels of security. Such attacks include fault injection (FI) as well as side-channel attacks (SCA) that might be used to deactivate crucial security controls in medical devices such as authentication and encryption [23, 66].

- *SCA*: These attacks occur due to the physical limitations of IoMT embedded systems. Moreover, this type of attack can also be used to recover the data hidden within the MCU, including control flow and passwords. In this attack, the attacker attempts to obtain secret keys from encryption protocols using communication timing, power consumption, fault attack, and other techniques on the system's medical devices while performing encryption procedures. It can encrypt and/or decrypt the exchanged data and access confidential information using these keys [23, 67].

- *Timing attacks*: These are security exploits where an intruder reveals security breaches in the computer and network system. They are particularly useful in IoMT devices with limited computing capabilities. In this case, the attacker attempts to compromise a cryptographic algorithm by evaluating the required time to perform the encryption/decryption process [20].

- *FI attacks*: Differential fault analysis can be used to either reveal hidden information or circumvent security mechanisms. This can be achieved by various methods, including supply voltage, clock glitches, and electromagnetic pulse attacks. The attacker can disrupt the circuit's functionality with varying degrees of precision based on the fault injection techniques utilized. An attack of this type can occur in any of the MCU's blocks [23].

### 6.4.7 Malware attacks

Malware software attacks on IoMT devices can include trojans, rootkits, botnets, worms, adware, spyware, viruses, back-doors, and many others [68, 69], which cause power dissipation, wireless network performance degradation, and financial loss in IoMT devices [70, 71]. Malware is built on exploiting a vulnerability, weakness, or security flaw in the software. This results in the potential to have a back door on a given IoMT device and/or system. Furthermore, the attacker may attempt to inject malicious software (malware) into the IoMT devices' memory or operating system. Moreover, it may lead to unauthorized access to IoMT devices, as well as patient's sensitive data leakage, disclosure, alteration, or deletion. It can be used to launch other forms of attacks that use IoT devices to create botnets (e.g., Mirai) or to deny any use of the services they provide (e.g., ransomware and DoS) [16, 20]. The most common types of malware attacks targeting medical devices and systems are listed below.

- *Botnet attacks*: Malware botnets compromise the system's data and other resources' confidentiality, authenticity, integrity, and availability. These attacks are designed to exploit medical device vulnerabilities and convert them into a botnet that waits for commands from the attacker to transmit false patient information. Therefore, botnets can launch a variety of attacks, including DDoS, identity theft, phishing, keylogging, reconnaissance, and bot proliferation [72]. The Mirai attacks, which have infected IoMT devices with malware to create botnets and perform distributed DoS attacks on medical servers, healthcare infrastructure, and so on, are examples of such an attack. Mirai can compromise implants, temperature sensors, smart pens, insulin pumps, infusions, monitors, and other IoMT devices in the medical domain if efficient security precautions are not in place. Consequently, these devices can be used to launch bot attacks against medical systems [20, 73]. Therefore, protecting the IoMT environment from malware attacks becomes critical.
- *Ransomware attacks*: These attacks can have an impact on medical devices, resulting in the denial of their services. It involves locking IoMT devices and demanding a ransom from their proprietors to unlock them [74]. IoMT ransomware is effective even though it is opportunistic, sensitive, and reversible. Consequently, intruders select scenarios in which users did not have enough time or were not in a position to reconfigure the device or target the ransomware impacts. In these situations, users seem more than ready to give the ransom. Medical devices, unfortunately, are attractive choices for ransomware [8]. Hence, locking the features of specific medical devices, including drug infusion pumps and pacemakers, can also have disastrous consequences, as patients can be seriously injured or even killed if such devices are not unblocked on time.

- *Worm attacks*: By exploiting the device's vulnerabilities, worm attacks replicate themselves vertically throughout a networked device. In the IoMT case, they are potentially the most dangerous and destructive type of malware. Furthermore, once infected by worms, the security of the whole IoMT system may be compromised because they can automatically spread throughout the system by exploiting existing security weaknesses. It should also be noted that worms can be combined with other types of malware attacks, including botnets and ransomware, to spread throughout the entire IoMT system [75, 76].
- *Remote access Trojan (RAT) attacks*: These attacks are designed to obtain secret, unauthorized entry as a back door to bypass all security procedures and protection mechanisms. RAT attacks occur when a targeted medical system's weakness or vulnerability is exploited. For instance, if a hacker gets remote control of an IoMT device, he can endanger the patient's life (e.g., a smart pacemaker may deliver a fatal shock to a given patient) [16].
- *Logic bomb attacks*: These attacks refer to the malicious software that logically explodes when a specific date or time is reached [77], causing severe damage to healthcare system components with IoMT devices.

## 6.5 TAXONOMY OF CURRENT SECURITY METHODS FOR IOMT

Various security measures have been developed to ensure data security [78] and privacy in the IoT ecosystem [79–81]. Moreover, such protocols are not designed with the IoMT's security criteria and risks in mind. The current security protocols proposed by researchers to protect the exchanged health information and data stored used in the IoMT communication environment are provided in this section. Current methods for ensuring the security of medical information in IoMT rely primarily on cryptographic methods counting access control via authenticated identity and encrypted data, in addition to key management, intrusion detection, and blockchain technology [9].

### 6.5.1 User/device access control

In IoMT systems, patient privacy is critical, and a malicious party must not be able to transfer any data to a particular patient [82]. To extend the lifetime of the IoMT communication environment, different available resources (e.g., medical devices) in the network must be granted access and privileges. Moreover, user access control schemes [83, 84] are required to differentiate between a malicious and original device, prevent malicious devices from entering the IoMT system, and grant access rights only to authorized users for the various resources and services available in IoMT environment. Table 6.1 lists several recent schemes designed to secure access control in the IoMT system.

*Table 6.1*   Current access control schemes for IoMT

| References | Description |
|---|---|
| [85] | A lightweight break-glass-based access control mechanism with two access modes: access based on the attribute for fine-grained access in normal situations and break-glass access for emergencies. |
| [86] | An IoMT's privacy protector data collection system prevents malicious activities and secures medical data storage from disclosing patients' privacy. |
| [87] | An access control method based on fog computing for the IoMT that improves protection for local mobile devices. In the proposed approach, the fine-grained control access is associated with fog implementation. |
| [88] | A security mechanism that guarantees user authentication and secure access to IoMT's services and resources. This access is protected cryptographically against tampering and provides secure access to IoMT devices. |
| [89] | A two-tiered flexible access control method developed for IoMT system's data storage can protect patients' privacy while also ensuring first-aid treatment in emergencies. |
| [90] | A secure and lightweight data sharing scheme for IoMT ensures mutual information protection and access. Furthermore, it protects the integrity of shared data. |
| [91] | A distance-bounding protocol for managing access control of implantable medical devices (IMD) uses both identity verification and proximity verification to enhance security. |

## 6.5.2 Authentication and encryption

The proposal of a secured authentication method for the IoMT environment is a crucial issue that raises several concerns (e.g., privacy, security, access control, and ownership transfer). Conventional authentication methods have not only high specificity but also several security breaches or computational complexity cost faults that make meeting the actual scene needs of IoMT more difficult [92, 93]. Consequently, it is necessary to develop provably secured and lightweight mutual authentication methods for IoMT devices to achieve secure communication and protect patients' privacy. Passwords, smart cards, biometrics, and other forms of identity authentication are frequently used. Furthermore, many authentication mechanisms have been published recently in the literature. Table 6.2 shows several authentication methods proposed for the IoMT environment.

## 6.5.3 Key management

Some studies have been recently interested in the generation and transmission of cryptographic keys used to protect medical data exchanged via an IoMT network. Due to sensor resource constraints, some proposed methods for biometric-based key establishment. Nevertheless, the existing solutions

*Table 6.2* Current authentication approaches for IoMT

| Approaches | References | Description |
|---|---|---|
| Biometric authentication | [94] | Implementation of biometric technology to develop smart healthcare through the IoMT, which includes a high capacity for data access. |
| | [95] | A secure and anonymous biometric-based user authentication method to guarantee communication security in smart healthcare applications. |
| | [96] | A biometric key-based authentication method for wireless body area network (WBAN) in the IoMT scenario. |
| Anonymous authentication | [97] | A privacy-preserving anonymous authentication mechanism provides users with data security and privacy while minimizing computing and communication resources. |
| | [98] | An improved anonymous authentication method for IoMT based on elliptic curve cryptography (ECC). |
| | [99] | A lightweight secure IoMT storage system uses an edge server to validate the integrity of sensitive physiology data and the patient's identity. |
| | [100] | A security architecture for IoMTs using lightweight ECC protocol for authentication and a policy-based framework for authorization. |
| Mutual authentication and key agreement schemes (MAKA) | [101] | A secure key agreement and lightweight mutual authentication system for IoMT can prevent sensor node capture, impersonation, and replay attacks. |
| | [92] | A secure and lightweight (MAKA) method for IoMT that prevents impersonation, replay, and stolen SN attacks while also providing secure mutual authentication, anonymity, and untraceability. |
| | [102] | A lightweight and provably secure (MAKA) mechanism provides key agreement and authentication for the entire public channel in IoMT. |
| | [103] | A mutual RFID authentication mechanism for IoMT scenarios to guarantee the security requirements of access control. |
| | [104] | A low-cost batch authentication system can identify each illegal, illegitimate RFID tag and reduce the overhead of authentication data transfer in IoMT. |

have several limitations, including success rate and resource consumption. Several proposed techniques for key management are shown in Table 6.3.

## 6.5.4 Intrusion detection systems (IDS)

An IDS can be categorized into two types: anomaly IDS and misuse IDS. The anomaly IDS mechanism identifies transactions that differ from acceptable behavior, whereas the misuse IDS detects attacks using system settings and

Table 6.3 Current key management methods for IoMT

| References | Description |
| --- | --- |
| [103] | An update mechanism for heterogeneous medical device authentication and session keys. The symmetric encryption algorithm for the session key and the signature of the elliptic curve encryption algorithm are used to authenticate the user's identity. |
| [31] | A biometric-based security system for IoMT increases secret key strength by applying bio-key generation methods for health information encryption. |
| [93] | A two-way identity authentication method in the IoMT context can solve the issue of device identity authentication while also securing the mechanism of updating authentication and session keys. |
| [105] | A biometric-based (ElectroCardioGram) method for symmetric cryptographic keys' generation and distribution in WBAN. |

Table 6.4 Current IDS for IoMT

| References | Description |
| --- | --- |
| [106] | A cross-tenant attack prevention and detection approach relies on SQL syntax analysis that meets the criteria of portability, compatibility, accuracy, and ease of integration. |
| [107] | A deep neural network can provide efficient and effective IDS in the IoMT ecosystem by classifying and predicting intruder attacks. |
| [108] | A trust-based intrusion detection method based on device behavioral profiling detects malicious devices in the IoMT environment, using the Euclidean distance difference of two behavioral profiles. |
| [109] | An intrusion detection mechanism based on multiple mobile agents for IoMT. Machine learning techniques and autonomous mobile agents are combined to detect and identify any unusual system behavior in this system. |

attack signatures, but it cannot identify new forms of attacks [106, 107]. Nevertheless, the main challenge for IDS mechanisms is the evolution of dynamic and random behavior of malicious software activity and the development of an adaptive method to manage this behavior. The transformation of the networks' behavior and the rapid expansion of different attacks prepared the path for analyzing different datasets produced over time and designing different dynamic strategies. We list some IDS methods for IoMT in Table 6.4.

## 6.5.5 Blockchain technology

Blockchain technology is considered a critical security enabler for the IoMT ecosystem. It can deal with the problem of distributed medical devices by providing multiplatform/services management, the confidentiality of

*Table 6.5* Current blockchain-based security protocols for IoMT

| References | Description |
|---|---|
| [110] | An IoMT-based security architecture that uses blockchain to ensure data transmission security between connected medical devices. |
| [112] | An authentication and authorization system for sharing medical data, incorporating both blockchain and edge computing to satisfy the scalability, security, and privacy requirements of a medical ecosystem. |
| [113] | A blockchain authentication key management mechanism for the IoMT ecosystem for securing key management between cloud servers, personal servers, and implantable medical devices (IMD). |
| [114] | A framework based on blockchain and edge computing to guarantee the data analysis process's confidentiality. The blockchain authenticates the IoMT devices, whereas the cloud service operators provide an access policy management mechanism for IoMT data. |
| [115] | A security and privacy mechanism based on the blockchain provides decentralized IoMT system-based service automation while maintaining system privacy and security. |
| [116] | A lightweight blockchain for IoMT maintains privacy and security in a smart healthcare framework. |

information exchanged, transaction forgery, non-trusted distributed authentication and authorization services, and non-traceable IoMT device transactions [110]. Several blockchain-based frameworks have been developed in this regard [111]. Table 6.5 summarizes the recent blockchain-based security methods for IoMT.

## 6.6 CONCLUSION

The increasing popularity of IoMT applications has many advantages. However, it is vulnerable to various attacks, concerns, and challenges explicitly aimed at patients' privacy as well as data integrity, confidentiality, and availability of IoMT devices that have restricted processing capabilities, storage space, and power capacity [117, 118]. In this study, we attempted to describe various security issues and challenges facing IoMT. In addition, we highlighted a categorization of current existing security mechanisms in the IoMT environment based on access control, authentication, key management, intrusion detection, and blockchain technology techniques. This work can help to explore the main privacy and security concerns in IoMT [119].

Furthermore, the different current proposed approaches are addressed to secure IoMT. Thus, it can serve to improve or design effective security mechanisms to protect sensitive medical data. New or unknown risks and features may emerge in the future due to the rapid development of technology and hacker skills. Moreover, securing the various wireless communication protocols [120] on which the IoMT relies is critical.

## REFERENCES

[1] Liu, J., Ma, J., Li, J., Huang, M., Sadiq, N., & Ai, Y. (2020). Robust watermarking algorithm for medical volume data in internet of medical things. *IEEE Access*, 8, 93939–93961.

[2] Wang, J., Wu, L., Wang, H., Choo, K. K. R., & He, D. (2020). An efficient and privacy-preserving outsourced support vector machine training for internet of medical things. *IEEE Internet of Things Journal*, 8(1), 458–473.

[3] Lokshina, I. V., & Lanting, C. J. (2018). Qualitative evaluation of IoT-driven eHealth: KM, business models, deployment and evolution. *International Journal of Interdisciplinary Telecommunications and Networking (IJITN)*, 10(4), 26–45.

[4] Sikarndar, M., Anwar, W., Almogren, A., Din, I. U., & Guizani, N. (2020). Iomt-based association rule mining for the prediction of human protein complexes. *IEEE Access*, 8, 6226–6237.

[5] Smys, S., Basar, A., & Wang, H. (2020). Hybrid intrusion detection system for internet of Things (IoT). *Journal of ISMAC*, 2(04), 190–199.

[6] Sun, L., Wang, H., Yong, J., & Wu, G. (2012, May). Semantic access control for cloud computing based on e-Healthcare. In *Proceedings of the 2012 IEEE 16th International Conference on Computer Supported Cooperative Work in Design (CSCWD)* (pp. 512–518). IEEE.

[7] Amanullah, M. A., Habeeb, R. A. A., Nasaruddin, F. H., Gani, A., Ahmed, E., Nainar, A. S. M., ... & Imran, M. (2020). Deep learning and big data technologies for IoT security. *Computer Communications*, 151, 495–517.

[8] Yaqoob, I., Ahmed, E., Rehman, M. H., Ahmed, A. I. A., Al-Garadi, M. A., Imran, M., Guizani, M. (2017). The rise of ransomware and emerging security challenges in the Internet of Things. *Computer Networks*, 129, 444–458.

[9] Li, X., Dai, H. N., Wang, Q., Imran, M., Li, D., & Imran, M. A. (2020). Securing internet of medical things with friendly-jamming schemes. *Computer Communications*, 160, 431–442.

[10] Abou-Nassar, E. M., Iliyasu, A. M., El-Kafrawy, P. M., Song, O. Y., Bashir, A. K., & Abd El-Latif, A. A. (2020). DITrust chain: towards blockchain-based trust models for sustainable healthcare IoT systems. *IEEE Access*, 8, 111223–111238.

[11] Aman, A. H. M., Hassan, W. H., Sameen, S., Attarbashi, Z. S., Alizadeh, M., & Latiff, L. A. (2021). IoMT amid COVID-19 pandemic: application, architecture, technology, and security. *Journal of Network and Computer Applications*, 174, 102886.

[12] Hatzivasilis, G., Soultatos, O., Ioannidis, S., Verikoukis, C., Demetriou, G., & Tsatsoulis, C. (2019, May). Review of security and privacy for the Internet of Medical Things (IoMT). In *2019 15th International Conference on Distributed Computing in Sensor Systems (DCOSS)* (pp. 457–464). IEEE.

[13] Alsubaei, F., Abuhussein, A., & Shiva, S. (2017, October). Security and privacy in the internet of medical things: taxonomy and risk assessment. In *2017 IEEE 42nd Conference on Local Computer Networks Workshops (LCN Workshops)* (pp. 112–120). IEEE.

[14] Sun, W., Cai, Z., Li, Y., Liu, F., Fang, S., & Wang, G. (2018). Security and privacy in the medical internet of things: a review. *Security and Communication Networks*, 2018.

[15] Kuila, S., Dhanda, N., Joardar, S., Neogy, S., & Kuila, J. (2019). A generic survey on medical big data analysis using internet of things. *In First International Conference on Artificial Intelligence and Cognitive Computing* (pp. 265–276). Springer, Singapore.

[16] Wazid, M., Das, A. K., Rodrigues, J. J., Shetty, S., & Park, Y. (2019). IoMT malware detection approaches: analysis and research challenges. *IEEE Access, 7*, 182459–182476.

[17] Yaqoob, T., Abbas, H., & Atiquzzaman, M. (2019). Security vulnerabilities, attacks, countermeasures, and regulations of networked medical devices—A review. *IEEE Communications Surveys & Tutorials, 21*(4), 3723–3768.

[18] Ray, P. P., Dash, D., & Kumar, N. (2020). Sensors for internet of medical things: State-of-the-art, security and privacy issues, challenges and future directions. *Computer Communications, 160*, 111–131.

[19] Putta, S. R., Abuhussein, A., Alsubaei, F., Shiva, S., & Atiewi, S. (2020). Security benchmarks for wearable medical things: stakeholders-centric approach. In *Fourth International Congress on Information and Communication Technology* (pp. 405–418). Springer, Singapore.

[20] Yaacoub, J. P. A., Noura, M., Noura, H. N., Salman, O., Yaacoub, E., Couturier, R., & Chehab, A. (2020). Securing internet of medical things systems: limitations, issues and recommendations. *Future Generation Computer Systems, 105*, 581–606.

[21] Somasundaram, R., & Thirugnanam, M. (2020). Review of security challenges in healthcare internet of things. *Wireless Networks*, 1–7.

[22] Islam, S. R., Kwak, D., Kabir, M. H., Hossain, M., & Kwak, K. S. (2015). The internet of things for health care: a comprehensive survey. *IEEE Access, 3*, 678–708.

[23] Nomikos, K., Papadimitriou, A., Stergiopoulos, G., Koutras, D., Psarakis, M., & Kotzanikolaou, P. (2020, August). On a Security-oriented Design Framework for Medical IoT Devices: The Hardware Security Perspective. In *2020 23rd Euromicro Conference on Digital System Design (DSD)* (pp. 301–308). IEEE.

[24] Kohli, L., Saurabh, M., Bhatia, I., Shekhawat, U. S., Vijh, M., & Sindhwani, N. (2021). Design and development of modular and multifunctional UAV with amphibious landing module. In *Data Driven Approach Towards Disruptive Technologies: Proceedings of MIDAS 2020* (pp. 405–421). Singapore: Springer.

[25] Kohli, L., Saurabh, M., Bhatia, I., Sindhwani, N., & Vijh, M. (2021). Design and Development of modular and multifunctional UAV with amphibious landing, processing and surround sense module. *Unmanned Aerial Vehicles for Internet of Things (IoT): Concepts, Techniques, and Applications*, eds. V. Mohindru, Y. Singh, R. Bhatt and A.K. Gupta (pp. 207–230).

[26] Garg, P., & Anand, R. (2011). Energy Efficient Data Collection in Wireless Sensor Network. *Dronacharya Research Journal, 3*(1), 41–45.

[27] Meelu, R., & Anand, R. (2010, November). Energy efficiency of cluster-based routing protocols used in wireless sensor networks. In *AIP Conference Proceedings* (Vol. 1324, No. 1, pp. 109–113). American Institute of Physics.

[28] Paliwal, K. K., Anand, R. & Garg, P. Energy efficient data collection in wireless sensor network-a survey. In 2011 *International Conference on Advanced Computing, Communication and Networks, 824–827*.

[29] Rakitin, S. R. (2009). Networked medical devices: essential collaboration for improved safety. *Biomedical instrumentation & technology, 43*(4), 332–338.

[30] Stellios, I., Kotzanikolaou, P., Psarakis, M., Alcaraz, C., & Lopez, J. (2018). A survey of iot-enabled cyberattacks: Assessing attack paths to critical infrastructures and services. *IEEE Communications Surveys & Tutorials, 20*(4), 3453–3495.

[31] Pirbhulal, S., Samuel, O. W., Wu, W., Sangaiah, A. K., & Li, G. (2019). A joint resource-aware and medical data security framework for wearable healthcare systems. *Future Generation Computer Systems, 95*, 382–391.

[32] Porras, J., Pänkäläinen, J., Knutas, A., & Khakurel, J. (2018, January). Security in the internet of things-a systematic mapping study. In *Proceedings of the 51st Hawaii International Conference on System Sciences*.

[33] Shackelford, S. J., Mattioli, M., Myers, S., Brady, A., Wang, Y., & Wong, S. (2018). Securing the Internet of healthcare. *Minnesota Journal of Law Science & Technology, 19*, 405.

[34] Baker, S. B., Xiang, W., & Atkinson, I. (2017). Internet of things for smart healthcare: Technologies, challenges, and opportunities. *IEEE Access, 5*, 26521–26544.

[35] Burhan, M., Rehman, R. A., Khan, B., & Kim, B. S. (2018). IoT elements, layered architectures and security issues: A comprehensive survey. *Sensors, 18*(9), 2796.

[36] Alsubaei, F., Abuhussein, A., & Shiva, S. (2019). Ontology-based security recommendation for the internet of medical things. *IEEE Access, 7*, 48948–48960.

[37] He, D., Chan, S., & Guizani, M. (2017). Drone-assisted public safety networks: The security aspect. *IEEE Communications Magazine, 55*(8), 218–223.

[38] Anand, S., & Sharma, A. (2020). Assessment of security threats on IoT based applications. *Materials Today: Proceedings*. https://doi.org/10.1016/j.matpr.2020.09.350

[39] Yang, C. W., Hwang, T., & Lin, T. H. (2013). Modification attack on QSDC with authentication and the improvement. *International Journal of Theoretical Physics, 52*(7), 2230–2234.

[40] Bostami, B., Ahmed, M., & Choudhury, S. (2019). False data injection attacks in internet of things. In *Performability in Internet of Things* (pp. 47–58). Springer, Cham.

[41] Liu, Y., Ning, P., & Reiter, M. K. (2011). False data injection attacks against state estimation in electric power grids. *ACM Transactions on Information and System Security (TISSEC), 14*(1), 1–33.

[42] Rahman, M. A., & Mohsenian-Rad, H. (2012, December). False data injection attacks with incomplete information against smart power grids. In *2012 IEEE Global Communications Conference (GLOBECOM)* (pp. 3153–3158). IEEE.

[43] Lin, J., Yu, W., Zhang, N., Yang, X., Zhang, H., & Zhao, W. (2017). A survey on internet of things: Architecture, enabling technologies, security and privacy, and applications. *IEEE Internet of Things Journal, 4*(5), 1125–1142.

[44] Spiekermann, S. (2019). *Ethical IT innovation: A value-based system design approach*. Auerbach Publications.

[45] Wang, H., Zhang, M., & Wang, J. (2010, March). Design and implementation of an emergency search and rescue system based on mobile robot and WSN. In *2010 2nd International Asia Conference on Informatics in Control, Automation and Robotics (CAR 2010)* (Vol. 1, pp. 206–209). IEEE.

[46] Kissel, R. (Ed.). (2011). *Glossary of key information security terms*. Diane Publishing.

[47] Grammatikis, P. I. R., Sarigiannidis, P. G., & Moscholios, I. D. (2019). Securing the Internet of Things: Challenges, threats and solutions. *Internet of Things, 5*, 41–70.

[48] Sindhwani, N., Bhamrah, M. S., Garg, A., & Kumar, D. (2017, July). Performance analysis of particle swarm optimization and genetic algorithm in MIMO systems. In *2017 8th International Conference on Computing, Communication and Networking Technologies (ICCCNT)* (pp. 1–6). IEEE.

[49] Sindhwani, N., & Singh, M. (2017, March). Performance analysis of ant colony based optimization algorithm in MIMO systems. In *2017 International Conference on Wireless Communications, Signal Processing and Networking (WiSPNET)* (pp. 1587–1593). IEEE.

[50] Sindhwani, N. (2017). Performance analysis of optimal scheduling based firefly algorithm in MIMO system. *Optimization*, 2(12), 19–26.

[51] Baig, Z. A., Sanguanpong, S., Firdous, S. N., Nguyen, T. G., & So-In, C. (2020). Averaged dependence estimators for DoS attack detection in IoT networks. *Future Generation Computer Systems*, 102, 198–209.

[52] Rathore, H., Al-Ali, A. K., Mohamed, A., Du, X., & Guizani, M. (2019). A novel deep learning strategy for classifying different attack patterns for deep brain implants. *IEEE Access*, 7, 24154–24164.

[53] Sun, Y., Lo, F. P. W., & Lo, B. (2019). Security and privacy for the internet of medical things enabled healthcare systems: A survey. *IEEE Access*, 7, 183339–183355.

[54] Andrea, I., Chrysostomou, C., & Hadjichristofi, G. (2015, July). Internet of things: Security vulnerabilities and challenges. In *2015 IEEE symposium on computers and communication (ISCC)* (pp. 180–187). IEEE.

[55] Aly, M., Khomh, F., Haoues, M., Quintero, A., & Yacout, S. (2019). Enforcing security in Internet of Things frameworks: A systematic literature review. *Internet of Things*, 6, 100050.

[56] Bogdanoski, M., Suminoski, T., & Risteski, A. (2013). Analysis of the SYN flood DoS attack. *International Journal of Computer Network and Information Security (IJCNIS)*, 5(8), 1–11.

[57] Harshita, H. (2017). Detection and prevention of ICMP flood DDOS attack. *International Journal of New Technology and Research*, 3(3), 263333.

[58] Vadlamani, S., Eksioglu, B., Medal, H., & Nandi, A. (2016). Jamming attacks on wireless networks: A taxonomic survey. *International Journal of Production Economics*, 172, 76–94.

[59] Proano, A., & Lazos, L. (2010, May). Selective jamming attacks in wireless networks. In *2010 IEEE International Conference on Communications* (pp. 1–6). IEEE.

[60] Ten, C. W., Manimaran, G., & Liu, C. C. (2010). Cybersecurity for critical infrastructures: Attack and defense modeling. *IEEE Transactions on Systems, Man, and Cybernetics-Part A: Systems and Humans*, 40(4), 853–865.

[61] McMahon, E., Williams, R., El, M., Samtani, S., Patton, M., & Chen, H. (2017, July). Assessing medical device vulnerabilities on the Internet of Things. In *2017 IEEE International Conference on Intelligence and Security Informatics (ISI)* (pp. 176–178). IEEE.

[62] Kumar, P., & Lee, H. J. (2012). Security issues in healthcare applications using wireless medical sensor networks: A survey. *Sensors*, 12(1), 55–91.

[63] Nam, J., Paik, J., Kang, H. K., Kim, U. M., & Won, D. (2009). An off-line dictionary attack on a simple three-party key exchange protocol. *IEEE Communications Letters*, 13(3), 205–207.

[64] Cho, J. S., Yeo, S. S., & Kim, S. K. (2011). Securing against brute-force attack: A hash-based RFID mutual authentication protocol using a secret value. *Computer Communications, 34*(3), 391–397.

[65] Butun, I., Österberg, P., & Song, H. (2019). Security of the Internet of Things: Vulnerabilities, attacks, and countermeasures. *IEEE Communications Surveys & Tutorials, 22*(1), 616–644.

[66] Kazemi, Z., Papadimitriou, A., Hely, D., Fazcli, M., & Beroulle, V. (2018, July). Hardware security evaluation platform for MCU-based connected devices: application to healthcare IoT. In *2018 IEEE 3rd International Verification and Security Workshop (IVSW)* (pp. 87–92). IEEE.

[67] Singh, A., Chawla, N., Ko, J. H., Kar, M., & Mukhopadhyay, S. (2018). Energy efficient and side-channel secure cryptographic hardware for IoT-edge nodes. *IEEE Internet of Things Journal, 6*(1), 421–434.

[68] Costin, A., & Zaddach, J. (2018). Iot malware: Comprehensive survey, analysis framework and case studies. *BlackHat USA*.

[69] Xiao, L., Li, Y., Huang, X., & Du, X. (2017). Cloud-based malware detection game for mobile devices with offloading. *IEEE Transactions on Mobile Computing, 16*(10), 2742–2750.

[70] Zhou, J., Cao, Z., Dong, X., & Vasilakos, A. V. (2017). Security and privacy for cloud-based IoT: Challenges. *IEEE Communications Magazine, 55*(1), 26–33.

[71] Karimipour, H., Geris, S., Dehghantanha, A., & Leung, H. (2019, May). Intelligent anomaly detection for large-scale smart grids. In *2019 IEEE Canadian Conference of Electrical and Computer Engineering (CCECE)* (pp. 1–4). IEEE.

[72] Yin, M., Chen, X., Wang, Q., Wang, W., & Wang, Y. (2019). Dynamics on hybrid complex network: Botnet modeling and analysis of medical IoT. *Security and Communication Networks, 2019*.

[73] Stone-Gross, B., Cova, M., Cavallaro, L., Gilbert, B., Szydlowski, M., Kemmerer, R., ... & Vigna, G. (2009, November). Your botnet is my botnet: analysis of a botnet takeover. In *Proceedings of the 16th ACM conference on Computer and communications security* (pp. 635–647).

[74] Zahra, S. R., & Chishti, M. A. (2019, January). Ransomware and internet of things: A new security nightmare. In *2019 9th International Conference on cloud Computing, Data Science & Engineering (Confluence)* (pp. 551–555). IEEE.

[75] Deogirikar, J., & Vidhate, A. (2017, February). Security attacks in IoT: A survey. In *2017 International Conference on I-SMAC (IoT in Social, Mobile, Analytics and Cloud)(I-SMAC)* (pp. 32–37). IEEE.

[76] Cooke, E., Jahanian, F., & McPherson, D. (2005). The Zombie Roundup: Understanding, Detecting, and Disrupting Botnets. *SRUTI, 5,* 6–6.

[77] Milosevic, J., Sklavos, N., & Koutsikou, K. (2016). Malware in IoT software and hardware. https://www.semanticscholar.org/paper/Malware-in-IoT-Software-and-Hardware-Milosevic-Sklavos/8467861c3a934681a427fef652358fa5bf2902cc

[78] Anand, R., Shrivastava, G., Gupta, S., Peng, S. L., & Sindhwani, N. (2018). Audio watermarking with reduced number of random samples. In *Handbook of Research on Network Forensics and Analysis Techniques* (pp. 372–394). IGI Global.

[79] Anand, R., Sinha, A., Bhardwaj, A., & Sreeraj, A. (2018). Flawed security of social network of things. In *Handbook of Research on Network Forensics and Analysis Techniques* (pp. 65–86). IGI Global.

[80] Gupta, A., Srivastava, A., Anand, R., & Tomažič, T., "Business Application Analytics and the Internet of Things: The Connecting Link. In New Age Analytics: Transforming the Internet through Machine Learning, IoT, and Trust Modeling". 249–273.

[81] Gupta, R., Shrivastava, G., Anand, R., & Tomažič, T. (2018). IoT-based privacy control system through android. In *Handbook of E-Business Security* (pp. 341–363). Auerbach Publications.

[82] Kim, D., Park, K., Park, Y., & Ahn, J. H. (2019). Willingness to provide personal information: Perspective of privacy calculus in IoT services. *Computers in Human Behavior, 92*, 273–281.

[83] Singh, L., Saini, M. K., Tripathi, S., & Sindhwani, N. (2008). An intelligent control system for real-time traffic signal using genetic algorithm. In *AICTE Sponsored National Seminar on Emerging Trends in Software Engineering* (Vol. 50).

[84] Saini, M. K., Nagal, R., Tripathi, S., Sindhwani, N., & Rudra, A. (2008). PC interfaced wireless robotic moving Arm. In *AICTE Sponsored National Seminar on Emerging Trends in Software Engineering* (Vol. 50).

[85] Yang, Y., Liu, X., & Deng, R. H. (2017). Lightweight break-glass access control system for healthcare internet-of-things. *IEEE Transactions on Industrial Informatics, 14*(8), 3610–3617.

[86] Luo, E., Bhuiyan, M. Z. A., Wang, G., Rahman, M. A., Wu, J., & Atiquzzaman, M. (2018). Privacyprotector: Privacy-protected patient data collection in IoT-based healthcare systems. *IEEE Communications Magazine, 56*(2), 163–168.

[87] Wang, X., Wang, L., Li, Y., & Gai, K. (2018). Privacy-aware efficient fine-grained data access control in Internet of medical things based fog computing. *IEEE Access, 6*, 47657–47665.

[88] Hossain, M., Islam, S. R., Ali, F., Kwak, K. S., & Hasan, R. (2018). An Internet of Things-based health prescription assistant and its security system design. *Future Generation Computer Systems, 82*, 422–439.

[89] Yang, Y., Zheng, X., Guo, W., Liu, X., & Chang, V. (2019). Privacy-preserving smart IoT-based healthcare big data storage and self-adaptive access control system. *Information Sciences, 479*, 567–592.

[90] Lu, X., & Cheng, X. (2019). A secure and lightweight data sharing scheme for Internet of medical things. *IEEE Access, 8*, 5022–5030.

[91] Camara, C., Peris-Lopez, P., De Fuentes, J. M., & Marchal, S. (2020). Access control for implantable medical devices. *IEEE Transactions on Emerging Topics in Computing, 9*(3), 1126–1138.

[92] Park, K., Noh, S., Lee, H., Das, A. K., Kim, M., Park, Y., & Wazid, M. (2020). LAKS-NVT: Provably secure and lightweight authentication and key agreement scheme without verification table in medical internet of things. *IEEE Access, 8*, 119387–119404.

[93] Cheng, X., Zhang, Z., Chen, F., Zhao, C., Wang, T., Sun, H., & Huang, C. (2019). Secure identity authentication of community medical internet of things. *IEEE Access, 7*, 115966–115977.

[94] Hamidi, H. (2019). An approach to develop the smart health using Internet of Things and authentication based on biometric technology. *Future Generation Computer Systems, 91*, 434–449.

[95] Deebak, B. D., Al-Turjman, F., Aloqaily, M., & Alfandi, O. (2019). An authentic-based privacy preservation protocol for smart e-healthcare systems in IoT. *IEEE Access, 7*, 135632–135649.

[96] Mahendran, R. K., & Velusamy, P. (2020). A secure fuzzy extractor based biometric key authentication scheme for body sensor network in Internet of Medical Things. *Computer Communications, 153*, 545–552.

[97] Jegadeesan, S., Azees, M., Babu, N. R., Subramaniam, U., & Almakhles, J. D. (2020). EPAW: Efficient privacy preserving anonymous mutual authentication scheme for wireless body area networks (WBANs). *IEEE Access, 8*, 48576–48586.

[98] Sowjanya, K., Dasgupta, M., & Ray, S. (2021). Elliptic curve cryptography based authentication scheme for Internet of medical things. *Journal of Information Security and Applications, 58*, 102761.

[99] Ding, R., Zhong, H., Ma, J., Liu, X., & Ning, J. (2019). Lightweight privacy-preserving identity-based verifiable IoT-based health storage system. *IEEE Internet of Things Journal, 6(5)*, 8393–8405.

[100] Karmakar, K. K., Varadharajan, V., Tupakula, U., Nepal, S., & Thapa, C. (2020, June). Towards a Security Enhanced Virtualised Network Infrastructure for Internet of Medical Things (IoMT). In *2020 6th IEEE Conference on Network Softwarization (NetSoft)* (pp. 257–261). IEEE.

[101] Xu, Z., Xu, C., Liang, W., Xu, J., & Chen, H. (2019). A lightweight mutual authentication and key agreement scheme for medical Internet of Things. *IEEE Access, 7*, 53922–53931.

[102] Li, J., Su, Z., Guo, D., Choo, K. K. R., & Ji, Y. (2021). PSL-MAAKA: Provably-secure and lightweight mutual authentication and key agreement protocol for fully public channels in internet of medical things. *IEEE Internet of Things Journal, 8(17)*, 13183–13195.

[103] Aghili, S. F., Mala, H., Kaliyar, P., & Conti, M. (2019). SecLAP: Secure and lightweight RFID authentication protocol for Medical IoT. *Future Generation Computer Systems, 101*, 621–634.

[104] Kang, J., Fan, K., Zhang, K., Cheng, X., Li, H., & Yang, Y. (2021). An ultra light weight and secure RFID batch authentication scheme for IoMT. *Computer Communications, 167*, 48–54.

[105] Sammoud, A., Chalouf, M. A., Hamdi, O., Montavont, N., & Bouallegue, A. (2020). A new biometrics-based key establishment protocol in WBAN: energy efficiency and security robustness analysis. *Computers & Security, 96*, 101838.

[106] Yassin, M., Talhi, C., & Boucheneb, H. (2019). ITADP: an inter-tenant attack detection and prevention framework for multi-tenant SaaS. *Journal of Information Security and Applications, 49*, 102395.

[107] Singh, P., et al. (2019). A visual cryptography scheme for secret hiding using pre-processing. *Proceedings of the 13th INDIACom; INDIACom-2019; IEEE Conference ID: 46181 2019 6th International Conference on "Computing for Sustainable Global Development"*, (pp. 958–961), 13th–15th March'2019.

[108] Meng, W., Li, W., Wang, Y., & Au, M. H. (2020). Detecting insider attacks in medical cyber–physical networks based on behavioral profiling. *Future Generation Computer Systems, 108*, 1258–1266.

[109] Thamilarasu, G., Odesile, A., & Hoang, A. (2020). An intrusion detection system for internet of medical things. *IEEE Access, 8*, 181560–181576.

[110] Kumari, K. A., Padmashani, R., Varsha, R., & Upadhayay, V. (2020). Securing Internet of Medical Things (IoMT) using private blockchain network. In *Principles of Internet of Things (IoT) Ecosystem: Insight Paradigm* (pp. 305–326). Springer, Cham.

[111] Dwivedi, A. D., Srivastava, G., Dhar, S., & Singh, R. (2019). A decentralized privacy-preserving healthcare blockchain for IoT. *Sensors, 19*(2), 326.

[112] Akkaoui, R., Hei, X., & Cheng, W. (2020). Edgemedichain: A hybrid edge blockchain-based framework for health data exchange. *IEEE Access, 8*, 113467–113486.

[113] Garg, N., Wazid, M., Das, A. K., Singh, D. P., Rodrigues, J. J., & Park, Y. (2020). BAKMP-IoMT: Design of blockchain enabled authenticated key management protocol for internet of medical things deployment. *IEEE Access, 8*, 95956–95977.

[114] Gao, Y., Lin, H., Chen, Y., & Liu, Y. (2021). Blockchain and SGX-enabled edge computing empowered secure IoMT data analysis. *IEEE Internet of Things Journal*.

[115] Egala, B. S., Pradhan, A. K., Badarla, V. R., & Mohanty, S. P. (2021). Fortified-chain: a blockchain based framework for security and privacy assured internet of medical things with effective access control. *IEEE Internet of Things Journal*.

[116] Seliem, M., & Elgazzar, K. (2019, June). BIoMT: Blockchain for the internet of medical things. In *2019 IEEE International Black Sea Conference on Communications and Networking (BlackSeaCom)* (pp. 1–4). IEEE.

[117] Kumar, A., Tripathi, S., & Raw, R. S. (2016). Bringing Healthcare to Doorstep using VANETs. In *3rd IEEE International Conference as INDIACom-2016* (pp. 4747–4750), 16–18 March, Delhi.

[118] Kumar, S., & Raw, R. S. (2020). Health Monitoring Planning for On-Board Ships Through Flying Ad Hoc Network. *Advanced Computing and Intelligent Engineering* (pp. 391–402) Springer.

[119] Anand, R., Sindhwani, N., & Saini, A. (2021). Emerging Technologies for COVID-19. *Enabling Healthcare 4.0 for Pandemics: A Roadmap Using AI, Machine Learning, IoT and Cognitive Technologies*, 163–188.

[120] Kirubasri, G., Sankar, S., Pandey, D., Pandey, B. K., Singh, H., & Anand, R. (2021, September). A Recent Survey on 6G Vehicular Technology, Applications and Challenges. In *2021 9th International Conference on Reliability, Infocom Technologies and Optimization (Trends and Future Directions) (ICRITO)* (pp. 1–5). IEEE.

Chapter 7

# Impact of Industry 4.0 and Healthcare 4.0 for controlling the various challenges related to healthcare industries

*Rekha Narang*
Geeta University, Panipat, India

*Sumit Zokarkar and Shweta Mogre*
Prestige Institute of Management and Research, Indore, India

*Ankit Trivedi*
Comp-Feeders Group of Institutions, Indore, India

## CONTENTS

## 7.1 INTRODUCTION

In the second decade of the 21st century, the world stands on the cusp of the Industry 4.0 paradigm, which has remarkably become a global emergence with a core of industrial transformation, revitalization, and development [1]. Industry 4.0 has made a revolution not only in the manufacturing industry but also in the healthcare industry. The name healthcare industry has been updated to 'Healthcare 4.0' according to Ref. [2] in which it is stated that Industry 4.0 has changed the way of treatment as well as diagnosis. The authors in [3] stated that the new relationship between patients and health

DOI: 10.1201/9781003239888-7

professionals has also changed. According to [4], the high risk of morality can be reduced by using the innovative method of digital technologies and keeping the patient in proper isolation. They have suggested some major technologies of Industry 4.0 that can help in solving the problem of virus-like COVID-19 by detecting its symptoms without any confusion regarding the disease [5, 6]. Their study talked about the health monitoring systems such as smartphones, smart bracelets, smart watches, and various sensors and wearable devices [7, 8] that involve in processing and analysis of data as well as continuous monitoring of the health conditions of patients with the use of instruments that can sense and transmit various measurements such as body temperature, blood pressure readings, heart rate, electrocardiogram, respiratory, and chest sounds.

Several technological changes have been observed by the healthcare industry around the world, beginning with Healthcare 1.0, in which doctors saved the affected person's data manually. Then Healthcare 2.0 arrived, wherein paper-based manual facts had been changed by electronic file. Healthcare 3.0 is superior to the point where wearable devices were brought [9].

The important technological feature that differentiates Healthcare 4.0 from the previous revolutions of healthcare is that a huge wide variety of gadgets of various kinds display an affected person's fitness to conduct other fitness-related activities driven via the internet of things (IoT), cyber-physical systems (CPS), and internet of services [10, 11] defines Healthcare 4.0 as a mix utility of IoT, artificial intelligence (AI), robot, and sensible sensing in healthcare to transform its cost chain. It aims at digitizing healthcare employers and offerings. We have seen that, in the context of rapid improvements in scientific equipment, medical development, data analysis (DA), and recording technology, people are becoming more and more interested in engineering methods for medical care.

Recent breakthroughs in virtual fitness technologies (e.g., digital fitness information, fitness tracking, and wearable devices) are not only effective and transformative for reengineering care approaches and improving fitness care outcomes such as first-class care and affected person's safety, but they can also have an essential socio-monetary impact, as nearly 20% of the US gross domestic product (GDP) is devoted to fitness fees. These technological advancements have generated numerous innovation possibilities as well as good-sized demanding situations for care transport, and they provide a threat to move beyond the traditional scope of healthcare engineering, consisting of manner development and technology implementation. There was developing attention that data technology, structure engineering gear, and organizational innovation play a vital role in overcoming the interrelated productivity and quality crises faced by health structures in the arena [12–14]. Such technologies and tools can aid healthcare structures in accomplishing the quadruple intention of improving the affected person's experience, populace health, fee manipulation, and clinician pride [15]. The Healthcare

Systems Engineering (HSE) community has a critical function to play in addressing these demanding situations. Industry 4.0 has transformed the production industry into a brand-new paradigm [16–18]. Smart and sustainable manufacturing technologies have significantly improved productivity, first-class quality, and/or customer satisfaction with strategy, products, and services. These modern changes can have a huge impact, and it has become easier now, not only in production but also in all areas of our society, including the healthcare sector, where these technological innovations have begun to be implemented. Fitness care shipping, like production, is at the sunrise of a paradigm trade to reach the new era, known as Fitness Care 4.0. A large number of analyses and solutions are continuously carried out in an exponential manner. Important data is generated and provided. Various equipments, sensors, and radio equipments have been installed and used in hospitals, clinics, nursing homes, pharmacies, and many different medical institutions.

The revolutionary upgradation of computing power, new equipment gaining knowledge, AI protocols, and algorithms have become increasingly important. Some new complex modeling and optimization techniques [19–23] have been developed, and cognitive effects are increasingly considered. Factor technology is being incorporated into the development of technological improvements. These innovations will greatly improve the social and technical skills of attention and, if properly designed, implemented, and used, will provide opportunities to improve care. Experience and effectiveness, community capabilities, and clinical pride are therefore the main benefits to the group and society as a whole.

Further in this chapter, we will cover the industrial revolutions, the pillars of Industry 4.0, the introduction to Healthcare 4.0 and major trending technologies, the impact of technological trends on healthcare, upcoming challenges, and quality assurance in healthcare.

## 7.1.1 Industry

Industries are organized economic activities concerned with the manufacture, extraction, and processing of raw materials, or construction. Over the years, various innovations in technology, modifications in socioeconomic behavior, and cultural aspects have revolutionized the industry. Technological changes, such as new energy sources, new materials, and new machines, have reformed industrial processes, whereas socioeconomic modifications, such as improved agricultural production, new currencies, new trading systems, and cultural transformation, have affected the perception of products and services, resulting in the revolutionization of both industries.

*The first industrial revolution*
The first industrial revolution came at the end of the 18th century (1760–1840) in Britain with the introduction of machines in industries. Labor

came to optimize the use of water as a power source. During this period, the term "factory" became very famous, and many industries, including the textile industry, benefited greatly from these changes.

*The second industrial revolution*

The second industrial revolution in the early part of the late 19th and early 20th centuries increased the efficiency of manufacturing companies with the use of steel and electricity. The electrification of factories helped make factory machinery more mobile. The large production of steel has changed the railways into the system.

*The third industrial revolution*

The third industrial revolution means the digital revolution that came in the late 1950s. It has changed analog and mechanical systems to digital ones. Manufacturers put more emphasis on electronic and computer technologies.

*The fourth industrial revolution, or Industry 4.0*

Industry 4.0, a fourth industrial revolution has emerged in the past few decades. The concept of CPS has been introduced. Manufacturers are now able to communicate with computers rather than operate them. This communication enables a manufacturing system in which pieces of machinery are augmented with Wi-Fi, sensors, and actuators to monitor, execute, and visualize the complete manufacturing process and make independent decisions.

### 7.1.2 Pillars of Industry 4.0

The concept of Industry 4.0, however, is not a simple one. Many technologies in Industry 4.0 are used in a variety of different contexts.

*IoT*

IoT [24–26] is a new trend in which all devices are connected to the existing infrastructure and can share information or exchange data between physical word and computer systems without any interaction of humans. IoT is enabling devices to communicate through the internet [27]. This helps the device to take instructions and data from the outer world and execute them. IoT has a variety of application domains such as smart appliances, smart manufacturing, smart farming, and smart healthcare. With a vast diversity of technology, the IoT finds its application in various sectors ranging from general consumer uses to large-scale industrial.

*AI*

It is the science and engineering of making intelligent machines, especially intelligent computer programs. It is related to the similar task of using computers to understand human intelligence [28], but AI does not have to confine itself to methods that are biologically observable [29]. In a simple form, AI is a combination of computer science and robust datasets to enable problem-solving. It also encompasses the sub-fields of machine learning (ML) and deep learning [30], which are frequently mentioned in conjunction with AI. These disciplines are comprised of AI algorithms that seek to create expert systems that can make predictions or classifications based on input data.

*Cloud computing (CC)*

Optimal management of big data is a critical success factor for the company as far as digitization of big data is concerned.. Cloud plays a very important role in the management of this big data. In CC [31], we store and access data and all the programs over the internet rather than on the hard drive of the computer.

*CPS*

CPS means a combination of cyber components as well as physical components. CPSs are "systems of collaborating computational entities which are in intensive connection with the surrounding physical world and its on-going processes, providing and using, at the same time, data-accessing and data-processing services available on the internet" [32]. Thus, CPSs can: (i) gather data from the surrounding environment, (ii) store, process, and analyze data, (iii) communicate with larger networks, and (iv) execute decisions based on processing [33, 34].

CPSs are most commonly used in the health industry. Now it is easier to real-time monitor and remote sense the physical conditions of the patients.

*DA*

A large amount of heterogeneous data is produced at a very fast speed in big data [35]. With Industry 4.0 now in the organization, data is being collected and monitored by big data analytics systems that utilize ML and AI techniques for the quick processing of tons of data generated by traditional and digital sources.

These technologies are used to process and interpret the data and give information to decision-makers to improve if needed. Industry 4.0 started in the manufacturing industry, but it has since expanded enormously to include Fashion 4.0, Agriculture 4.0, Education 4.0, and Healthcare 4.0.

The various pillars of Industry 4.0 are shown in Figure 7.1

## 7.2 HEALTHCARE 4.0

The aforementioned technologies are driving changes in all segments of the industry [36, 37]. Initially, it affected the manufacturing sector, but it is now affecting other sectors as well, such as healthcare, which has been called Healthcare 4.0.

A healthcare system comprises all the health-improving activities. For example, it includes all such establishments, groups of people, and activities whose primary intent is to encourage and retain health. Previously, many

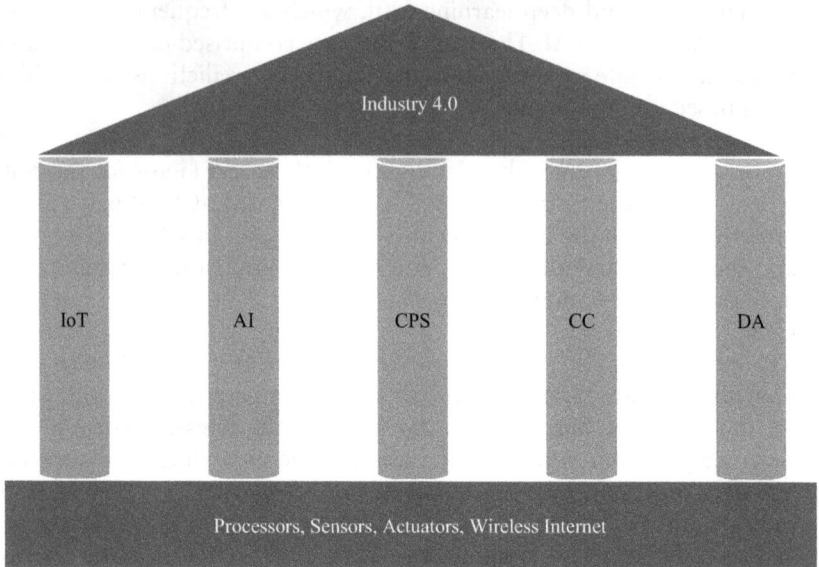

*Figure 7.1* Pillars of Industry 4.0.

technological innovations have changed healthcare systems, such as magnetic resonance imaging (MRI), computed tomography (CT) scan, and light amplification by stimulated emission of raidation (LASER) surgery.

Today, the healthcare industry is experiencing significant transformation due to technological innovation. Various healthcare frontrunners are interested to invest in transforming the healthcare industry. Many innovative techniques are changing the interaction way or medium of patients with health professionals, e.g., telemedicine, online consulting, the internet of medical things (IoMT), and mobile apps.

## 7.2.1 Technology trends in Healthcare 4.0

(i)  *Wearable technology and IoMT*

Wearable technologies popularly known as wearables are electronic devices that are worn by any person (usually close to the skin) to monitor their physical activities. It allows the non-stop monitoring of human physical activities and behaviors, in addition to physiological and biochemical parameters in the course of everyday life. The maximum normally measured statistics encompass important signs and indicators such as heart rate, blood strain, and body temperature, in addition to oxygen saturation, posture, and bodily sports through the use of electrocardiogram (ECG), Bacillus Calmette-Guerin (BCG), and different devices. Potentially, wearable image or video gadgets could provide extra medical information. Wearable gadgets can be connected to shoes, eyeglasses, rings, clothing, gloves, and watches. In addition, wearable devices might also evolve to be pores and skin-attachable gadgets. Sensors may be embedded into the surroundings, along with chairs, vehicle seats, and mattresses. A phone is commonly used to gather information and transmit it to a far-flung server for garage and analysis. There are fundamental types of wearable devices that can be used for studying gait styles. Some devices have been developed for healthcare specialists to screen walking patterns, along with the accelerometer, multi-attitude video recorders, and gyroscopes. Different gadgets have been developed for health consumers, together with on-wrist pass time trackers (which includes Fitbit) and mobile smartphone apps. Wearable devices and information evaluation algorithms are frequently used together to carry out gait assessment responsibilities in extraordinary situations.

Some wearable technology applications are designed for the prevention of sicknesses and preservation of fitness, which includes weight management and physical interest tracking. Wearable gadgets are also used for affected person control and disorder control. The wearable programs can without delay impact medical selection-making. Some accept as true that wearable technology may improve the care of affected people while decreasing the cost of care, which includes patient rehabilitation outside of hospitals.

The big records generated by using wearable gadgets are both an undertaking and a possibility for researchers who can observe more AI techniques on that data in the destiny.

(ii)  *IoMT*

It is also referred to as a healthcare IoT. It is an international infrastructure such as the collection of medical gadgets and packages that are interconnected through records and verbal exchange technology. Various sensor devices like oxygen saturation sensor, temperature sensor, ECG/electroencephalogram (EEG)/electromyogram (EMG) sensor, pressure sensor, humidity sensor, breathing sensor, and blood-stress sensor continuously monitor the health of the patient. The IoMT senses the sufferers' health repute after which it transfers the medical records to doctors and care holders with the assistance of far-off cloud facts centers. This fact is most customarily used for sickness diagnosis and medical care. The beneficial data mined from the scientific database is used for preventing and protecting the affected person's fitness at some stage in an emergency. But, the primary assignment in IoMT is a way to operate with essential packages, in which some of the connected devices generate a huge amount of medical facts.

The significant change that IoMTs are resulting to healthcare is decreasing the duration from vital measurement to problem detection and treatment. For IoMT-enabled insulin pumps, it calculates and executes medicine doses with accuracy, with due patient intervention, and with connected blood glucose monitors with sensors under the skin.

Although IoMT is still evolving and building new devices for patient care, the available IoMT devices may be broadly divided into the following categories:

*General fitness trackers*

They are also called consumer-grade wearables. These come in the form of smartwatches, wristbands, smart apparel, etc. They are mostly connected to smartphone-based applications for collecting and processing data. They use sensitive biosensors to monitor the physical activities of the user along with medical parameters such as heart rate (pulse rate) and blood pressure, and then assess general fitness based on that.

*Clinical grade wearables*

These are also wearable gadgets with biosensors, but they are recognized and certified by a regulatory authority for specific purposes. These devices require consultation and prescription from physicians before being applied to any patient. Ambulatory blood pressure monitors, Holters, smart BP cuffs, smart glucometers, etc., come under this type.

*Remote monitoring devices*

Remote monitoring devices provide a facility to keep track of patient health. In the case of chronic or acute diseases, the patient requires monitoring even after being discharged from the hospital. With the use of IoMT devices, doctors can observe patients continuously and ensure that proper medication is being done.

*Smart pills*

A smart pill is a special kind of sensor that is sent inside the patient's body in the form of a pill. After reaching inside the body, it gets activated and sends data to a device worn by the patient, from which data gets transmitted to a smartphone app. The doctors get easy reach to the data and treatment can be decided accordingly. It is very helpful in case of mental illness or multiple illnesses. After the drug dissolves within the human body, the biosensor is discharged from the pill into the gastrointestinal (GI) tract naturally.

*Point of care (POC) devices*

POC devices are like self-serving kiosks, similar to ATMs, where patients can get preliminary services such as doctor's appointments, registration, and test reports. POCs can be implemented in two ways: the first is inside the hospital premises to automate the outpatient department (OPD) and inpatient department (IPD) workflow and the second is at remote locations for providing better access to preliminary medical services. POCs can also help in conducting the preliminary screening through IoMT-enabled testing devices. It will reduce the time, effort, and cost required for diagnosis and treatment.

*Clinical monitors*

Clinical monitors are smart devices used by physicians for recording observations and patient data in electronic form. These electronic

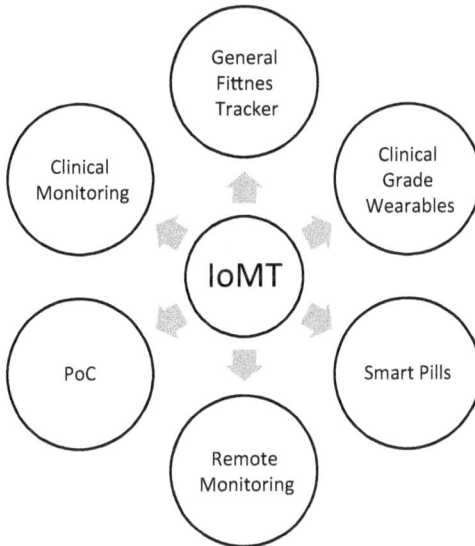

*Figure 7.2* IoMT devices.

records are saved in the cloud for further review or future reference. An example of a clinical monitor could be a digital stethoscope that records the heart sound and transfers it to the cloud for storage and replay when needed.

Various IoMT devices are shown in Figure 7.2.

(iii) *AI and data analytics*

It is quite a tough task for the healthcare industry to select among the affordability, accessibility, and effectiveness of their offerings. In a perfect global, hospital therapy might be absolutely handy, cheap, and effective. Luckily, AI has the capability to assist the industry to emerge as extra available, cheap, and powerful. AI structures can assist in decreasing the prices by means of completing time-eating responsibilities that human beings once did, which could permit healthcare professionals to focus on more complicated or patient-targeted obligations. AI can also be used to permit sufferers to apply self-provider terminals when appropriate, permitting clinics or hospitals to apply assets in approaches that supply the best effect on sufferers' fitness. Accenture found in its study that 20% of clinical demand would be met by AI systems.

Also, $150 billion per year was saved by the healthcare industry by using top AI programs till 2026. Moreover, AI structures are being advanced to assist medical officers in examining statistical information very effectively. For example, computerized axial tomography (CAT) scans are analyzed in fractions of seconds by using AI software. It reduces the amount of time an affected person has to wait for their consequences. One can get an idea of the benefits of AI through healthcare executives. As per the PWC Health Research Institute, approximately 40% of healthcare executives are investing in AI, ML, and predictive analytics. The ability of AI to enhance medical services is producing extensive quantities of capital to finance this era. By the end of 2021, the entire investment by the public and private sectors in healthcare AI is projected to attain $6.6 billion. AI has the capacity to deliver customized care as nicely, mainly on the subject of prescribing remedies for patients. For instance, AI software can analyze a large number of clinical studies to discover better treatment strategies based totally on significant parameters of the affected persons' like age group.

(iv)  *Augmented reality (AR) and virtual reality (VR)*

AR and VR are other innovative techniques that have changed the healthcare sector. It is predicted that the value of healthcare based on AR and VR techniques will be increased from $933 million to $3.2 billion from 2018 to 2023. AR and VR have a number of uses in healthcare, which include supporting each patient and expert. VR, for instance, is assisting scientific specialists to discover ways to carry out dangerous approaches while not having to place sufferers at risk. In the course of complex methods, AR is providing help to doctors and surgeons to minimize the chance of mistakes. AR and VR have treatment applications for sufferers. For patients affected by dementia or Alzheimer's, AR and VR are being used to recreate the stories that allow them to relive a particular memory or general intervals of their lives that have been happy. VR is also being used as a remedy tool to assist patients to overcome their painful and worrying histories, which may be extremely difficult to cope with.

(v)  *Telemedicine*

Interaction between patients and health professionals has changed nowadays. Several modern solutions are converting the way patients communicate with health professionals or fitness experts. From locating a doctor to attending the appointment, new solutions are facilitating people's right of entry to health experts. Virtual appointments with Health Professionals are one example of telehealth technology. These kinds of digital appointments provide assistance to patients from a village or inaccessible areas, wherein access to healthcare has been historically limited. It enables such needy patients to visit doctors. Similarly, patients with mobility challenges can also use this technology to see doctors or medical experts. Due to so many advantages, most people are shifting towards this technology. From 2015 to 2018, users of this technology have increased from 1 million to 7 million. Doctolib is one of the major players in the European telemedicine field. It provides assistance to the user in finding and booking appointments with general physicians, doctors, and specialists. All of these modifications are contributing to extra-affected person empowerment and improved service within the industry. The rapid development in customer-friendly devices and technologies will change the scenario of healthcare services. It will affect the healthcare infrastructure, the caregiver, service providers, and physicians in a greater sense. These developments will improve the quality of healthcare service resulting in a better quality of life. The major impacts of technological developments on healthcare systems are discussed next.

## 7.3  IMPACT OF TECHNOLOGICAL DEVELOPMENTS ON HEALTHCARE SYSTEMS

*Restoration*
In healthcare systems, post-operative recovery is very crucial in terms of time and cost. It could be optimized for both time and money by using clinical-grade wearable sensors. IoMT devices would help the caregivers by providing values of critical metrics and alerting them to react in time. Furthermore, a sensor can be attached with telemedicine to boost the recovery time.

*Understanding patterns of new diseases*
There are many complex diseases where symptoms and biological parameters do not exactly match. There is a need to understand the pattern of the patient's symptoms and his vital parameters. Here the remote monitoring devices can help the physicians to understand that at the time when the patient had symptoms – what were the values of vital parameters at that time? The application of AI and data analytics can transform healthcare patterns for the better. Further, with the help of big data, new trends and patterns can be discovered, which will help doctors come up with customized medication plans that may be easy and economical with enhanced customer experience.

The major dissimilarity between healthcare and other industry is that the former handles critical data, thereby requiring watchful and timely decisions.

*Wider accessibility*
Various recent events including the worldwide pandemic (COVID-19) have highlighted the insufficiency of medical infrastructure. With the help of better connectivity and remote patient monitoring, medical services can be accessed by a wider population. POC kiosks can help remote patients to fetch diagnostics at their convenience and proper advice. These technologies will also reduce the time occupation of healthcare.

*Enhanced quality*
With the availability of better quality and large-size data, physicians and healthcare providers can make quality medication plans. In the case of chronic diseases, accurate information about patient symptoms and biological parameters will lead to a quality assessment of disease progression that may result in the management of medication. In the case of designing

infrastructures, categorized information about the patient requirements will help to enhance the quality of medical facilities.

*Personalized care*

Another big advantage of having access to individual patient data is personalization and emphasizing the "customer experience." The medication plan can be decided based on the individual patient's situation instead of the general disease progression theory.

*Cost reduction*

These technological developments may also reduce the cost of healthcare due to the availability of wider accessibility and better quality services. Automated processes and self-service model facilities also reduce the cost of diagnostics.

## 7.4 CHALLENGES OF TECHNOLOGY IN HEALTHCARE

Digital has now become common in the healthcare sector. It applies to all activities, from patient admissions to prescription management to remote monitoring of their health conditions. Revolutionary changes in the network-driven digital technological tools have not only provided tremendous growth in industrial development but also shaped the healthcare sector. On the one hand, it provides various accelerating opportunities, and on the other hand, there exist some challenges and risks too.

*Data processing*

Data processing is an action performed on datasets, which includes collection, storage, aggregation, and update, to make them meaningful [38, 39]. The healthcare industry generates a large pool of data that includes medical data of patients, diagnostic reports, all claims-related data, hospital administrative data, and financial statements, and it needs an hour for the systematic process of these datasets to make it worthy for various decision-making purposes. New digital tools in the healthcare sector, such as cloud technology, AI, IoT, and wireless connectivity, are now being used by hospitals and healthcare units to render qualitative healthcare services, but it is complex for them to implement them in every corner of the healthcare system as there exist some challenges with regards to data processing, i.e., data storage, data cleaning, data synchronization, and data visualization.

*Data storage*

Data in the healthcare industry originate from varied sources and have different aspects that make it heterogeneous and unstructured in nature that needs to be processed and stored in an effective manner so that quick decisions can be drawn from it. But due to its complexity, data files that are being shared over network devices cover a large space, and its processing becomes quite slow within the memory slots of the medical equipment, causing devices to become unresponsive for a few seconds.

*Data cleaning*

Data cleaning is the process of scanning and deleting the inappropriate data files that are no longer in use and become a reason for inaccurate results. Hospital, path labs, and patient-related data generated by E-medical equipment like digital thermometers, ECG machines, and pulse oximeters stored in device systems need to be scrubbed to ensure precision and perfectness, but the volume of files makes its cleaning process critical, resulting in delayed customer services.

*Data visualization*

Data visualization is the process of analyzing the bulk of data and sharing the results in a visual report form. Diagnostic reports and medical examination results generated by medical equipment would be of no use if they are not visualized and interpreted properly by medical practices and healthcare professionals, which requires analytical skills and statistical DA techniques to understand the charts, graphs, and images; sometimes, when using digital types of equipment, it shows blur images, errors or blank report due to poor battery backup or interconnectivity that leads to misinterpretation.

*Data synchronization*

The application of modern digital tools in the healthcare system provides reliable and productive services. Electronic medical records (EMRs) has been used by the majority of the hospital for this purpose but synchronization of patient data among health facilities is still a problem that is caused due to the sharing of high volume heterogeneous data over the network from source to destination.

*Cybersecurity*

Cybersecurity is a set of practices developed to secure networks, computer systems, and personal data from unauthorized access, or misuse from an unknown party. Cybersecurity aims at perils minimization from cyber-attacks and protecting businesses and individuals. Due to the rising invention of network-connected medical devices, cybersecurity is necessary for the normal functioning of companies. Healthcare organizations include hospital information systems such as E-Health Record systems, automated order booking, prescription remote patient monitoring devices, and infusion pumps that need to be secured well.

The common type of cybersecurity-related challenges include:

- Direct security – Access to a computer or device from an unauthorized person can be risky when leaving a computer unattended when not present or not encrypted with codes.
- Phishing emails – In the modern era, all kinds of information are received, sent, and maintained within email systems, and phishing leads to security incidents by allowing hackers to steal sensitive or proprietary information from the recipient when opening a malicious link or attachments [40].

- Legacy systems – The software and hardware systems that become not in trend after a certain period of time include outdated medical devices, operating systems, or versions of software. It becomes more challenging for healthcare in many organizations to upgrade if they do not have enough budget for cybersecurity.
- Malware – Remotely accessed network devices and medical equipment have risky data for the hospital as sensitive data can be stolen by malware attacks on this connection.
- Unauthorized access (internal) – Confidential health data when leaked by internal resources of an organization or unauthorized access becomes a serious problem.
- Spoofing – When hackers find a way to change a website's URL with a website of the hospital that looks the same and credentials are entered by anyone hacked, it is spoofing. Cyberattacker develops websites similar to the name of reputed healthcare organizations to mislead users and patients to access sensitive information.
- Unencrypted data – It is a cyber theft in which data from computers or wireless devices within healthcare institutions are stolen by hackers and can be utilized by them if not encrypted, causing problems to the organization.
- Manipulated data – Sometimes hackers are not interested in changing the original data. It becomes difficult to trace and incurs a huge cost because the altered data looks just like the old data.

## 7.5 DIGITAL USER EXPERIENCE

Going digital in healthcare has experienced an exponential hike due to the high diffusion of mobile technology around the world. It provides ease to a large portion of potential users, i.e., doctors, nurses, medical practitioners, and healthcare workers. They feel these in multiple ways that are described on various grounds like experience over smart healthcare apps and portals, electronic health record (EHR), digital medical devices, user interface, network access, system integration, and cost-effectiveness.

- Experience over smart healthcare apps and websites – For providing preventive and readily healthcare services, hospitals and healthcare service providers allow the users to choose their smart health apps and websites, where a user can easily book a doctor appointment and get records and data. However, because it is operative on wireless mode, it requires credentials to login for safety purposes, sometimes users face login issues due to poor connectivity. Apps are easily compatible with all models of mobiles device, and websites should have a suitable home page with feasible information at the top for quick access.

- Experience over EHR: The electronic health record is a database maintained in one place using the computer system for keeping patients' related information, past medical records that can be easily accessed and makes healthcare operations effective; however, sometimes users feel difficulty in accessing the data over it because of changes in recording policy, work procedure, and alteration made on a frequent basis, which needs to be properly communicated to all the respective users of it.
- User interface – Unattractive user interfaces of medical devices being used in healthcare contexts become challenging sometimes due to lack of visibility color aspects and navigation in the mobile site, and hence it increases the chance of errors in information reading that can be risky for the health of the patient. To minimize such problems, the device should be user-friendly enough and easy to operate.
- Network accessibility – For the smooth functioning of digital devices, the internet connections should be strong enough, but due to the lack of poor network quality, devices become disconnected or stop reviewing data on a real-time basis, which becomes a strong reason for work breakdown.
- System integration – Medical devices that are in regular use must be able to exchange information with other devices also. Mobile devices must be connected to the hospitals' or organizations' personal LAN to access clinical information; otherwise, users face hurdles in using it.
- Digital medical devices – Medical devices used for patient care and diagnostics, such as X-ray, CT scan, MRI scan, an ECG machine, ultrasound, nebulizers, dialysis machine, incubators, and pulse oximeter, have complex functions before using it to patient application. The nurses and lab attendants require some specialized training as it can have an adverse effect on patients when used by inexperienced ones.
- Cost-effectiveness – Installation of medical devices in a hospital, lab, or for personal use requires a huge amount of investment due to its high cost and some of the small business units in healthcare. Users face so many issues to afford it.

## 7.6 QUALITY ASSURANCE

The healthcare system consists of various actors like service organizations (hospitals and clinics), receivers (patients), intermediaries (insurance companies) regulatory authorities, and solution vendors. The key challenge before them is to have good quality software that generates accurate and realizable results.

Quality assurance testing is the process of assuring quality for the services related to healthcare and results obtained from the various devices. It is an assessment of whether something is good enough and whether it is suitable for its purpose.

There are some parameters that justify the quality parameters like accuracy, reliability, safety, risk-free system, efficiency, and effectiveness [41].

*Accuracy* – Accuracy is the first parameter while using the device. It is necessary for the best medical and clinical practices. For getting accurate results, users should have operating precautions. While using it, connectivity should be properly verified and batteries in thermometers should be replaced periodically as and when required.

*Reliability* – The medical types of equipment that are taken into consideration must produce less dispersive readings many a time, the separate device produces separate results which do not become the reason for doubt.

*Safety and risk-free system* – The medical devices that are part of the latest technological advancements like IoT, AI, AR, and VR include the various modern features if a preventive measure is not adhered to on time by the users or interested ones. So it can be a reason for huge loss to the entire healthcare system. Patients' safety from the perils like cybercrimes, data loss, fire, and electricity should be the priority to make service qualitative.

*Efficiency and effectiveness* – Efficiency and effectiveness in healthcare are always at the top as digital healthcare devices provide an edge to hospitals and medical professionals as it reduces time to make services flexible but sometimes device speed becomes affected due to poor network, low server quality, low signal, connectivity, and data load, and hence these devices call for protective use so that we can generate effective results out of them.

## 7.7 CONCLUSION

The revolving growth in industrial activities using smart technologies, like the IoT, wireless connectivity, cryptography, relational databases, VR, and AR, has shown industrial manufacturing units away following the trend from Industry 1.0 to 4.0 and also given the path to the healthcare sector to move in the same direction as Healthcare 1.0 to 4.0. In the same way, this study is highlighting the healthcare sector with the various opportunities and pitfalls arising from these inventions, pointing out shared experiences from the user about the medical equipment, and suggesting corrective measures so that various advancements in healthcare could be easily directed toward providing the people healthier life by the use of hi-tech medical devices [42]. Speedily use of the digital tool with IoMT, biosensors, cloud storage, and customized and automatically initiated medicinal treatments [43] have transformed the doctors' and medical practitioners' journey from ward visits to virtual treatment residing in their remote clinics with the help of telehealth services, also saving time and provides cost-effective healthcare services.

# REFERENCES

[1] Bongomin, O., Yemane, A., Kembabazi, B., Malanda, C., Chikonkolo Mwape, M., Sheron Mpofu, N., & Tigalana, D. (2020). Industry 4.0 disruption and its neologisms in major industrial sectors: A state of the Art. *Journal of Engineering*. DOI: 10.1155/2020/8090521.

[2] Li, J., & Carayon, P. (2021). Health care 4.0: A vision for smart and connected health care. *IISE Transactions on Healthcare Systems Engineering, 11*(3), 171–180.

[3] Celani, G. (2020). Shortcut to the fourth industrial revolution: The case of Latin America. *International Journal of Architectural Computing, 18*(4), 320–334.

[4] Javaid, M., Haleem, A., Vaishya, R., Bahl, S., Suman, R., & Vaish, A. (2020). Industry 4.0 technologies and their applications in fighting COVID-19 pandemic. *Diabetes & Metabolic Syndrome: Clinical Research & Reviews, 14*(4), 419–422.

[5] Vitabile, S., Marks, M., Stojanovic, D., Pllana, S., Molina, J. M., Krzyszton, M., ... & Salomie, I. (2019). Medical Data Processing and Analysis for Remote Health and Activities Monitoring. In *High-Performance Modelling and Simulation for Big Data Applications*, eds. J. Kolodziej, H. Gonzalez-Velez (pp. 186–220). Springer, Cham.

[6] Jain, S., Kumar, M., Sindhwani, N., & Singh, P. (2021). SARS-Cov-2 Detection using Deep Learning Techniques on the basis of Clinical Reports. In *2021 9th International Conference on Reliability, Infocom Technologies and Optimization (Trends and Future Directions) (ICRITO)* (pp. 1–5).

[7] Kohli, L., Saurabh, M., Bhatia, I., Sindhwani, N., & Vijh, M. (2021). Design and Development of Modular and Multifunctional UAV with Amphibious Landing, Processing and Surround Sense Module. In *Unmanned Aerial Vehicles for Internet of Things (IoT) Concepts, Techniques, and Applications*, eds. V. Mohindru, Y. Singh, R. Bhatt, R.K. Gupta (pp. 207–230).

[8] Kohli, L., Saurabh, M., Bhatia, I., Shekhawat, U. S., Vijh, M., & Sindhwani, N. (2021). Design and Development of Modular and Multifunctional UAV with Amphibious Landing Module. In *Data Driven Approach Towards Disruptive Technologies: Proceedings of MIDAS 2020*, eds. T.P. Singh, R. Tomar, T. Choudhury, T. Perumal, H.F. Mahdi (pp. 405–421). Springer, Singapore.

[9] Hathaliya, J. J., Tanwar, S., Tyagi, S., & Kumar, N. (2019). Securing electronics healthcare records in healthcare 4.0: a biometric-based approach. *Computers & Electrical Engineering, 76*, 398–410.

[10] Chung, M., & Kim, J. (2016). The internet information and technology research directions based on the fourth industrial revolution. *KSII Transactions on Internet and Information Systems (TIIS), 10*(3), 1311–1320.

[11] Hathaliya, J. J., Tanwar, S., Tyagi, S., & Kumar, N. (2019). Securing electronics healthcare records in healthcare 4.0: A biometric-based approach. *Computers & Electrical Engineering, 76*, 398–410.

[12] Xu, M., David, J. M., & Kim, S. H. (2018). The fourth industrial revolution: Opportunities and challenges. *International Journal of Financial Research, 9*(2), 90–95.

[13] Saini, M. K., Nagal, R., Tripathi, S., Sindhwani, N., & Rudra, A. (2008). PC Interfaced Wireless Robotic Moving Arm. In *AICTE Sponsored National Seminar on Emerging Trends in Software Engineering* (Vol. 50).

[14] Kaplan, G., Bo-Linn, G., Carayon, P., Pronovost, P., Rouse, W., Reid, P., & Saunders, R. (2013). Bringing a systems approach to health. *NAM Perspectives*. https://doi.org/10.31478/201307a

[15] Cassel, C. K., & Saunders, R. S. (2014). Engineering a better health care system: A report from the President's Council of Advisors on Science and Technology. *Jama*, *312*(8), 787–788.

[16] Bichler, M., Frank, U., Avison, D., Malaurent, J., Fettke, P., Hovorka, D., ... & Thalheim, B. (2016). Theories in business and information systems engineering. *Business & Information Systems Engineering*, *58*(4), 291–319.

[17] Rüßmann, M., Lorenz, M., Gerbert, P., Waldner, M., Justus, J., Engel, P., & Harnisch, M. (2015). Industry 4.0: The future of productivity and growth in manufacturing industries. *Boston Consulting Group*, *9*(1), 54–89.

[18] Liao, Y., Deschamps, F., Loures, E. D. F. R., & Ramos, L. F. P. (2017). Past, present and future of Industry 4.0-a systematic literature review and research agenda proposal. *International Journal of Production Research*, *55*(12), 3609–3629.

[19] Sindhwani, N., & Bhamrah, M. S. (2017). An optimal scheduling and routing under adaptive spectrum-matching framework for MIMO systems. *International Journal of Electronics*, *104*(7), 1238–1253.

[20] Anand, R., & Chawla, P. (2016, March). A review on the optimization techniques for bio-inspired antenna design. In *2016 3rd International Conference on Computing for Sustainable Global Development (INDIACom)* (pp. 2228–2233). IEEE.

[21] Sindhwani, N., & Singh, M. (2017, March). Performance analysis of ant colony based optimization algorithm in MIMO systems. In *2017 International Conference on Wireless Communications, Signal Processing and Networking (WiSPNET)* (pp. 1587–1593). IEEE.

[22] Sindhwani, N. (2017). Performance analysis of optimal scheduling based firefly algorithm in MIMO system. *Optimization*, *2*(12), 19–26.

[23] Anand, R., & Chawla, P. (2014). Bandwidth Optimization of a Novel Slotted Fractal Antenna Using Modified Lightning Attachment Procedure Optimization. In *Smart Antennas, Latest Trends in Design and Application* (pp. 379–392). DOI: 10.1007/978-3-030-76636-8_28.

[24] Gupta, A., Srivastava, A., Anand, R., & Tomažič, T. (2020). Business Application Analytics and the Internet of Things: The Connecting Link. In *New Age Analytics: Transforming the Internet through Machine Learning, IoT, and Trust Modeling*, eds. G. Shrivastava, S.L. Peng, H. Bansal, K. Sharma, M. Sharma (pp. 249–273). CRC Press.

[25] Anand, R., Sinha, A., Bhardwaj, A., & Sreeraj, A. (2018). Flawed Security of Social Network of Things. In *Handbook of Research on Network Forensics and Analysis Techniques*, eds. G. Shrivastava, P. Kumar, B.B. Gupta, S. Bala, N. Dey (pp. 65–86). IGI Global.

[26] Gupta, R., Shrivastava, G., Anand, R., & Tomažič, T. (2018). IoT-Based Privacy Control System through Android. In *Handbook of E-business Security*, eds. J.M.R.S. Tavares, B.K. Mishra, R. Kumar, N. Zaman, M. Khari (pp. 341–363). Auerbach Publications.

[27] Singh, P., et al. (2019). Voice Control Device using Raspberry Pi. In *SOUVENIR, IEEE Conference, Amity International Conference on Artificial Intelligence (AICAI'19)*, Amity University Dubai, Dubai International Academic City, IEEE, UAE Section. February 4–6, 2019.

[28] Ratnaparkhi, S. T., Singh, P., Tandasi, A., & Sindhwani, N. (2021). Comparative Analysis of Classifiers for Criminal Identification System Using Face Recognition. In *2021 9th International Conference on Reliability, Infocom Technologies and Optimization (Trends and Future Directions) (ICRITO)* (pp. 1–6).

[29] Singh, P, Pareek, V., & Ahlawat, A.K. (2017). Designing an energy efficient network using integration of KSOM, ANN and data fusion techniques. *International Journal of Communication Networks and Information Security (IJCNIS)*, 9 (3), 466–474.

[30] Sindhwani, N., Verma, S., Bajaj, T., & Anand, R. (2021). Comparative analysis of intelligent driving and safety assistance systems using YOLO and SSD model of deep learning. *International Journal of Information System Modeling and Design (IJISMD)*, 12(1), 131–146.

[31] Ahmed, A., Abdul Hanan, A., Omprakash, K., Lobiyal, D. K., & Raw, R. S. (2017). Cloud Computing in VANETs: Architecture, Taxonomy and Challenges. In *IETE Technical Review* (Vol. 35, pp. 523–547). India & USA: Taylor & Francis.

[32] Monostori, L. (2014). Cyber-physical production systems: Roots, expectations and R&D challenges. *Procedia Cirp, 17*, 9–13.

[33] Thoben, K. D., Wiesner, S., & Wuest, T. (2017). "Industrie 4.0" and smart manufacturing-a review of research issues and application examples. *International Journal of Automation Technology, 11*(1), 4–16.

[34] Anand, R., Singh, B. & Sindhwani, N. (2009). Speech perception & analysis of fluent digits' strings using level-by-level time alignment. *International Journal of Information Technology and Knowledge Management, 2*(1), 65–68.

[35] Juneja, S., Juneja, A., & Anand, R. (2020). Healthcare 4.0-digitizing healthcare using big data for performance improvisation. *Journal of Computational and Theoretical Nanoscience, 17*(9-10), 4408–4410.

[36] Kumar, A., Tripathi, S., & Raw, R. S. (2016). Bringing Healthcare to Doorstep using VANETs. In *3rd IEEE International Conference as INDIACom-2016*, ISSN (0973-7529), 16-18 March, Delhi, pp. 4747–4750.

[37] Singh, P., Raw, R. S., Khan, S. A., Mohammed, M. A., Aly, A. A., & Le, D. -N. (2021). "W-GeoR: Weighted geographical routing for VANET's Health monitoring applications in urban traffic networks. *IEEE Access*. DOI: 10.1109/ACCESS.2021.3092426.

[38] Singh, P. et al. A visual cryptography scheme for secret hiding using preprocessing. In Proceedings of the 13th INDIACom; INDIACom-2019; IEEE Conference ID: 46181 2019 6th International Conference on "Computing for Sustainable Global Development", pp. 958–961, 13th–15th March'2019, Bharati Vidyapeeth's Institute of Computer Applications and Management (BVICAM), New Delhi, India.

[39] Garg, P., & Anand, R. Energy Efficient ata collection in wireless sensor network. *Dronacharya Research Journal, 3*(1), 41–45.

[40] Anand, R., Shrivastava, G., Gupta, S., Peng, S. and Sindhwani, N. (2018). Audio watermarking with reduced number of random samples. In *Handbook of Research on Network Forensics and Analysis Techniques*, eds. G. Shrivastava, P. Kumar, B.B. Gupta, S. Bala, N. Dey (pp. 372–394). IGI Global.

[41] Juneja, S., Juneja, A., & Anand, R. (2019, April). Reliability Modeling for Embedded System Environment compared to available Software Reliability Growth Models. In *2019 International Conference on Automation, Computational and Technology Management (ICACTM)* (pp. 379–382). IEEE.

[42] Anand, R., Sindhwani, N., & Saini, A. (2021). Emerging Technologies for COVID-19. *Enabling Healthcare 4.0 for Pandemics: A Roadmap Using AI, Machine Learning, IoT and Cognitive Technologies*, eds. A. Juneja, V. Bali, S. Juneja, V. Jain and P. Tyagi (pp. 163–188).

[43] Singh, P. et al. (2020). Source of Treatment Selection for different States of India and Performance Analysis using Machine Learning Algorithms for Classification. In *International Journal Series Book of Advances in Intelligent Systems and Computing*, Springer; volume: soft computing: theories and applications. 2020. ISSN: 2194-5357. http://www.springer.com/series/11156. May'2020.

# Chapter 8

# A review on healthcare data privacy and security

*Rahul and Sahithi Bommareddy*
Delhi Technological University, Delhi, India

*Monika*
Shaheed Rajguru College of Applied Sciences for Women,
University of Delhi, Delhi, India

*Javed Ahmad Khan*
Govt. Girls Polytechnic Ballia, UP, India

*Rohit Anand*
DSEU, G.B.Pant Okhla-1 Campus (formerly GBPEC), New Delhi, India

## CONTENTS

DOI: 10.1201/9781003239888-8

## 8.1 INTRODUCTION

As defined in the dictionary suggests, health is the state of being physically, mentally, and socially fit. If any one of these is compromised, then we can deem a person to be unhealthy. Healthcare is usually a form of treatment or intervention for a person who is not unwell. It requires a registered medical representative to deem someone to be not well. In the Healthcare Industry, there should be various fields to be filled out by a patient, so that the diagnosis is effective. For this, every hospital must maintain a database. Healthcare databases usually contain the information that healthcare workers enter simultaneously after every visit. Apart from this, the routine laboratory results, surgery details, and emergency visits are also included. Electronic Health Records, also known as EHRs, are used to store the details of the patients in the Database [1]. It is maintained and linked to the official Identity cards issued by the Indian government or any other governing body of a country. It is the electronic version of the complete health report of the person. This can be transferred to the various medical facilities whenever required.

A total analysis of this can be given which leads to a better and accurate diagnosis. Digital Information security in Healthcare Act 2018 was devised by the Indian Government as per the government order given by the GOI, an act to incorporate establishment of National and State Health Authorities and Health Information Exchanges; to standardize and regulate the processes related to the gathering, storing, transmission, and use of digital health data; to ensure reliability, data privacy, degree of confidentiality and security of digital health data and such other matters related and incidental thereto [1]. In connection with the DISHA Act, there was another bill devised by the Ministry of Electronics and Information technology that categorizes data revelation into three main categories. It is India's first comprehensive act that provides and ensures security for the data of every Indian Citizen. Though this Healthcare database is very informative, there can also be a negative side to this Data Breach Scandals [2].

During the COVID pandemic itself, there has been a scandal. In this, over ten thousand patients' COVID reports have been leaked all over the internet through multiple government domains. This is something that accidentally took place in Delhi but deliberately took place in Karnataka. In the state of Karnataka, COVID reports had been deliberately leaked through government portals to monitor the COVID patients to tackle the situation. Though this was an unethical thing to do in terms of data privacy, some of the reasons for data privacy breaches and compromisation is the use of cloud solutions, phishing, and ransomware threats. This chapter provides a sketch of the laws implemented in various countries, the regulatory aspect, the known threats to data security, cloud computing and the role of cloud computing in the healthcare industry, and finally blockchain technology emerging in the healthcare industry.

## 8.2 RELATED WORK

There are publications on the data security over the past few years in the healthcare industry. Among these topics, there was research published in the year 2018 by Bruno M.C Silva and others in which they proposed a novel data encryption technique for healthcare systems, particularly in mobile health systems [3] to overcome the challenges like phishing, message interception, and evaluation. According to them, the most ideal solution is to avoid these threats by using cryptography. In 2019, another research article was published on Hospital Information Systems in addition to HIPAA compliance which was given by Scholars Mbonihankuye and other researchers [4]. In this, they have mentioned that there are 6 defensible actions against threats to the healthcare industry concerning data- Detect, Deny, Disrupt, Degrade, Deceive, and Contain [5].

According to the survey of Ashish Singh & Kakali Chatterjee in 2020 regarding the Security and privacy issues of the electronic healthcare systems, it has been stated that EHS is the new paradigm in the healthcare system [6]. They have very correctly stated that the three fundamental security requirements- Confidentiality, uprightness, and Availability need to be followed to protect instances where the system would be susceptible to many threats such as service hijacking, data leak, and phishing. The modern healthcare system of architecture was discussed and through this, some effective techniques were explored. In connection to this, the duo has produced another research article on truth-based access control models for securing electronic healthcare systems (EHS). In this, they targeted a very important issue which is the cloud-based EHS.

In the review of the work of Adarsh Kumar, Rajalakshmi Krishnamurthi, Anand Nayyar, Kriti Sharma, Vinay Grover, and Eklas Hossain, blockchain technology, because of its versatility, is applicable in every subfield [1]. As the blockchain data healthcare 4.0 process suggests, it works based on high integration and interoperability. As block utilization lies at an outstanding 80%, this makes the previously stated proposed system reliable. This theory started when Gross and miller JR. devised a theory on ethical implementation with blockchain technology [7]. In the big data security and privacy in healthcare review, Karim Abou El Mehdi and others emphasized the increasing integration of data generation technologies [8]. Nowadays, as big data is such a big concern and aim for most companies in the computer science sector, a few technologies were discussed- Authentication, Encryption. Data Masking and Access Control. Some of the important laws are there on big data privacy concerns. Such laws which were made all over the world have been discussed in this review paper as well. Under India's name, two laws were mentioned, the IT Act and the IT (Amendment) Act. This strives to implement reasonable security practices by providing compensation to the people affected by the wrongful gain or loss. In 2019, Maria Prokofieva and Shah J. Miah of Australia threw light on blockchain in healthcare [9]. They have documented that blockchain is decentralized in nature and the permissionless nature of it might offer a unique solution which is quite ironic. However, supporting their documentation, they have shown a proper way of developing the measures against counterfeit drugs. This also gives rise to providing access to the patients by managing the consent and integrating the consent procedure.

As per the review on Blockchain technology in the researches, Seyednima Khezr and others have appropriately stated that because of the digitization in healthcare there have been a titanic amount of electronic records on patients [10]. Blockchain is one such technology that provides a list of records that are interconnected with each other with the help of cryptography which ensures the security and data privacy of the patients. Following the research done on Cardiovascular disease Classification by using Different algorithms cited by Rahul et al., it has been researched that data has to be obtained through private methods which call for a need for data privacy especially in the healthcare industry [11]. In Ref. [12], S.Juneja et al. have discussed about the increasing use of big data in healthcare industry.

A comprehensive review on data security in cloud computing was authored by Abraham Ekow Dadzie. In this, he mentioned the characteristics of cloud computing- On-demand self-service, Broad Network Access, Resource Pooling, Rapid Elasticity, all of which are very important for data security in the healthcare sector. According to this, research cloud computing is seen as a fast-developing area that can instantly supply extensible service with the proper usage of hardware and software virtualization. According to the article on the future of cloud computing: opportunities and challenges by Narendra Rao Tadapaneni, cloud computing is the medium of simplification of data security and storage as well. Though there are user issues and reliability issues raised by several individuals [13], they are still significantly desperate for the technology that is offered.

## 8.3 THE REGULATORY ASPECT FOR PRESERVING SECURITY IN THE HEALTHCARE

Over the decades, there have been some regulatory measures taken by the governments of various countries all over the world. Table 8.1 shows the most important laws or regulatory initiatives taken by some of the most advanced countries in the world.

Table 8.1 Legal initiatives, year of existence and the place of implementation

| Law/Initiative | Year of existence | Place of Implementation |
|---|---|---|
| Digital Information Security in Healthcare Act (DISHA) | 2018 | India |
| Personal Data Protection Bill | 2019 | India |
| Information Technology Act | 2000 | India |
| HIPAA Act | 1996 | USA |
| Genetic Information Nondiscrimination Act | 2008 | USA |
| Oregon Genetic Privacy Act | 2001 | Oregon, USA |
| Confidentiality of Medical Information Act (CMIA) | 2013 | California, USA |
| Health Information Privacy Code | 2020 | New Zealand |
| Patient Data Protect | 2018 | UK |
| Electronic Records Development and the Implementation Programme (ERDIP) | 2000 | UK |
| Personally Controlled Electronic Health Records Act | 2012 | Australia |
| Health Identifier Act | 2010 | Australia |
| Personal Health Information Protection Act | 2004 | Canda |
| Legislation Concerning Privacy | 2000 | Canada |

Digital Information Security in Healthcare Act, popularly known and abbreviated as DISHA was initiated by the Ministry of Health and Family welfare in the year 2018. The objective of this act was to provide privacy and to protect integrity in the health data along with standardization, security, and privacy. Through this act, healthcare data can be regulated, stored, transmitted, and accessed upon proper authorization and is also associated with personally identifiable information [14, 15].

Along with this, the Personal Data Protection (PDP) bill came into existence in 2019 intending to make a secure database and store it efficiently thereby reducing as many scandals in data privacy as possible. This was passed by the Ministry of Electronics and Information Technology on December 11, 2019. This was enacted by the Parliament of India with the initiative of Ravi Shankar Prasad, the minister of Electronics and Information. The main motive of the bill was to control how personal information can be used by the government itself along with various organizations, businesses, and companies. Those citizens who use personal data to e-Health apps to monitor their healthcare facilities have to follow the data protection principles. They should ensure that the information is to be used in a fair and legally transparent manner.

The Healthcare Insurance Portability and Accountability Act of 1996 was approved by the former President of the United States, Bill Clinton. It was enacted by the 104th United States congress. According to HIPAA, there is a requirement to make national standards in the healthcare industry to protect the sensitive patient information that is restricted to unauthorized personnel without the consent of the patient. There are four main purposes of HIPAA. The first one is the assurance of healthcare portability thereby eliminating the job lick because of pre-existing medical conditions. The second purpose is to reduce healthcare fraud and abuse. The third one is to enforce standards for health information and the last motive is to guarantee the extent of security and privacy of health information [15].

Genetic Information Nondiscrimination Act, popularly known as GINA was introduced in 2008 which was aimed to protect the Americans based on what their ethnicity is. This applies to the fields of health insurance and employment. In a diverse country like the USA, there is a possibility of misuse of such personal information.

The Health Information Privacy Code of 2020 was released in New Zealand. The main importance of this code is to set specific rules for the agencies and companies in the healthcare sector. There is a disclosure by health agencies and it holds the health information. The privacy act of 1993 was to promote and protect individual privacy. The 2020 act is in addition to the 1993 Privacy act. It encompasses three primary rights- the right to own data records, the right to change incomplete records, and subject to Privacy Act exemptions.

**Data Protection**

| Data Protection | Data Security | Data Privacy |
|---|---|---|
| Data Retention | Encryption | Policies |
| Backup/ Restore | Access Control | Legislation |
| Data Replication | Authentication | Data Governance |
| Physical Infrastructure | Breach recovery | Best Practice |

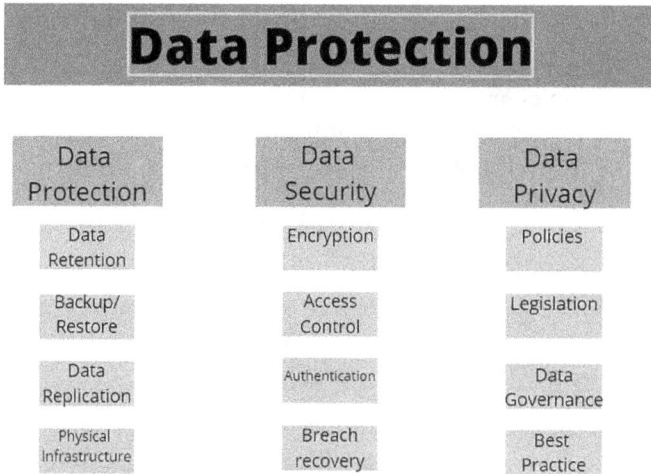

Figure 8.1 Classification of data protection and the ways of data protection.

As per the UK Data Protection Act, the citizens have the right to erase the data or reuse the data using a different service. It allows you to predict the behavior or interest of a particular person and helps automate the decision-making process. Table 8.1 shows the various legal initiatives, year of existence and the place where it was implemented. Figure 8.1 shows the classification of data protection and the ways in the data protection can be obtained

## 8.4 KNOWN THREATS AND RISKS TO DATA SECURITY

### 8.4.1 Cyberattacks

In 2020, in the month of November and December, there was a 39% rise in cyberattacks. Attackers in India have also been increasing because of the increase in digitalization. It has been a well-known theory that such attackers usually target the data that has significant value like customer's financial data records in health records and tax files.

### 8.4.2 Insider threats

Insider threats are difficult for any industry and multinational companies as well. In the healthcare sector, insider information can be accessed because of promoting a database or to give an update of the medical conditions going on. Some of the popular insider threat problems that arise are careless workers, inside agents, feckless third-party associates, disgruntled employees, and malicious insiders [1].

### 8.4.3 Phishing

Phishing is the act of sending emails on purpose by acting to be from well reputable companies and stealing some important personal health information either for third-party websites or to place those for the public and sell it for a database. Phishing attacks are increasing day by day all over the world. The pharmaceutical industry in the healthcare sector is worth $1.2 trillion. It records as the hardest hit or affected industry by phishing attacks. According to a renowned review website, 40 million patients' healthcare records had been breached [15].

### 8.4.4 Distributed denial-of-service threats

A DDoS attack is a modified DoS attack that starts from multiple locations. This makes room for more ambiguity for the hacker to track the source. This is a pre-planned scandal that happens on a greater scale. This poses a serious problem for the healthcare providers who need to access the patients' concerns. DDOS is against the network without taking permission which costs around 10 years in prison and up to a $500,000 fine as well. It results in the bombardment of simultaneous data requests to a central server. According to HHS data, there were 320% more healthcare providers in 2016 than in 2015 by hackers.

### 8.4.5 Identity theft

In healthcare scandals, some common identity theft threats are imposed. This can be because a deceased person's identity, which is not used anymore, can be undertaken by a criminal. In addition to identity theft, there can be cases of medical fraud as well. The medical industry does have an appalling track for safeguarding public information and data security. In 2020 alone, there were 20 million identity theft cases registered. A new identity theft case is registered every second. The number of identity thefts has also increased and is tripling each year.

### 8.4.6 Loss of data

Data loss is often a threat to the healthcare industry [16]. All the data records in the healthcare sector are equally important. It can be illegal to lose a certain information.

### 8.4.7 Weak link in security infrastructure

The weakest link of security infrastructure is us, humans. This is because today's WiFi networks are often unsecured in the cybersecurity system.

This not only imposes threats to the individuals but also to the entire system. The most vulnerable element is us, humans. Without ensuring a framework of security measures for the employees, any such company cannot guarantee the security measures. Cybersecurity strategies must be implemented.

### 8.4.8 Viruses and worms

These contagious viruses and worms are one of the most prominent causes of healthcare threats. They usually occur when the software is opened and subsequently the virus is copied and is multiplied. Viruses and worms can be threats from any source. They can be from an email from a third-party medical representative or even from a spy patient. Worms and viruses can often infect through downloadable or executable files. There can also be non-executable files like word documents. Worms can also enter through a network or internet connection.

### 8.4.9 Botnets

Botnets are used by the hackers to access the connections and the networks. They are used to perform DDoS and steal the data. The botnet is derived from the words health, robot [17] and network. It is used negatively with a malicious outcome that can harm many people. The Healthcare industry can pose a threat by the Botnets which can act as a primary source for such attacks [15]. Botnets are usually the collection of internet-connected devices which can range from computers to smartphones to internet of things devices. They are widely used in today's times [18].

### 8.4.10 Ransomware

Ransomware is the biggest threat to healthcare organizations. The first ransomware attack was in 2016. Ransomware is a malicious software that can infect the system which attacks by displaying a message and a fee to be paid. Ransomware is one such threat that has a modern technique of being able to infect a machine and also sniffing out the machines connected to that particular network. This class of malware is usually a money-making strategy. It doesn't need to be a method in which there is a procedure to steal information but can also be used as a way to get the money from the government or the company. According to Emsisoft, over 2000 US government healthcare services were affected in 2020. Figure 8.2 shows the drastic increase in the number of data scandal cases registered.

**Data Scandals**

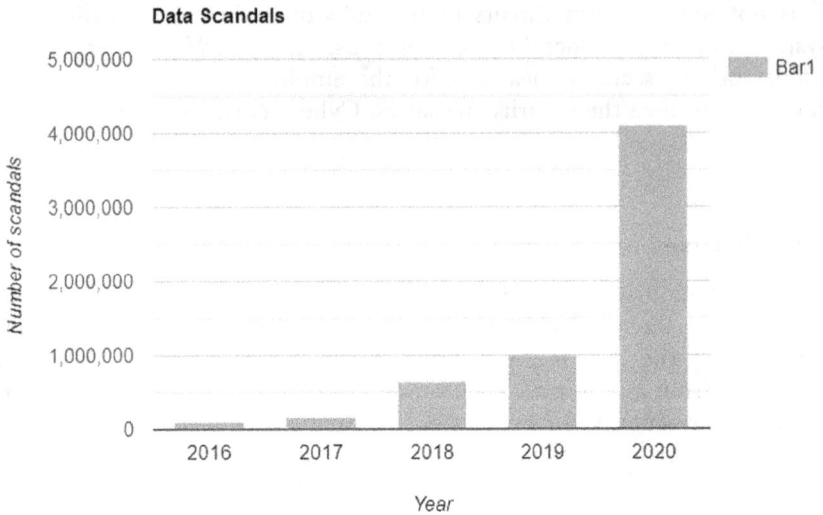

Figure 8.2 Drastic increase in the number of data scandal cases registered.

## 8.5 CLOUD COMPUTING AND HEALTHCARE

Cloud computing is an expert of delivery of different services through the Internet. Many features like data storage, networking and server databases can also be accessed. There are 3 types of cloud computing:

A. Infrastructure as a service
B. Platform as a service
C. Software as a service

With the increase in the data potential and need for data storage in health-care, safety and privacy concerns [19] have been overwhelming for data analysts. Due to digitization, healthcare has adopted certain cloud services. According to a report by West Monroe in Becker's Hospital Review, 35% of the healthcare organizations that were surveyed helped 50% of that data in the cloud. Hence cloud computing is such a wise method for the stored data in the cloud architecture. Because of cloud computing, there are many advantages:

1. Cost efficiency
2. Interoperability ease of access
3. Telemedicine capabilities
4. Mobility
5. Highspeed
6. Backup and restoration

Cloud Computing is one resource that is cost-efficient and it provides a desirable quality for the cost provided. It is a perfect solution for scaling.

## 8.5.1 Cloud models in healthcare

According to the United States of America's NIST, cloud computing can be deployed by using four particular models.

### 8.5.1.1 Public cloud

Public cloud is the cloud service provider that makes the resources like applications and storage available to the public. Usually, they are available to be availed on the oasis of paying when the payment is needed. Amazon Elastic Compute Cloud (Amazon EC2) is one such web service that helps distribute the public resources at a resizable capacity in the cloud. Its specialty is to obtain the data from the cloud and configure the capacity with as minimum friction as possible.

### 8.5.1.2 Private cloud

This is a type of cloud the infrastructure makes available only for a particular organization. There is a security barrier for the organization where people outside a particular organization cannot access. The proprietary network helps to host the particular services to a group of people. HP Datacenter is a private cloud that helps to accelerate the transformation with the data center infrastructure. Through this service, center security and agility are guaranteed.

### 8.5.1.3 Community cloud

The cloud infrastructure can be shared by several organizations with a common objective and outlook. This is suitable to exchange information based on policies and conditions for the entire industry. It can also be based on the safeguarding rules issued by the government. Anything on a common level can be stored in this community cloud.

Google Apps for the government was the first cloud platform to be used by the federal government in the US. As the government is spending millions of dollars on security concerns, this gives a chance to safeguard the issues in the future.

### 8.5.1.4 Hybrid cloud

Hybrid cloud consists of a hybrid variety of more than one cloud which consists of public, private, or community. In this type of model, the organization can manage its resources in its data center and also provide them to third parties externally.

Blackline is an American software company that develops cloud-based services. For financial service companies, availability and compliance are very important. Security [20] is also an important thing. To maintain the reputation of the company, blackline used the Verizon facility to gain control [21] on the property of plans and projects and sensitive data while they were networking.

## 8.5.2 Opportunities in healthcare via cloud computing

### 8.5.2.1 Management aspect

As the cost of cloud computing is really low, the vast data on the patients' records can be stored in the system. The Healthcare industry can also get an on-premise solution about this information technology solution of cloud computing regarding the patient's records. Though there would have to be jobs in the healthcare sector for IT professionals to achieve cloud computing, Cloud computing also maintains the flexibility of the organization thereby modulating the requirement of the industry. With the rapid changes in the healthcare industry, data is primarily dependent on the individuals for the proper treatment [1].

### 8.5.2.2 Technology aspect

For the countries without a centralized monitoring system, every hospital would have to initiate an IT department to continue the service. So they need not have internal staff for the hospitals. Instead the IT application is shared with a third-party provider to access the services from them. This makes sure that the company needs to hire the staff and maintain the IT aspects of the service at their own risk. With the availability of flexibility and cost-effectiveness of the infrastructure, cloud computing has justified its name of green computing [22].

### 8.5.2.3 Legal aspect

As data protection and privacy is a great deal for healthcare industries, the customer needs to reach the full trust capacity to commit with a company that provides cloud computing services. Many laws and acts safeguard the use protection of customer data. The government with the ministry of electronics and communication has also devised the acts that help to safeguard data security.

### 8.5.2.4 Security aspect

Health centres usually revolve around safe security measures that can be reliable. The cloud computing is something that has always provided a greater resistance. Though cloud computers like Google, Amazon, and others are improving the cloud computing services, there still have been various issues. Many studies are being devoted to resolve this security issue.

### 8.5.3 Challenges in healthcare via cloud computing

#### 8.5.3.1 Management aspect

The number of merits account for the demerits also. The main purpose of this article is "security and data privacy in the healthcare sector". Data security and privacy are compromised to an extent. Due to the lack of trust, inertia from the organization, and change in the governance from time to time, the sensitive data is sometimes misused, threatened to be misused, and violated of the safety laws.

#### 8.5.3.2 Technology aspect

In this aspect, the challenges arise due to the use of cloud computing for resource exhaustion and uncertainty of the performance. Through cloud computing, bugs also arise on a bigger scale. Due to the resources provided at a low cost and with computing resources made available, there are a lot of challenges faced. To maintain a profit, the third-party companies or healthcare companies themselves can make sure to cut the corners in the value delivery system. Many customers do not have access to the architecture because the cloud-providing service companies often leave out the users from making changes or accessing the architecture. With cloud computing, data lock-in is risky. Cloud users have to move the data around because of the fast changes in cloud computing services. One such incident arose in January of 2012 when Google discontinued its service of Google Health [1].

GH was an initiative to create a repository of health records to connect with healthcare providers directly. Sixers were given the notice to move that particular data to another service in a year. This creates a sense of ambiguity and guarantees failure to commit to a particular company. Even today, the cloud computing disability of transferring the data to the cloud is a big hassle. It will not be able to download or upload the massive amounts of data. Therefore it is hard trying to use cloud computing.

#### 8.5.3.3 Security aspect

Cloud computing is one field that invites data risks of all types. Many instances, where there were network breaks, hacks, natural disasters, poor key encryption management, and many more others, were associated with cloud computing. Privilege abuse is one more important challenge cloud computing faces today. It is usually accessible to everyone who wishes to avail of the service, but such threats can lead to some more critical problems. There have also been cases where the third parties could access the discarded information of a customer as well. To secure the cryptographic keys, there must be a proper key management system in place. Through the separation of duties, dual functioning of control and split knowledge, etc are more secure ways to manage encryption keys [1].

### 8.5.3.4 Legal aspect

Data privacy laws in the healthcare sector are very crucial. Legal action is also very easily taken when some laws are breached. If the company does not have strong terms and conditions, they can be sued and in loss severely. Many legal issues make cloud computing even more difficult to rely on. Some laws like contract law, data jurisdiction, and privacy have also been included. These are the most important of them all.

There are many laws as discussed above like the US Health Insurance Portability and Accountability Act which considers such issues to safeguard particular data breaches, especially in the healthcare sector. The Canadian Act of Personal Information Protection and Electronic Document also limits the power of such organizations to use the data without notice. Some countries also provide the safeguards to healthcare industries and patients themselves. Some even can change what can be on their health profile as well. After all, it is the patient's responsibility to choose what he wants to see. According to a survey, consumers are at more potential risks for fraud. Figure 8.3 shows the cloud computing security classification and the contributing factors of it.

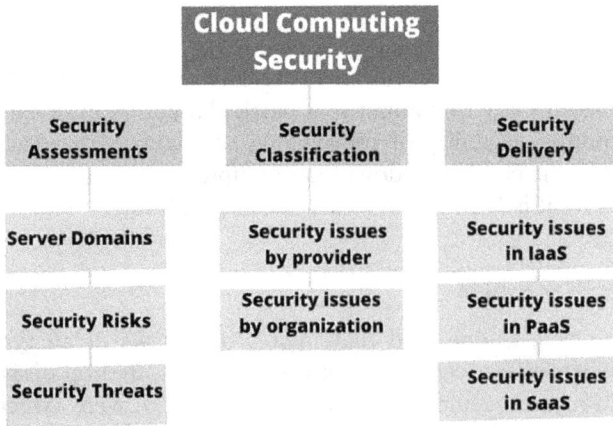

*Figure 8.3* Cloud computing security classification and its contributing factors.

### 8.5.4 Cloud computing scandals

Many companies like eBay and Apple are prone to cloud computing scandals. What is more important is the degree of breach of the data of some of the most important information like credit cards and bank accounts. In 2014, cloud computing scandals were a pretty popular thing. Over 145 million customers are being affected by the security breach that resulted in the stealing of passwords. However, the security breach did not reach the payment gateway of the company at that time which protected the hackers from getting into the company's customer financial database system.

Apple also faced a similar problem in mid-2014 where the iCloud was affected. It had been reported that cloud accounts had been broken into and inappropriate pictures had been released. This is the chance of data security threats that cloud services face.

### 8.5.5 Cloud security alliance

CSA is one of the globally leading organizations which is dedicated to raising an awareness thereby helping to secure the cloud computing environments. It came into action in 2008 when there was a need to adopt the methods for the safe use of cloud computing. Cloud security alliance had researched various parts of the cloud standards, education tools, and certifications. After all considerations, there were some of the policies implemented.

In the healthcare industry, trust is very important for the customers. They have devised a Cloud Trust Protocol in which cloud service asks about the elements of transparency. This ensures that there are no security breaches or ransoms of any type which can jeopardize millions of patients' details. According to the Cloud controls Matrix also known as CCM which is a cyber tool, all the key aspects are covered in cloud security. There are sixteen domains and each domain is broken up into subdomains called control objectives.

CSA is a third-party independent assessment to help maintain the standards. According to CSA, there are three levels of the CSA star which is a self-assessment phase.

### 8.5.6 Problems in cloud computing

Many of the cloud service providers do not provide customer support but they have been improving it in the past few years. With Google giving extra data after the used up base data, the response time for it to provide the updated version has been noted approximately as four hours. Even the Google takeout service by Google Co. requires 24 hours to provide access to the app or compressed version of the customized cloud files. Ideal cloud support should have a live chat option, better technical support during long hours, and a good service discontinuation relief period [18].

## 8.6  BEST PRACTICES FOR CYBER SECURITY IN HEALTHCARE

### 8.6.1  Devising cybersecurity strategies

Cybersecurity strategy is there to help the patient or healthcare provider. In the healthcare industry, all the devices and settings are to be configured and there can be only a few devices that work for the company and that can process company information. Some techniques which include cybersecurity strategies are: by encrypting the application data, by using malware detectors and defenders to screen the email accounts and attachments, to use strong passwords, to manage device configurations, and authorization for installation of new software other than the company's requirement.

### 8.6.2  Data encryption (DE)

Data are to be protected by encryption. This is the most important and useful method used by the healthcare organizations. DE is a process of unscrambling the information and using the algorithm as a key to decrypt the encrypted information. Healthcare providers make the information to be attacked harder by providing encryption. HIPAA does not require organizations to implement data encryption measures in their healthcare but many healthcare providers do implement encryption in the workflow. It is important to prevent the unauthorized access and to prevent access to sensitive health information.

### 8.6.3  Cyber security awareness training

Healthcare staff should be more educated as they are the primary contacts for any encrypted data to be misused. It is important as the human element remains one of the biggest threats to security across all industries. Human error can result in something as simple as a data misplacement to a whole disastrous scandal with expensive consequences. Security training is important as it equips the healthcare staff with the necessary inputs and consequences which helps them make better decisions as healthcare providers and frontline workers. It is important to educate them regarding the consequences and use appropriate caution to handle the data.

### 8.6.4  Adopting the right cybersecurity defenses

Data usage controls are one way to adopt the right cybersecurity defense. This helps us to access and monitor the controls of the staff. For example, in the UK government, healthcare is a public industry where the National Health Service workers are given a chip containing a memory reader generating a new password every time where they can track the IP address [18].

## Cloud Computing divisions percentage

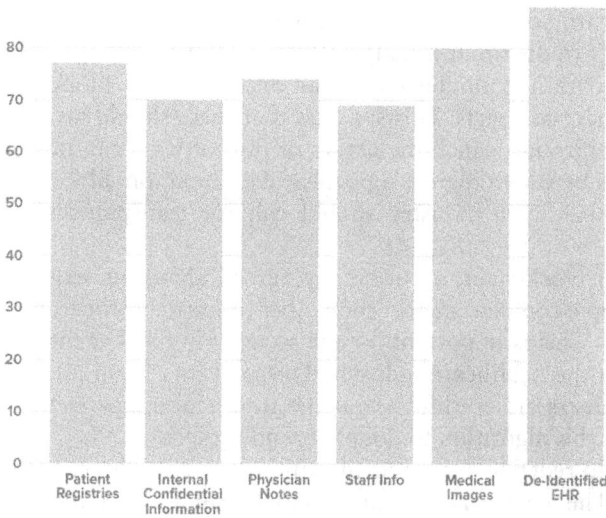

*Figure 8.4* Cloud computing divisions in the healthcare sector for various services.

Therefore a secure network should be used to access the data ethically. This makes sure that the sensitive data is safeguarded. This chip tracks the movements of the healthcare workers and can easily be protected. There should be some awareness campaigns regarding the data usage controls for the employees from time to time. Figure 8.4 shows the cloud computing divisions in the healthcare sector for various services.

## 8.7 ALTERNATIVES FOR DATA PROTECTION IN HEALTHCARE

### 8.7.1 Blockchain

Blockchain technology is one of the most emerging technologies in all fields. There have also been strong health care applications emerging from blockchain technologies. It is amazing how it has provided so many important opportunities and applications. Through this, it has shown the potential to revolutionize technology.

Though there have been so many scandals in recent times regarding healthcare and information records, healthcare has played a massive role in generating data regarding the electronic records of patients. Analyzing this data is as tricky as safeguarding it. The rise of blockchain helps dissolve the issue of storing and distributing data while safeguarding it against potential threats. It has been giving out studies on securing the privacy, integrity, and security of the data and the patients associated with it. Blockchain technology serves as a distributed ledger technology. This helps it to connect peer to peer and carry forward some of the transactions. The data can be stored publicly and privately to distribute amongst the users. It helps to lay a set of rules to access the data and double-check the authorization. Blockchain shines because of smart contracts. This specifies that there should be a customized set of rules through which the actors of the software can interact with the other actors by which there is a process of automation. Blockchain technology in the healthcare industry should call for transparency and security [18].

In the network of blockchain, an originally agreed algorithm exists, in which groups of people compete against each other to finish off the transaction on the network. This is important for the security in blockchain technology as well as in the healthcare industry. This prevents fraud and also ensures that data miners are truthful about the transaction. For example, bitcoin functions on this algorithm to double-spend protection.

Blockchain helps to redefine data modeling and helps to make many current developments. The emerging blockchain-based healthcare technologies are categorized into four layers.

*Data sources* – This is the primary foundation of the blockchain layer where the data sources are extracted. This can include the results from clinical trials, laboratories, or even the ones on social media. It can also consist of medical images [23]. They can be generated by the patient as well.

*Blockchain Technology* – It refers to the blockchain technology devised for the healthcare industry on the whole. The protocols, functions, networks, services, hash functions, and platforms are the members of this layer.

*Healthcare Applications* – Some of the healthcare applications are used in the medical product ecosystem that depends upon the medicines prescribed and sold. It also consists of the management of the data in the database which pulls up the medical records and also modifies if essential. Throughout this, a medical practitioner would be able to access the files of the patients and a patient would be able to transfer the file from one hospital to another.

*Stakeholders* – The stakeholder of this workflow would be patients, medical practitioners, cloud computing companies, regulators, hospital medical staff, its staff, the government, the patients, and the public.

### 8.7.1.1 Where blockchains are used in healthcare

Information exchange in healthcare is pretty massive. But there are so many problems and obstacles revolving around the whole idea like cloud

# Industry Wise Blockchain Solution

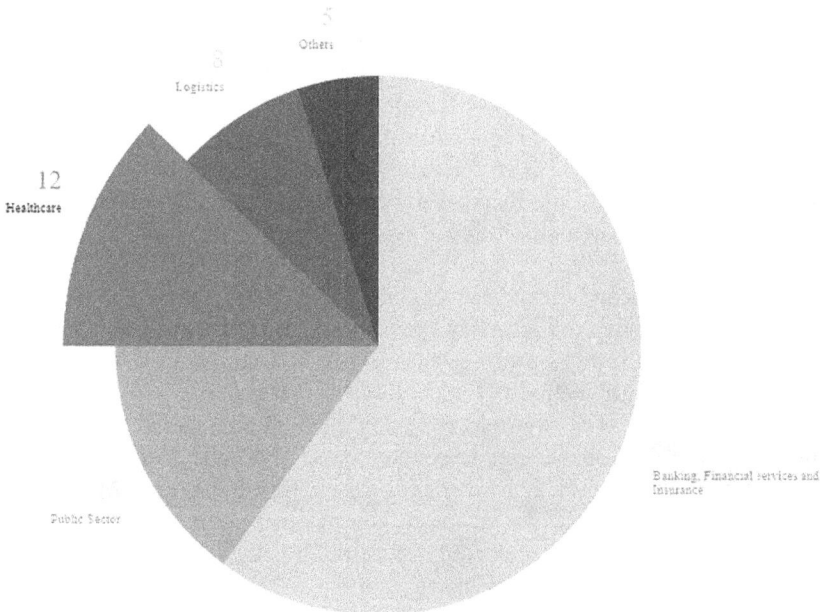

Others

5

Logistics

8

12

Healthcare

Banking, Financial services and Insurance

Public Sector

*Figure 8.5* Pie chart shows a split of the sector-wise blockchain solution.

technology and mobile application development. Blockchain provides a pretty straightforward outlook to those threats and allows winning over those challenges. It is important to make this easily accessible. Blockchain helps to solve this problem by using distributed technology. Distributed technology helps to track the assets and ensure transparency, security, and trust. Thus with the blockchain, there is not a need to store the entire data in the chain. Therefore, blockchain links the data with a hash function or cryptographic encryption. This allows the data transfer to take place only between both parties with the consent to view. Editing also can be accessed only by the owner. Blockchain is different in which healthcare has thousands of X-rays, prescriptions, and reports which are very crucial for the patient database. Those files are usually stored in pdf or tiff files. They should be easily accessible to the healthcare providers. Blockchain works on the validation logic of shared control and hence the blocks cannot be transferred or duplicated except by the authorized personnel. Figure 8.5 shows a pie-chart that shows a splitting of the sector-wise blockchain solution. We see that healthcare constitutes of 12% of the total industry.

### 8.7.1.2 Master patient index (MPI)

This is a medical database that contains important details like DOB, social security number, name, gender, address, and many other important details. MPI is used to represent each patient. It should not be accessed by unauthorized activity and the patients also do not have the right to modify information in some cases. MPI can be the identity of every patient uniquely. MPI is to be well organized and the institution is responsible for the data access. MPI is the index created in the electronic health act systems. MPIs are the universal indices where the medical patient index is confined to a particular hospital to track down the hospital-related significant details. EHRs also access the MPIs.

Data in healthcare can often be mismatched or entered incorrectly. Mismatches are when the information is entered incorrectly, that is with the DOB or gender. If many systems are involved, the data cannot be verified at all. Thus blockchain helps to break down these systems and make them more decentralized. For example, the patients' data are hashed to the ledger and the content will be unique for each patient. This ensures access to certain parts of the system. It also makes sure that certain parties can view certain information only. For example, the patients can view the details of the procedure, bills, insurance coverage, and all. The attending doctor will be able to access x-rays prescriptions and data. The laboratory physicians will be able to access the MPIs through authorization only.

### 8.7.1.3 Remote patient monitoring

A remote patient monitoring device is an IoT-based system [24–26] that helps to initiate tele-monitoring and helps to monitor the patients' health at home. This technique is a set of technology that helps to provide and track the patients' health with a proper diagnosis. The data can be used and retrieved at a distance. This is a technique which is very convenient, especially during the COVID-19 pandemic.

This helps the monitoring of the patient to be made easier and provides status updates at the respective times. There is a total collection of medical data. This makes sure that there is data updation through IoT devices, sensors, and mobile devices [27, 28]. Blockchain helps in the storage and retrieval of data. This is essential for the data [17]. Ethereum is a blockchain-based cryptocurrency platform for providing software. RPM works on the principle of IoT which is used by many of the devices worn on the patients for monitoring. The IoT devices collect and disseminate the data collected by such devices. Through this, there is protected health information that can be accessed through the RPM devices. These devices follow the regulations of HIPAA. Similarly in India, we can also provide them following DISHA and PDP Act. IoT devices are those which record and transmit information. The security of such devices is more important. There is a requirement for the contract of RPM and they would send the results back to the healthcare providers. Thus there is a need for the facilitation of medical interventions. There is a need for the security in this intervention. For this, each intervention is stored in separate blocks of the blockchain. These are private blockchains that have security features to ensure a safe and protected environment for the patients' information as well [1].

## 8.8 CONCLUSION

Summing the whole chapter, blockchain helps for the Conceptual Evolution based on concept development and benefit-based application. It also works on promoting decentralization as we discussed in the facts above. This provides more optimized [29, 30] and secure access to the database, in this case by the patients and the healthcare workers [31]. It helps in the advancement of technology by paying heed to the healthcare ecosystems through which data can be more secured. It helps to make sure that the predictions are ready for real-life problems. It helps to build architectural stability as well by assigning blocks and hashing them from each other. Blockchain has a positive impact on the efficiency process of the process and the system. The most important aspect is the data management of the system which helps in safely handling the data, protecting it, and also storing it effectively. Therefore to safeguard against all the threats discussed and all the technologies existing in the healthcare industry, the Blockchain system is safe in terms of data efficiency, privacy and security.

## REFERENCES

[1] Kumar, A., Krishnamurthi, R., Nayyar, A., Sharma, K., Grover, V., & Hossain, E. (2020). A novel smart healthcare design, simulation, and implementation using healthcare 4.0 processes. *IEEE Access, 8*, 118433–118471.

[2] Pardini, K., Rodrigues, J. J., Diallo, O., Das, A. K., de Albuquerque, V. H. C., & Kozlov, S. A. (2020). A smart waste management solution geared towards citizens. *Sensors, 20*(8), 2380.

[3] Silva, B. M., Rodrigues, J. J., Canelo, F., Lopes, I. M., & Lloret, J. (2019). Towards a cooperative security system for mobile-health applications. *Electronic Commerce Research, 19*(3), 629–654.

[4] Mbonihankuye, S., Nkunzimana, A., & Ndagijimana, A. (2019). Healthcare data security technology: HIPAA compliance. *Wireless Communications and Mobile Computing, 2019*. https://doi.org/10.1155/2019/1927495

[5] Singh, P., et al. (2019). A visual cryptography scheme for secret hiding using preprocessing. In *Proceedings of the 13th INDIACom; INDIACom-2019; IEEE Conference ID: 46181 2019 6th International Conference on "Computing for Sustainable Global Development"*, pp. 784–787, 13th–15th March'2019, Bharati Vidyapeeth's Institute of Computer Applications and Management (BVICAM), New Delhi, India.

[6] Singh, A., & Chatterjee, K. (2017). Cloud security issues and challenges: A survey. *Journal of Network and Computer Applications*, 79, 88–115.

[7] Gross, M. S., & Miller Jr, R. C. (2019). Preserving privacy & promoting learning: Technology to empower Belmont 2.0. *Available at SSRN 3390979*. https://dx.doi.org/10.2139/ssrn.3390979

[8] Abouelmehdi, K., Beni-Hessane, A., & Khaloufi, H. (2018). Big healthcare data: Preserving security and privacy. *Journal of Big Data*, 5(1), 1–18.

[9] Jain, S., Sindhwani, M., Anand, R., & Kannan, R. (2021). COVID Detection Using Chest X-Ray and Transfer Learning. In *ISDA* (pp. 933–943). https://doi.org/10.1007/978-3-030-96308-8_87

[10] Khezr, S., Moniruzzaman, M., Yassine, A., & Benlamri, R. (2019). Blockchain technology in healthcare: A comprehensive review and directions for future research. *Applied Sciences*, 9(9), 1736. https://doi.org/10.3390/app9091736

[11] Ray, P., Kharke, R. B., & Chauhan, S. S. (2021). Cardiovascular Disease Classification Using Different Algorithms. In *Inventive Communication and Computational Technologies*, eds. G. Ranganathan, J. Chen, A. Rocha (pp. 189–201). Springer, Singapore.

[12] Juneja, S., Juneja, A., & Anand, R. (2020). Healthcare 4.0-digitizing healthcare using big data for performance improvisation. *Journal of Computational and Theoretical Nanoscience*, 17(9–10), 4408–4410.

[13] Ahmed, A., Abdul Hanan, A., Omprakash, K., Lobiyal, D. K., & Raw, R. S. (2017). Cloud Computing in VANETs: Architecture, Taxonomy and Challenges. In *IETE Technical Review* (Vol. 35, pp. 523–547). India & USA: Taylor & Francis.

[14] Boddy, A., Hurst, W., Mackay, M., El Rhalibi, A., Baker, T., & Montañez, C. A. C. (2019). An investigation into healthcare-data patterns. *Future Internet*, 11(2), 30.

[15] Bouck, Z., Pendrith, C., Chen, X. K., Frood, J., Reason, B., Khan, T., … & Bhatia, R. S. (2019). Measuring the frequency and variation of unnecessary care across Canada. *BMC Health Services Research*, 19(1), 1–11.

[16] Sansanwal, K., Shrivastava, G., Anand, R., & Sharma, K. (2019). Big Data Analysis and Compression for Indoor Air Quality. In *Handbook of IoT and Big Data* (pp. 1–21). CRC Press.

[17] Saini, M. K., Nagal, R., Tripathi, S., Sindhwani, N., & Rudra, A. (2008). PC Interfaced Wireless Robotic Moving Arm. In *AICTE Sponsored National Seminar on Emerging Trends in Software Engineering* (Vol. 50).

[18] Meinke, A., Hawighorst, M., Wagner, A., Trojan, J., & Schweiker, M. (2017). Comfort-related feedforward information: occupants' choice of cooling strategy and perceived comfort. *Building Research & Information*, 45(1–2), 222–238.

[19] Sindhwani, N., Verma, S., Bajaj, T., & Anand, R. (2021). Comparative analysis of intelligent driving and safety assistance systems using YOLO and SSD model of deep learning. *International Journal of Information System Modeling and Design (IJISMD)*, 12(1), 131–146.

[20] Anand, R., Shrivastava, G., Gupta, S., Peng, S. L., & Sindhwani, N. (2018). Audio Watermarking With Reduced Number of Random Samples. In *Handbook of Research on Network Forensics and Analysis Techniques* (pp. 372–394). IGI Global.

[21] Singh, L., Saini, M. K., Tripathi, S., & Sindhwani, N. (2008). An Intelligent Control System for Real-Time Traffic Signal Using Genetic Algorithm. In *AICTE Sponsored National Seminar on Emerging Trends in Software Engineering* (Vol. 50).

[22] Juneja, A., Bajaj, S., Anand, R., & Sindhwani, N. (2020). Improvising green computing using multi-criterion decision making. *Journal of Advanced Research in Dynamical and Control Systems*, 12(03), Special Issue, 1161–1165.

[23] Goyal, B., Dogra, A., Khoond, R., Gupta, A., & Anand, R. (2021, September). Infrared and Visible Image Fusion for Concealed Weapon Detection using Transform and Spatial Domain Filters. In *2021 9th International Conference on Reliability, Infocom Technologies and Optimization (Trends and Future Directions)(ICRITO)* (pp. 1–4). IEEE.

[24] Anand, R., Sinha, A., Bhardwaj, A., & Sreeraj, A. (2018). Flawed Security of Social Network of Things. In *Handbook of Research on Network Forensics and Analysis Techniques* (pp. 65–86). IGI Global.

[25] Gupta, A., Srivastava, A., Anand, R., & Tomažič, T. (2020). Business Application Analytics and the Internet of Things: The Connecting Link. In *New Age Analytics* (pp. 249–273). Apple Academic Press.

[26] Gupta, R., Shrivastava, G., Anand, R., & Tomažič, T. (2018). IoT-Based Privacy Control System through Android. In *Handbook of E-business Security* (pp. 341–363). Auerbach Publications.

[27] Kohli, L., Saurabh, M., Bhatia, I., Shekhawat, U. S., Vijh, M., & Sindhwani, N. (2021). Design and Development of Modular and Multifunctional UAV with Amphibious Landing Module. In *Data Driven Approach towards Disruptive Technologies: Proceedings of MIDAS 2020*, eds. T.P. Singh, R. Tomar, T. Choudhury, T. Perumal, H.F. Mahdi (pp. 405–421). Springer Singapore.

[28] Kohli, L., Saurabh, M., Bhatia, I., Sindhwani, N., & Vijh, M. (2021). Design and Development of Modular and Multifunctional UAV with Amphibious Landing, Processing and Surround Sense Module. In *Unmanned Aerial Vehicles for Internet of Things (IoT) Concepts, Techniques, and Applications*, eds. V. Mohindru, Y. Singh, R. Bhatt and A.K. Gupta (pp. 207–230).

[29] Sindhwani, N., & Bhamrah, M. S. (2017). An optimal scheduling and routing under adaptive spectrum-matching framework for MIMO systems. *International Journal of Electronics*, 104(7), 1238–1253.

[30] Sindhwani, N., & Singh, M. (2020). A joint optimization based sub-band expediency scheduling technique for MIMO communication system. *Wireless Personal Communications*, 115(3), 2437–2455.

[31] Anand, R., Sindhwani, N., & Saini, A. (2021). Emerging Technologies for COVID-19. In *Enabling Healthcare 4.0 for Pandemics: A Roadmap Using AI, Machine Learning, IoT and Cognitive Technologies*, eds. A. Juneja, V. Bali, S. Juneja, V. Jain, P. Tyagi, (pp. 163–188).

Chapter 9

# Breast cancer detection using microwave imaging

*Ajay Kumar and Man Mohan Singh*
Meerut Institute of Engineering and Technology, Meerut, India

*Ramesh Kumar Verma*
Bundelkhand Institute of Engineering and Technology, Jhansi, India

*Subodh Kumar Tripathi*
Meerut Institute of Engineering and Technology, Meerut, India

## CONTENTS

### 9.1 INTRODUCTION

Breast cancer is common cancer in women; the mortality rate occurring due to breast cancer in women is very high compared to the other types of cancer. The main causes of breast cancer are age, dissimilarity, and reduction of breastfeeding. These are the major causes of breast cancer in high-resource countries, but it is increasing in all countries now [1]. The American Cancer Society shows that in 2019, 40,000 women and 500 men passed away due to breast cancer, and more than 260,000 women and 2,700 men were diagnosed with new breast cancer in the United States [2]. The main causes of mortality are unawareness as well as delay in treatment. A cancer diagnosis at an early stage is a key point for the success of the treatment. For breast cancer diagnosis, several methods are widely used, such as X-ray, ultrasound, and magnetic resonance imaging (MRI).

X-ray scanning is most broadly used for the diagnosis of breast cancer. The main disadvantage of X-ray scanning is the risk of exposure to radiation [3–5]. Due to the large number of scanning, breast shows harmful side effects, and sometimes overtreatment is required. During the breast examination, the breast should be as flat as possible, which provides pain to the patient. The flat breast is required during X-ray scanning because cancer and dense tissues are shown as a white image, whereas fat tissues are shown in the form of a black image. In ultrasound, the basic waves used are sound waves (>20 kHz) to see the internal body structure. In ultrasound, the transducer sends the sound signals inside the body and after the reflection echoes signals are received, these echoes are helpful in designing a sound image. This method is painless and safe in terms of radiation exposure due to the low resolution of sound waves. Due to low resolution, the ultrasound is incompetent to distinguish between virulent and benign breast tumors [6]. Although MRI is based on radio waves that generate a strong magnetic field to make images inside the body, MRI is basically used for the detection of small abnormalities compared to X-ray and ultrasound. However, the testing cost by MRI is relatively very high.

Due to the limitations of the existing diagnosis techniques, researchers are working on the alternative microwave imaging (MI) diagnosis technique [7, 8]. MI-based breast cancer diagnosis attracts researchers due to its low cost, simplicity, and less harmful radiations as compared to the current/existing techniques [9, 10]. The MI for breast cancer detection is highly sensitive and able to detect minor breast tumors because it differentiates normal and cancerous tissues by their electrical properties [10]. The aim of this article is to provide a review of MI design techniques to detect breast cancer. The literature survey covers methods, algorithms, and imaging systems [11, 12].

## 9.2 PROPERTY OF BREAST TISSUES AT MICROWAVE

The microwave involves special properties for the detection of breast cancer. This technique avoids discomfort and provides a cost-effective solution compared to X-ray and MRI. To avoid the limitations of conventional techniques, researchers are moving towards the MI technique. The working principle of MI is based on the dielectric property of the breast tissues, i.e., the dielectric property of the cancerous cell differs from the normal cell. The microwave image technique detects hidden and small abnormalities in the tissues. The working of the MI system is classified into two parts. First, breast imaging is set up to gather the reflected motions from the breast. The received data by the MI system is further processed via some algorithm to reconstruct the image of the object [13]. The knowledge of the dielectric property of the normal tissues and cancer tissues is required to understand the behavior of electromagnetic waves inside the tissues. The incident waves are reflected from the breast tissue, which is able to draw an image of the breast that shows malignant and healthy tissues. The accuracy for the detection of infectious tissues and healthy tissues depends on many factors, such as the number of elements arranged/setup, number of samples, type of sample, depth of measurement, environmental use, and algorithm for data execution [14–18].

Several types of research based on dielectric constant in the malignant and standard breast tissues have been done. In 1994, Joines et al. [19] measured the electric conductivity and permittivity of the normal and malignant tissues in the frequency range of 50 MHz to 900 MHz. At all these frequencies, the conductivity and permittivity of the malignant tissues are higher as compared to the normal tissues. Furthermore, in 2016, Fornes-Leal et al. [20] characterized the dielectric constant of healthy and malignant muscles by the frequency of 0.5–18.0 GHz. The measurement was performed on 20 patient samples using open-ended coaxial probe techniques. The experimental calculations show that the cancerous sample consists of 8.8% higher dielectric constant and 10.6% higher conductivity as compared to healthy tissues. Similarly, Hesabgar et al. [21] calculated the dielectric property of standard and malignant breast tissues at the frequency of 100–1.0 MHz. The electrical permittivity and conductivity of the samples are measured using a custom-made experimental setup using an inverse finite element basis. The conductivity and permittivity of the cancerous tissues and normal tissues were found in a ratio of 3.5:1 and 10.9:1, respectively. Furthermore, in 2018, Cheng et al. [22] evaluated the dielectric properties of normal, benign tumor, and malignant cancer tissue for the frequency band of 0.5 GHz to 8 GHz. The conductivity and dielectric constant of the cancerous tissue are high compared to the benign tumor and normal tissues. In the next year, Hussein et al. [23] measured the dielectric constant of normal and cancer cells in the frequency range of 200 MHz–13.6 GHz using an open-ended coaxial probe technique. From the results, the dielectric constant of the cancer cell is found to be high as compared to the normal tissues. Furthermore, in the same year, Kuwahara et al. [24] measured the complex permittivity of cancer in the breast at the frequency of the microwave range. From the experiment evaluation, it has been found that for greater than 80% of cancer cases, the dielectric constant and conductivity are higher, but in the remaining 20% of cases, the dielectric constant of the mammary gland is higher.

## 9.3 DETECTION OF BREAST CANCER USING MI

The recognition of breast cancer based on MI has numerous advantages with respect to the other techniques, such as low cost, non-ionization, and a comfortable mechanism for detection [25]. The MI techniques have high sensitivity and the ability to detect a small tumor, where the recognition is based on the electrical properties of normal tissues and malignant tissues [25].

The recognition technology is based on the hypothesis that the electrical properties, i.e., conductivity and permittivity, of healthy tissues and malignant tissues differ at microwave frequencies [26, 27]. Based on MI, several types of research have been done. In 2010, for breast cancer recognition, an ultra-wideband (UWB) antenna was designed by Adnan et al. [28]. The antenna is a combined structure of a circular radiating patch with a ground plane. The patch feeding is done by using a vertical plate. The antenna covered 3.5–8.0 GHz bandwidth with 8.0 dBi gain, best suited to detect cancer using MI. In the same year, Zhurbenko et al. [29] designed a 3-D MI system to detect breast cancer. In this design for cancer detection, 32 trans-receiving channels are utilized that operate at 0.3–3.0 GHz frequency. The system takes around 100 minutes to generate a single image using a single frequency algorithm. The image could be improved by using single or multiple frequency reconstruction algorithms. Furthermore, Klemm et al. [30] designed an antenna array for MI-based breast cancer detection. The UWB antenna was designed by cutting the slot in the radiating patch. To detect cancer in the breast, 31 antennas are placed in the neighborhood of the breast phantom. This type of system is able to recognize a 7.0 mm diameter tumor within the breast at any location within the breast.

In 2012, Wang et al. [31] designed a UWB multiple input multiple output (MIMO) antenna to detect breast tumor. The required antenna is fabricated on an FR4 substrate with a patch of circular shape and a circular slot cut from the ground plane. The required antenna is used for the UWB MIMO antenna design, which covered 2.3–12.2 GHz frequency band with high isolation. In the next year, Latif et al. [32] designed a UWB monopole antenna for breast tumor detection. The antenna is designed by an elliptical patch with a partial ground plane, which covered 1.0–4.0 GHz frequency band. In this model, glycerine is used for designing the breast model, which has electrical parameters similar to breast tissue, and an antenna is utilized for MI. In 2014, Kahar et al. [33] designed a UWB monopole antenna for breast tumor detection. The antenna is designed by a regular dodecagon-shaped radiating patch and a partial ground plane. The antenna measured the breast tumor by MI. From the simulation, it is observed that at the tumor, a high current distribution is observed. Furthermore, in the same year, Ünal et al. [34] designed a UWB bow-tie antenna to detect cancer in breasts. For MI-based breast cancer detection, a half-spherical antenna array is placed surrounding the breast. The antenna covered 1–8 GHz bandwidth. For tumor detection, an image is formed using a delay-and-sum algorithm that can measure up to 2.0 mm of tumor located at a 40.0 mm depth inside the three-layer phantom mode. In 2015, Bahrami et al. [35] used 16 flexible antenna arrays for breast cancer detection. For that, monopole and spiral antennas covered 2.0–4.0 GHz bandwidth with single and two polarizations at both antennas, respectively. The flexible arrays of the antenna are placed on the phantom of the breast, similar to the bra pattern for breast cancer detection.

In 2015, Islam et al. [36] designed a metamaterial-based antenna for microwave breast cancer detection. The antenna is fabricated on the FR4 substrate by a strip loaded with modified split-ring resonators. The antenna consists of a slotted ground plane with a strip line feed. The antenna covered 3.4–12.5 GHz bandwidth with a maximum gain of 5.16 dBi at 10.15 GHz frequency. For MI, the antenna is placed near the breast phantom for breast phantom detection. In the detection of the phantom, two antennas are located near the phantom of the breast to measure the mutual connection. In the same year, Katbay et al. [37] designed a miniature antenna to detect cancer in breasts. The antenna is fabricated on a Plexiglas substrate with a meander line and partial ground plane. The antenna is placed in the breast phantom for tumor detection. During the simulation, antennas are placed on a serum with and without tumor. For tumor care, the steel balls are placed inside the serum. Furthermore, for breast cancer detection, a MI technique was used by Abbosh et al. [38]. For cancer detection in the breasts, an array of antennas is placed surrounding the breast. The antenna sends the frequency signal from 2.5 to 6 GHz toward the breasts, and the signal is received by using a monostatic radar approach. In this approach, the false detection is removed by subtracting the consequent images. Breast cancer detection was done by ÇalÕúkan et al. [39] by creating a microstrip patch antenna. The antenna is fabricated on the FR4 substrate by cutting a slot in the patch with the modified ground plane. The designed antenna resonates at 2.4 GHz resonance frequency. The antenna performances (like current density, electric field, and magnetic field) are measured on the breast structure with and without tumors. In the same year, Afyf et al. [40] designed a coplanar waveguide (CPW)-fed flexible slotted antenna to detect cancer in breasts. The antenna resonated at 3 GHz with 550 MHz bandwidth and achieved around 1.0 dB gain. The antenna is placed in contact with the human skin for the detection of cancer in breasts. Furthermore, in the next year, Mahmud et al. [41] designed a directive antenna for MI applications. The slotted Vivaldi antenna was designed by cutting slots into the fins. The slots in the ground plane increase the gain and electrical length. The antenna covered 3.9–9.15 GHz bandwidth with gain and efficiency of 6.8 dBi and 88%, respectively. A breast phantom with two antennas is used for tumor detection. The data is received through the healthy and unhealthy breast phantom models; it helps to identify the tumor inside the breast.

In 2016, Afifi et al. [42] designed a ring resonator for broken bones as well as breast cancer detection. The ring resonator is used for tumor identification by material characterization. The ring resonator forms 1-D and 2-D images for bone fracture and breast tumor detection, respectively. Similarly, Narkhede et al. [43] developed an array of microwave annular antenna systems to detect cancer in the breast. This is a UWB monopole antenna array system in the range of 2.2–12 GHz for performing the proper detection of cancer in the breast of any woman. An assembly of 12 antennas has been designed for the proper working of this system. Furthermore, Medina et al. [44]

have done experimental MI by the comparison of confocal and holography to detect breast cancer. This technique has been applied to UWB radars to achieve high performance. It has an accuracy of up to 7.5 mm radii tumor and provides an accurate position. Both the algorithms work together to get high performance, which has also been seen through the experiment. These techniques have been working in the range of 5–15 GHz to perform the proper detection of cancer. Alborova et al. [45] designed an experimental model to detect cancer in the breasts. In this model, a helical antenna is used for measuring the S11 parameter. For that model, two phantom models are used: one model is based on without dielectric, and the other is based on the dielectric. The breast model is considered in such a way that its dielectric properties are similar to those of biotic tissues. The antenna is placed in front of the phantom and behind the phantom, also an absorbing material is placed to reduce the clutter. The antenna measurements were done at 5.6–6.6, 14–15, and 21–22 GHz frequency bandwidths. The images are processed using RASCAN-Q software for inhomogeneous biological tissue detection.

In 2016, AFYF et al. [46] designed a UWB flexible antenna for breast cancer detection. The antenna provides 2.4 GHz bandwidth at 3 GHz resonance frequency. An inhomogeneous multi-layer breast phantom model is used for measuring antenna performance in the human body. Song et al. [47] designed a UWB antenna for breast cancer detection. The antenna was designed on Duroid RT 6010LM substrate with Bow-tie shaped patch and square slot ground plane. It covered 6–17 GHz frequency bandwidth. For breast tumor detection, a 4 × 4 antenna array is used to reconstruct the image and location of the tumor in the phantom model. In the next year, Mirza et al. [48] designed a microwave sensor to detect cancer in breasts. The antenna is designed on a rectangular ground plane with a circular patch. In the antenna, two vertical plates are used for feeding into the patch. For breast cancer detection, a phantom model was designed by using a plastic container with low dielectric fatty tissues, and the tumor is detected by using the UWB antenna at the frequency of 4–8 GHz.

In 2017, Ouerghi et al. [49] breast cancer was detected using a circular patch antenna array. The circular antenna resonates at 2.45 GHz resonance frequency. For the breast MI system, an 8-antenna array is used in circular pattern. In these antennas, with the help of the electric and magnetic fields, breast models are studied. Similarly, a UWB system was designed by Fouad et al. [50] for breast cancer/tumor detection. For detection of the tumor, an antipodal Vivaldi antenna was designed using radiating elements, transition, and feedline. The antenna covered 2.3 GHz to more than 11 GHz bandwidth. The combination of two antennas is placed horizontally at 90° along the breast phantom. This type of system is able to detect 5 mm-diameter tumors, Furthermore, Wang et al. [51] designed an antenna array MI system for breast cancer/tumor detection. The UWB omnidirectional antenna covered 4.97–11.73 GHz frequency band. For breast cancer detection, 24 antennas are placed on the phantom model. The signals received by the antennas are evaluated by the delay-and-sum algorithm using MATLAB. This system is available to detect a 5 mm diameter tumor inside the breast and cancer in the breast system. Song et al. [52] designed a system based on a complementary metal oxide semiconductor integrated with a 4 × 4 antenna array. In that system, a circuit monocycle pulse is generated by a complementary metal oxide semiconductor (CMOS) circuit that is transmitted and received by the antenna array. The signal that is received by the antenna is converted into a digital signal by CMOS sampling circuit. With the help of an antenna array, the signal is extracted at various positions on the breast phantom. In this model, a confocal imaging algorithm is utilized to extract the signal from the phantom, which helps to create a breast image. This system is able to detect $1.0 \text{ cm}^3$ cancer inside the phantom.

Furthermore, in 2017, Islam et al. [53] designed a slotted patch antenna for tumor detection. The antenna is designed by cutting a slot from the patch and ground plane to enhance the gain and produce the omnidirectional radiation pattern. The antenna provides 117% (3.1–12 GHz) bandwidth with an average gain (efficiency) of 4.7 dBi (98%). The antenna is able to detect the tumor inside the phantom model with the MI method. In the next year, Mohamed et al. [54] designed a defected ground structure (DGS) ring resonator for breast cancer detection. It is designed on Roger 4003 substrate. The working principle is dependent on the material properties, i.e., the resonance frequency is shifted in the presence of tumor. Furthermore, a holographic MI (HMI)-based breast cancer detection system was designed by Asghar et al. [55], which operates in 5.05–8.23 GHz bandwidth. In this system for breast cancer detection, a phantom model with 18 bow-tie antennas is used. Out of these 18 antennas, 8 antennas are utilized as transmitters and the remaining 14 antennas work as receivers. In this technique, holographic microwave simulation was done for tumor, and its size detection was done using MATLAB. Similarly, Tasnim et al. [56] designed an imaging technique-based system for breast tumor detection. For that system, six directive Vivaldi antennas are used, which covered 3.04–3.30 GHz bandwidth with a maximum gain of 4.1 dB. In these antennas, one antenna transmits the signal while the other receives the signal. The received signals are processed using MATLAB to detect the tumor images. The tumor measurement setup and its 3-D radiation pattern are shown in Figure 9.1 (a) and (b).

In 2018, Inum et al. [57] designed a microstrip antenna for brain tumor detection. The antenna is designed by a square patch, and its performance is improved by using an electromagnetic band gap (EBG) structure. The EBG-based antenna structure provides 5.84% and 16.53% improved bandwidth and gain, respectively. The antenna provides a specific absorption rate (SAR) within a specific limit. The tumor is detected inside the human phantom model using the MI algorithm. In the same year, Jamlos et al. [58] arranged a UWB antenna array for brain tumor detection.

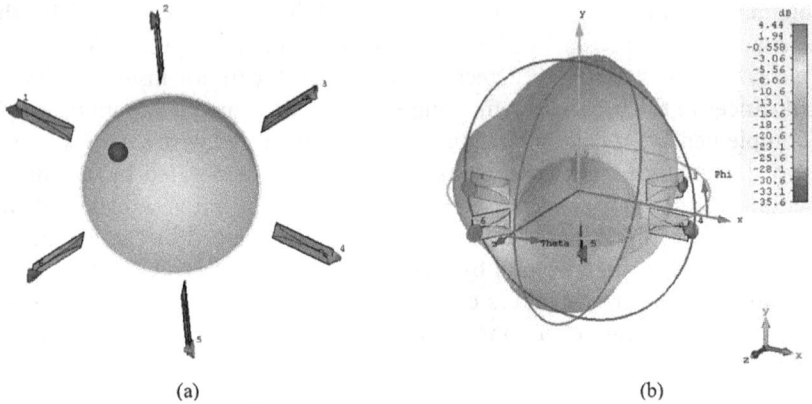

(a)                                                    (b)

*Figure 9.1* (a) Tumor measurement setup and (b) 3D radiation pattern of the phantom model [56].

The antenna is designed on Taconic (TLY-5) dielectric substrate with $4 \times 1$ circular radiating patch. The antenna operates in 1.2–10.8 GHz bandwidth with a gain between 5.2 and 14.5 dB. For tumor location identification, the antennas are placed at nine different locations in the phantom model. The received signals from the phantom are observed with and without tumor. These signals are further processed using MATLAB by iteratively corrected delay, multiply, and sum algorithm. Similarly, Amdaouch et al. [59] designed a UWB antenna for breast tumor detection. The antenna is designed by a square ring with partial ground plane, which covered 3.0–12.0 GHz bandwidth. For tumor detection, the antenna is placed on the human breast model, and with the help of power absorbed by normal and malignant tissue, the tumor is detected. In 2019, a confocal MI technique was used by Hammouch et al. [60] for tumor detection and location identification. First, a UWB antenna was designed for 3.1–14.0 GHz band, and after that, a confocal MI algorithm was applied for creating the image of the tumor. The results show the feasibility of the breast tumor. In the same year, Geetharamani et al. [61] designed a metamaterial-based THz antenna for breast cancer detection. The antenna is designed by the combined structure of a rectangular patch with a complementary split ring resonator. The equation with an equivalent circuit is also incorporated into the design. The antenna operates at the frequency of 1.0 THz with a gain of 20 dBi. With the help of simulation and measurement, the tumor was detected within the human breast, and based on the UWB microstrip antenna, a breast tumor detection system was designed by Kaur et al. [62]. The antenna is a three-layer structure that consists of active and passive patches on the top and middle layers. The bottommost layer of the structure consists of a feedline, and the upper layer of the feed consists of a plus-shaped slot in the ground plane, which covered 4.9–10.9 GHz bandwidth.

The antenna scans breast phantom at different locations at different times. Based on S-parameters, the image of the tumor is identified.

In 2019, Srinivasan et al. [63] designed a textile antenna for breast cancer detection. The flexible antenna is designed on jeans material with slot loaded on patch and ground plane designed by copper conducting material. The antenna resonates at 2.4 GHz frequency. With the help of this antenna, breast cancer is detected with and without tumor. Furthermore, Samsuzzaman et al. [64] designed a Vivaldi antenna array for breast tumor detection. The antenna is designed by cutting fins on the radiating patch with the addition of an elliptical patch. The elliptical patch is responsible for enhancing the directivity and gain. The Vivaldi antenna provides 120% (2.50–11 GHz) bandwidth with 7.2 dBi gain. For breast MI, 16 antennas are placed surrounding the phantom. In this antenna arrangement, one antenna works as a transmitter, and the remaining antennas work as receivers. The imaging performance of the tumor is investigated using MERIT source software, which identifies the tumor inside the image. Likewise, Wang [65] designed an HMI algorithm for breast tumor detection. A realistic breast and data acquisition model was designed using MATLAB software, and their performances were measured [66–68] using the multi-frequency HMI method. In this model, single and multi-frequency HMI models are utilized to evaluate the performance in terms of sensitivity, accuracy, and effectiveness [69]. In terms of the single frequency model, the multi-frequency model provides detailed information about tumors more accurately. Similarly, for breast cancer detection, a metamaterial-loaded high gain antenna was designed by Islam et al. [70]. The antenna is designed on a metasurface. The Vivaldi patch works as a radiating element; 12 metasurfaces are placed below the radiating element; and the tapered slot is printed in the ground plane. For matching the impedance, several slots are also created and the antenna covered 8.5 GHz (2.70–11.20 GHz) bandwidth. The antennas are placed in a cylindrical arrangement along the phantom model. The data received by the antennas are processed using MATLAB by the iteratively corrected delay multiply and sum algorithm. The system is capable of detecting multiple tumor objects.

In 2020, Hossain et al. [71] designed a UWB antenna array for breast cancer tumor detection. The antenna is designed by a slotted semicircle patch with partial ground plane. The antenna covered 2.30–11.00 GHz bandwidth with a maximum gain of 5.8 dBi. For tumor detection, a 16-antenna array is placed on the breast phantom model. Of those antennas, one is used as a transmitter, and the remaining are used as receivers. With the help of those phantom models, data is found with and without tumor, and with the help of iteratively corrected delay and sum image reconstruction algorithm, tumor detection is performed. In the same year, Kaur et al. [72] designed a dielectric resonator antenna for breast tumor detection using MI techniques. In this tumor, a 4.3–12.6 GHz dielectric resonator antenna is placed parallel to the breast phantom (with and without tumor)

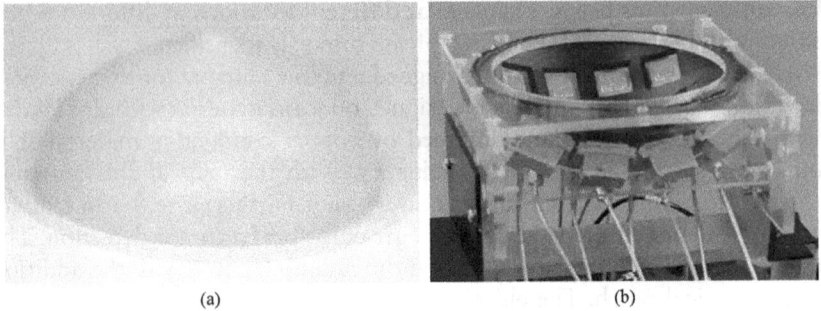

*Figure 9.2* (a) Breast phantom model and (b) breast cancer measurement system [73].

and rotates at 10° intervals to the azimuth (0–2$\pi$) and elevation angle (0–$\pi$). For that model, a total of 1,080 back scatterings were received and processed for tumor detection. Similarly, Alibakhshikenari et al. [73] designed a metamaterial-inspired antenna array for breast cancer detection using the MI technique. The antenna is designed using a square-shaped, concentric-rings-shaped patch with a feedline. In this technique, an array of antennas is placed surrounding the sample breast, and in this arrangement, at a time, only one antenna works as a transmitter, and the remaining antennas work as receivers. The antenna covered 2–12 GHz band with gain and efficiency of 4.8 dBi and 18%, respectively. The antenna array surrounding the breast exhibits an average of 30 dB isolation. From the band of frequencies, it is observed that a shorter wavelength provides better resolution. The prototype of the breast phantom model and its measurement setup are shown in Figure 9.2 (a) and (b).

Likewise, in 2020, Niranjan Kumar et al. [74] designed a UWB monopole antenna for breast cancer detection. The MI technique is basically used for breast cancer detection. It has many advantages compared to conventional techniques such as X-ray radiography and tomography. The MI techniques provide a deep examination. In these techniques, a UWB antenna was designed by cutting a square slot in the middle of the patch and placing another square slot cut in the corner of the patch. The antenna covered 141% (3.22–11.92 GHz) bandwidth with a gain of 1.4–6.43 dBi. Breast cancer is detected by the dielectric constant of the breast tissues. Ahadi et al. [75] designed a square-shaped monopole antenna for breast cancer detection. The UWB antenna covered 3.8–9.0 GHz frequency band. For breast cancer detection (10 and 5 mm tumor), 16 UWB antennas are placed in the form of a hemispherical arrangement. In this arrangement, two tumors are detected at different locations of up to 5.0 mm tumor. The phantom with holding device and cancer measurement setup are shown in Figure 9.3 (a) and (b).

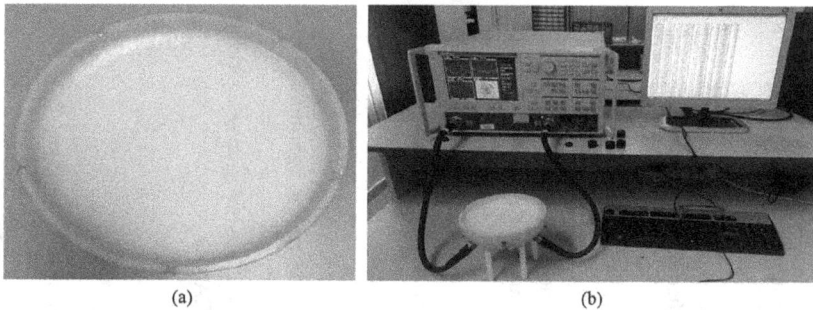

*Figure 9.3* (a) Breast phantom model and (b) breast cancer measurement setup [75].

## 9.4 CHALLENGES OF USING MI

There are numerous issues that hamper the MI technique in a practical scenario. Such issues are discussed here. The MI system should be portable for cancer patients for malignant tissue measurement. For this, WU and Amineh developed a low-cost portable imaging system for 3-D imaging [76], and similarly, Hiroshima University developed a portable system for breast cancer scanning as well as natural disaster applications [77]. Furthermore, the operating frequency also plays an important role in cancer imaging. We know that as frequency increases, better resolution is achieved, but it also increases the penetration into the tissues. In terms of imaging, 3-D imaging provides a more accurate shape compared to 2-D imaging. The 2-D imaging provides only two dimensions of the images, but 3-D images show the actual size of the cancer/tumor. The image of cancer depends on an array of MI sensors, i.e., antennas. The larger number of antennas (antenna array) increases the coupling [78–87], which is responsible for the inverse problem. The calculation of antenna numbers depends on the theory (degree of freedom) for MI [88]. For cancer detection, frequency hopping, i.e., the use of multiple frequencies, is able to construct better images [89]. The multiple frequencies reduce the effect of nonlinearity for that algorithm so that it is not trapped in local minima. For designing a better MI system, several research groups are working with clinical trials to arbitrate the effectiveness of the system. The MI research for tumor/cancer detection is based on humanity and not on financial gain, but all research needs funding. For cancer detection research, several government agencies and universities are providing funds for the development of the cancer imaging system. The aim of this research is basically to design a low-cost imaging system to detect cancer in breasts. The research based on breast cancer/tumor is summarized in Table I, which shows the comparison in terms of operating frequencies, design software, number of antennas, tumor size, and image extraction algorithms.

Table 9.1 Summary of various research articles based on breast cancer detection

| Reference | Year | Author | Operating frequency (GHz) | No of antennas | Software | Tumor size | Image algorithm |
|---|---|---|---|---|---|---|---|
| [28] | 2010 | Adnan | 3.5–8.0 GHz | — | FEM | — | — |
| [29] | 2010 | Zhurbenko et al. | 0.3–3.0 GHz | 32 | MOM | 5.0 mm | Image reconstruction algorithm |
| [30] | 2010 | Klemm et al. | 6.0 GHz | 31 | — | 7.0 mm | Modified delay and sum algorithm |
| [31] | 2012 | Wang et al. | 2.3–12.2 GHz | — | FEM | — | — |
| [32] | 2014 | Latif et al. | 1.0–6.0 GHz | 02 | FEM | — | — |
| [33] | 2014 | Kahar et al. | 3.1–10.6 GHz | 01 | FEM | 5.0 mm | SAR |
| [34] | 2014 | Ünal et al. | 1.0–8.0 GHz | 07 | CST | 2.0 mm | Delay-and-sum algorithm |
| [35] | 2015 | Bahrami et al. | 2.0–4.0 GHz | 16 | FEM | — | Delay and sum algorithm |
| [36] | 2014 | Islam et al. | 3.4–12.5 GHz | 02 | CST | — | — |
| [37] | 2015 | Katbay et al. | 2.45 GHz | — | CST | 1 cm | — |
| [38] | 2015 | Abbosh et al. | 2.5–6.0 GHz | 08 | CST | — | Delay and summation algorithm |
| [39] | 2015 | Caliskan et al. | 2.45 GHz | — | FEM | — | — |
| [40] | 2015 | Affi et al. | 2–4.0 GHz | — | CST | — | — |
| [41] | 2016 | Mahmud et al. | 3.9–9.15 GHz | 02 | CST | 10.0 mm | Source software |
| [42] | 2016 | Affi et al. | 9.29 GHz | — | CST | — | Inverse scattering algorithm |
| [43] | 2016 | Narkhede et al. | 2.2–12.0 GHz | 12 | HFSS | — | — |
| [44] | 2016 | Medina et al. | 1.8–20.0 GHz | — | — | 15.0 mm | Confocal and holography algorithms |
| [45] | 2016 | Alborova et al. | 5.6–6.6 GHz; 14.0–15.0 GHz; 21.0–22.0 GHz | — | — | 10 mm | RASCAN-Q |
| [46] | 2016 | Afyf et al. | 2.0–4.0 GHz | — | CST | — | — |
| [47] | 2016 | Song et al. | 8.0–17.0 GHz | 49 | — | 10.0 mm | — |
| [48] | 2017 | Mirza et al. | 4.0–8.0 GHz | 01 | FEM | 4.0 mm | 3D inversion algorithm |
| [49] | 2017 | Ouerghi et al. | 2.45 GHz | 08 | FEM | 10 mm | — |
| [50] | 2017 | Fouad et al. | 2.3–11.0 GHz | 02 | CST | 5.0 mm | Subtract and add algorithm |

| Ref | Year | Author | Frequency | Samples | Tool | Resolution | Algorithm |
|---|---|---|---|---|---|---|---|
| [51] | 2017 | Wang et al. | 4.97–11.73 GHz | — | CST | 5.0 mm | Delay and sum algorithm |
| [52] | 2017 | Song et al. | 3.0–10.0 GHz | 16 | — | 1.0 cm³ | Confocal imaging algorithm |
| [53] | 2018 | Islam et al. | 3.1–12.0 GHz | — | CST and FEM | — | — |
| [54] | 2018 | Mohammed et al. | 9.65 GHz | — | CST | — | Image construction using MATLAB |
| [55] | 2018 | Asghar et al. | 5.05–8.23 GHz | 18 | FEM | 1.5 mm | MATLAB |
| [56] | 2018 | Tasnim et al. | 3.04–3.30 GHz | 06 | CST | — | Beam former algorithm |
| [57] | 2018 | Inum et al. | 7.3 GHz | — | CST and FEM | — | Microwave imaging algorithm |
| [58] | 2019 | Jamlos et al. | 1.2–10.8 GHz | 9 | — | — | Improved delay and sum imaging algorithm |
| [59] | 2018 | Amdaouch et al. | 3.0–12.0 GHz | 01 | CST | 4.0 mm | — |
| [60] | 2019 | Nirmine et al. | 3.1–14.0 GHz | — | — | — | CMI |
| [61] | 2019 | Geetharamani et al. | 1.0 THz | 02 | CST | — | — |
| [62] | 2019 | Kaur et al. | 4.9–10.9 GHz | 03 | CST | 4.0 mm | Delay and sum process using MATLAB |
| [63] | 2019 | Dhamodharan et al. | 2.4 GHz | — | FEM | — | — |
| [64] | 2019 | Samsuzzaman et al. | 2.5–11.0 GHz | 16 | CST | 1.8 mm | Microwave radar-based imaging toolbox software |
| [65] | 2019 | Wang et al. | 1.0–4.0 GHz | 16 | — | 5.0 mm | MATLAB |
| [70] | 2019 | Islam et al. | 2.7–11.2 GHz | 16 | CST | — | Iteratively correlated delay multiply and sum algorithm |
| [71] | 2020 | Hossain et al. | 2.3–11.0 GHz | 16 | Sat Env | 2.5 mm | Iteratively corrected delay and sum image reconstructed algorithm |
| [72] | 2021 | Kaur et al. | 4.3–12.6 GHz | — | CST | 5.0 mm | Delay and sum algorithm |
| [73] | 2020 | Alibakhshikenari et al. | 2.0–12.0 GHz | 06 | CST | 5.0 mm | Reconstruction algorithm |
| [74] | 2020 | Niranjan Kumar et al. | 3.22–11.92 GHz | 02 | FEM | — | — |
| [75] | 2020 | Mojtaba | 3.8–9.0 GHz | 16 | — | 5 and 10 mm | Delay multiply and sum algorithm |

## 9.5 CONCLUSION

The deaths due to breast cancer are the second cause of cancer death in women worldwide. There are different techniques used for cancer detection, i.e., X-ray, ultrasound, and MRI, but there are some limitations to these techniques, like cost, accuracy, and uncomforted. These restrictions are overwhelmed with the use of MI. Based on MI, several types of research have been done. In this article, a summarized view of the various MI techniques is covered for breast cancer/tumor detection. This review article covered the imaging method, trans-receiver elements, and algorithm. From the literature survey, it is visualized that breast cancer and other types of tumors are able to be detected with the use of MI. However, for cancer imaging, it requires high sensitivity and resolution sensors [90–95] for high-quality images.

Furthermore, the breast cancer/tumor detection system faces some restrictions and challenges such as multiple antennas with multiple feeding techniques; a requirement of a liquid that matches the impedance between antenna and skin for reducing the signal-to-noise ratio; a requirement of complex coding data from the antennas for drawing the image of cancer/tumor; and high cost due to the use of equipments like multiple antennas, vector network analyzer, signal generator, and oscillator, but still, the systems using MI are cost-effective compared to other related systems.

In the past few years, the MI system has gone for a clinical trial and subsequently its various shortcomings have been observed. There are several industrial agencies involved in generating the system using MI for breast cancer systems, such as Medfield Diagnostics and Micrima, and after several years of clinical trials, better cancer/tumor images are achieved.

## REFERENCES

[1] Murawa, P., Murawa, D., Adamczyk, B., & Połom, K. (2014). Breast cancer: Actual methods of treatment and future trends. *Reports of Practical Oncology and Radiotherapy*, 19(3), 165–172.
[2] Cokkinides, V., Albano, J., Samuels, A., Ward, M., & Thum, J. (2005). American cancer society: Cancer facts and figures. Atlanta: American Cancer Society.
[3] Humphrey, L. L., Helfand, M., Chan, B. K., & Woolf, S. H. (2002). Breast cancer screening: A summary of the evidence for the US Preventive Services Task Force. *Annals of Internal Medicine*, 137(5_Part_1), 347–360.
[4] US Preventive Services Task Force. (2002). Screening for breast cancer: Recommendations and rationale. *Annals of Internal Medicine*, 137(5), 344.
[5] US Preventive Services Task Force. (2009). Screening for breast cancer: US Preventive Services Task Force recommendation statement. *Annals of Internal Medicine*, 151(10), 716–726.

[6] Gupta, A., Anand, R., Pandey, D., Sindhwani, N., Wairya, S., Pandey, B. K., & Sharma, M. (2021). Prediction of breast cancer using extremely randomized clustering forests (ERCF) technique: Prediction of breast cancer. *International Journal of Distributed Systems and Technologies (IJDST)*, 12(4), 1–15.

[7] Saini, M. K., Nagal, R., Tripathi, S., Sindhwani, N., & Rudra, A. (2008). PC Interfaced Wireless Robotic Moving Arm. In *AICTE Sponsored National Seminar on Emerging Trends in Software Engineering* (Vol. 50).

[8] Singh, L., Saini, M. K., Tripathi, S., & Sindhwani, N. (2008). An Intelligent Control System For Real-Time Traffic Signal Using Genetic Algorithm. In *AICTE Sponsored National Seminar on Emerging Trends in Software Engineering* (Vol. 50).

[9] Nikolova, N. K. (2011). Microwave imaging for breast cancer. *IEEE Microwave Magazine*, 12(7), 78–94.

[10] Chaudhary, S. S., Mishra, R. K., Swarup, A., & Thomas, J. M. (1984). Dielectric properties of normal & malignant human breast tissues at radiowave & microwave frequencies. *Indian Journal of Biochemistry & Biophysics*, 21(1), 76–79.

[11] Saroha, R., Singh, N., & Anand, R. Echo cancellation by adaptive combination of normalized sub band adaptive filters. *International Journal of Electronics and Electrical Engineering*, 2(9), 1–10.

[12] Malik, S., Singh, N., & Anand, R. (2012). Compression artifact removal using SAWS technique based on fuzzy logic. *International Journal of Electronics and Electrical Engineering*, 2(9), 11–20.

[13] Kwon, S., & Lee, S. (2016). Recent advances in microwave imaging for breast cancer detection. *International Journal of Biomedical Imaging*, 2016.

[14] Lazebnik, M., McCartney, L., Popovic, D., Watkins, C. B., Lindstrom, M. J., Harter, J., ... & Hagness, S. C. (2007). A large-scale study of the ultrawideband microwave dielectric properties of normal breast tissue obtained from reduction surgeries. *Physics in Medicine & Biology*, 52(10), 2637.

[15] Halter, R. J., Zhou, T., Meaney, P. M., Hartov, A., Barth Jr, R. J., Rosenkranz, K. M., ... & Paulsen, K. D. (2009). The correlation of in vivo and ex vivo tissue dielectric properties to validate electromagnetic breast imaging: Initial clinical experience. *Physiological Measurement*, 30(6), S121.

[16] Porter, E., & O'Halloran, M. (2017). Investigation of histology region in dielectric measurements of heterogeneous tissues. *IEEE Transactions on Antennas and Propagation*, 65(10), 5541–5552.

[17] Juneja, S., Juneja, A., & Anand, R. (2020). Healthcare 4.0-digitizing healthcare using big data for performance improvisation. *Journal of Computational and Theoretical Nanoscience*, 17(9–10), 4408–4410.

[18] Sansanwal, K., Shrivastava, G., Anand, R., & Sharma, K. (2019). Big data analysis and compression for indoor air quality. In *Handbook of IoT and Big Data* (pp. 1–21). CRC Press.

[19] Joines, W. T., Zhang, Y., Li, C., & Jirtle, R. L. (1994). The measured electrical properties of normal and malignant human tissues from 50 to 900 MHz. *Medical Physics*, 21(4), 547–550.

[20] Fornes-Leal, A., Garcia-Pardo, C., Frasson, M., Beltrán, V. P., & Cardona, N. (2016). Dielectric characterization of healthy and malignant colon tissues in the 0.5–18 GHz frequency band. *Physics in Medicine & Biology*, 61(20), 7334.

[21] Hesabgar, S. M., Sadeghi-Naini, A., Czarnota, G., & Samani, A. (2017). Dielectric properties of the normal and malignant breast tissues in xenograft mice at low frequencies (100 Hz–1 MHz). *Measurement, 105*, 56–65.

[22] Cheng, Y., & Fu, M. (2018). Dielectric properties for non-invasive detection of normal, benign, and malignant breast tissues using microwave theories. *Thoracic Cancer, 9*(4), 459–465.

[23] Hussein, M., Awwad, F., Jithin, D., El Hasasna, H., Athamneh, K., & Iratni, R. (2019). Breast cancer cells exhibits specific dielectric signature in vitro using the open-ended coaxial probe technique from 200 MHz to 13.6 GHz. *Scientific Reports, 9*(1), 1–8.

[24] Kuwahara, Y., Nakada, Y., Nozaki, A., & Fujii, K. (2019, July). Measurement and Analysis of Complex Permittivity of Breast Cancer in Microwave Band. In *2019 41st Annual International Conference of the IEEE Engineering in Medicine and Biology Society (EMBC)* (pp. 2929–2932). IEEE.

[25] Chaudhary, S. S., Mishra, R. K., Swarup, A., & Thomas, J. M. (1984). Dielectric properties of normal & malignant human breast tissues at radio-wave & microwave frequencies. *Indian Journal of Biochemistry & Biophysics, 21*(1), 76–79.

[26] Fear, E. C., Hagness, S. C., Meaney, P. M., Okoniewski, M., & Stuchly, M. A. (2002). Enhancing breast tumor detection with near-field imaging. *IEEE Microwave Magazine, 3*(1), 48–56.

[27] Aldhaeebi, M. A., Alzoubi, K., Almoneef, T. S., Bamatraf, S. M., Attia, H., & Ramahi, O. M. (2020). Review of microwaves techniques for breast cancer detection. *Sensors, 20*(8), 2390.

[28] Adnan, S., Abd-Alhameed, R. A., See, C. H., Hraga, H. I., Elfergani, I. T., & Zhou, D. (2010). A compact UWB antenna design for breast cancer detection. *PIERS Online, 6*(2), 129–132.

[29] Zhurbenko, V., Rubæk, T., Krozer, V., & Meincke, P. (2010). Design and realisation of a microwave three-dimensional imaging system with application to breast-cancer detection. *IET Microwaves, Antennas & Propagation, 4*(12), 2200–2211.

[30] Klemm, M., Leendertz, J. A., Gibbins, D., Craddock, I. J., Preece, A., & Benjamin, R. (2010). Microwave radar-based differential breast cancer imaging: Imaging in homogeneous breast phantoms and low contrast scenarios. *IEEE Transactions on Antennas and Propagation, 58*(7), 2337–2344.

[31] Wang, L., & Huang, B. (2012). Design of ultra-wideband MIMO antenna for breast tumor detection. *International Journal of Antennas and Propagation*, 2012.

[32] Latif, S., Flores-Tapia, D., Pistorius, S., & Shafai, L. (2014). A planar ultra-wideband elliptical monopole antenna with reflector for breast microwave imaging. *Microwave and Optical Technology Letters, 56*(4), 808–813.

[33] Kahar, M., Ray, A., Sarkar, D., & Sarkar, P. P. (2015). An UWB microstrip monopole antenna for breast tumor detection. *Microwave and Optical Technology Letters, 57*(1), 49–54.

[34] Ünal, I., Türetken, B., & Canbay, C. (2014). Spherical conformal bow-tie antenna for ultra-wide band microwave imaging of breast cancer tumor. *Applied Computational Electromagnetics Society Journal, 29*(2), 124–133.

[35] Bahramiabarghouei, H., Porter, E., Santorelli, A., Gosselin, B., Popović, M., & Rusch, L. A. (2015). Flexible 16 antenna array for microwave breast cancer detection. *IEEE Transactions on Biomedical Engineering, 62*(10), 2516–2525.

[36] Islam, M. M., Islam, M. T., Samsuzzaman, M., & Faruque, M. R. I. (2015). A negative index metamaterial antenna for UWB microwave imaging applications. *Microwave and Optical Technology Letters, 57*(6), 1352–1361.

[37] Katbay, Z., Sadek, S., Lababidi, R., Perennec, A., & Le Roy, M. (2015, June). Miniature antenna for breast tumor detection. In *2015 IEEE 13th International New Circuits and Systems Conference (NEWCAS)* (pp. 1–4). IEEE.

[38] Abbosh, A. M., Mohammed, B., & Bialkowski, K. (2015, September). Differential microwave imaging of breast pair for tumor detection. In *2015 IEEE MTT-S 2015 International Microwave Workshop Series on RF and Wireless Technologies for Biomedical and Healthcare Applications (IMWS-BIO)* (pp. 63–64). IEEE.

[39] Çalışkan, R., Gültekin, S. S., Uzer, D., & Dündar, Ö. (2015). A microstrip patch antenna design for breast cancer detection. *Procedia-Social and Behavioral Sciences, 195*, 2905–2911.

[40] Afyf, A., Bellarbi, L., Errachid, A., & Sennouni, M. A. (2015, March). Flexible microstrip CPW sloted antenna for breast cancer detection. In *2015 International Conference on Electrical and Information Technologies (ICEIT)* (pp. 292–295). IEEE.

[41] Mahmud, M. Z., Islam, M. T., Samsuzzaman, M., Kibria, S., & Misran, N. (2017). Design and parametric investigation of directional antenna for microwave imaging application. *IET Microwaves, Antennas & Propagation, 11*(6), 770–778.

[42] Afifi, A. I., & Abdel-Rahman, A. B. (2016, December). Ring Resonator for Breast Cancer and Broken Bones Detection. In *2016 Asia-Pacific Microwave Conference (APMC)* (pp. 1–4). IEEE.

[43] Narkhede, A. S., Gandhi, A., & Prajapati, J. (2016, June). Annular antenna system for Microwave Imaging for Breast Cancer Detection. In *2016 IEEE Indian Antenna Week (IAW 2016)* (pp. 21–24). IEEE.

[44] Medina, Y., Augusto, M., & Paz, A. V. (2016, October). Microwave Imaging for Breast Cancer Detection: Experimental Comparison of Confocal and Holography Algorithms. In *2016 IEEE ANDESCON* (pp. 1–4). IEEE.

[45] Alborova, I. L., & Anishchenko, L. N. (2016, August). Experimental modeling of breast cancer detection by using radar aids. In *2016 Progress in Electromagnetic Research Symposium (PIERS)* (pp. 4635–4638). IEEE.

[46] Afyf, A., Bellarbi, L., Achour, A., Yaakoubi, N., Errachid, A., & Sennouni, M. A. (2016, May). UWB thin film flexible antenna for microwave thermography for breast cancer detection. In *2016 International Conference on Electrical and Information Technologies (ICEIT)* (pp. 425–429). IEEE.

[47] Song, H., Kubota, S., Xiao, X., & Kikkawa, T. (2016, September). Design of UWB antennas for breast cancer detection. In *2016 International Conference on Electromagnetics in Advanced Applications (ICEAA)* (pp. 321–322). IEEE.

[48] Mirza, A. F., See, C. H., Danjuma, I. M., Asif, R., Abd-Alhameed, R. A., Noras, J. M., ... & Excell, P. S. (2017). An active microwave sensor for near field imaging. *IEEE Sensors Journal, 17*(9), 2749–2757.

[49] Ouerghi, K., Fadlallah, N., Smida, A., Ghayoula, R., Fattahi, J., & Boulejfen, N. (2017, September). Circular antenna array design for breast cancer detection. In *2017 Sensors Networks Smart and Emerging Technologies (SENSET)* (pp. 1–4). IEEE.

[50] Fouad, S., Ghoname, R., Elmahdy, A. E., & Zekry, A. E. (2017). Enhancing tumor detection in IR-UWB breast cancer system. *International Scholarly Research Notices, 2017.*

[51] Wang, F., Arslan, T., & Wang, G. (2017, October). Breast cancer detection with microwave imaging system using wearable conformal antenna arrays. In *2017 IEEE International Conference on Imaging Systems and Techniques (IST)* (pp. 1–6). IEEE.

[52] Song, H., Azhari, A., Xiao, X., Suematsu, E., Watanabe, H., & Kikkawa, T. (2017). Microwave imaging using CMOS integrated circuits with rotating 4×4 antenna array on a breast phantom. *International Journal of Antennas and Propagation, 2017.*

[53] Islam, M. T., Samsuzzaman, M., Rahman, M. N., & Islam, M. T. (2018). A compact slotted patch antenna for breast tumor detection. *Microwave and Optical Technology Letters, 60*(7), 1600–1608.

[54] Mohamed, A. A. E., Hussein, H. M., Atallah, H. A., & Abdel-Rahman, A. B. (2018, March). Breast cancer detection using compact defected ground structure (DGS) ring resonator. In *2018 35th National Radio Science Conference (NRSC)* (pp. 489–494). IEEE.

[55] Asghar, I., Khan, A. A., & Brown, A. K. (2018, September). Multistatic Holographic Imaging for Breast Cancer Detection. In *2018 15th European Radar Conference (EuRAD)* (pp. 14–17). IEEE.

[56] Tasnim, F., Jannat, F., Kibria, S., Alam, M. S., Ahsan, T., Alam, T., ... & Islam, M. T. (2018, October). Electromagnetic performances analysis of a microwave imaging system (MIS) for breast tumor detection. In *2018 International Conference on Innovations in Science, Engineering and Technology (ICISET)* (pp. 442–446). IEEE.

[57] Inum, R., Rana, M., Shushama, K. N., & Quader, M. (2018). EBG based microstrip patch antenna for brain tumor detection via scattering parameters in microwave imaging system. *International Journal of Biomedical Imaging, 2018.*

[58] Jamlos, M. A., Mustafa, W. A., Husna, N., Idrus, S. S., Khairunizam, W., Zunaidi, I., ... & Shahriman, A. B. (2019, June). Ultra-Wideband Confocal Microwave Imaging for Brain Tumor Detection. In *IOP Conference Series: Materials Science and Engineering* (Vol. 557, No. 1, p. 012002). IOP Publishing.

[59] Amdaouch, I., Aghzout, O., Naghar, A., Alejos, A. V., & Falcone, F. J. (2018). Breast tumor detection system based on a compact UWB antenna design. *Progress In Electromagnetics Research M, 64,* 123–133.

[60] Hammouch, N., & Ammor, H. (2019, October). Microwave imaging for early breast cancer detection using CMI. In *2019 7th Mediterranean Congress of Telecommunications (CMT)* (pp. 1–5). IEEE.

[61] Geetharamani, G., & Aathmanesan, T. (2019). Metamaterial inspired THz antenna for breast cancer detection. *SN Applied Sciences, 1*(6), 1–9.

[62] Kaur, G., & Kaur, A. (2020). Breast tissue tumor detection using "S" parameter analysis with an UWB stacked aperture coupled microstrip patch antenna having a "+" shaped defected ground structure. *International Journal of Microwave and Wireless Technologies, 12*(7), 635–651.

[63] Srinivasan, D., & Gopalakrishnan, M. (2019). Breast cancer detection using adaptable textile antenna design. *Journal of Medical Systems*, *43*(6), 1–10.

[64] Samsuzzaman, M., Islam, M. T., Islam, M. T., Shovon, A. A., Faruque, R. I., & Misran, N. (2019). A 16-modified antipodal Vivaldi antenna array for microwave-based breast tumor imaging applications. *Microwave and Optical Technology Letters*, *61*(9), 2110–2118.

[65] Wang, L. (2019). Multi-frequency holographic microwave imaging for breast lesion detection. *IEEE Access*, 7, 83984–83993.

[66] Sindhwani, N., Bhamrah, M. S., Garg, A., & Kumar, D. (2017, July). Performance analysis of particle swarm optimization and genetic algorithm in MIMO systems. In *2017 8th International Conference on Computing, Communication and Networking Technologies (ICCCNT)* (pp. 1–6). IEEE.

[67] Sindhwani, N., & Singh, M. (2017, March). Performance analysis of ant colony based optimization algorithm in MIMO systems. In *2017 International Conference on Wireless Communications, Signal Processing and Networking (WiSPNET)* (pp. 1587–1593). IEEE.

[68] Sindhwani, N. (2017). Performance Analysis of optimal scheduling based firefly algorithm in MIMO system. *Optimization*, *2*(12), 19–26.

[69] Juneja, S., Juneja, A., & Anand, R. (2019, April). Reliability Modeling for Embedded System Environment compared to available Software Reliability Growth Models. In *2019 International Conference on Automation, Computational and Technology Management (ICACTM)* (pp. 379–382). IEEE.

[70] Islam, M. T., Samsuzzaman, M., Kibria, S., Misran, N., & Islam, M. T. (2019). Metasurface loaded high gain antenna based microwave imaging using iteratively corrected delay multiply and sum algorithm. *Scientific Reports*, *9*(1), 1–14.

[71] Hossain, A., Islam, M. T., Islam, M., Chowdhury, M. E., Rmili, H., & Samsuzzaman, M. (2020). A planar ultrawideband patch antenna array for microwave breast tumor detection. *Materials*, *13*(21), 4918.

[72] Kaur, G., & Kaur, A. (2021). Monostatic radar-based microwave imaging of breast tumor detection using a compact cubical dielectric resonator antenna. *Microwave and Optical Technology Letters*, *63*(1), 196–204.

[73] Alibakhshikenari, M., Virdee, B. S., Shukla, P., Parchin, N. O., Azpilicueta, L., See, C. H., ... & Limiti, E. (2020). Metamaterial-inspired antenna array for application in microwave breast imaging systems for tumor detection. *IEEE Access*, 8, 174667–174678.

[74] Srikanth, B. S., Gurung, S. B., Manu, S., Gowthami, G. N. S., Ali, T., & Pathan, S. (2020). A slotted UWB monopole antenna with truncated ground plane for breast cancer detection. *Alexandria Engineering Journal*, *59*(5), 3767–3780.

[75] Ahadi, M., Nourinia, J., & Ghobadi, C. (2021). Square monopole antenna application in localization of tumors in three dimensions by confocal microwave imaging for breast cancer detection: Experimental measurement. *Wireless Personal Communications*, *116*(3), 2391–2409.

[76] Wu, H., & Amineh, R. K. (2019). A low-cost and compact three-dimensional microwave holographic imaging system. *Electronics*, *8*(9), 1036.

[77] Song, H., Sasada, S., Kadoya, T., Okada, M., Arihiro, K., Xiao, X., & Kikkawa, T. (2017). Detectability of breast tumor by a hand-held impulse-radar detector: Performance evaluation and pilot clinical study. *Scientific Reports*, *7*(1), 1–11.

[78] Gangwar, A. K., & Alam, M. S. (2018). CSRR based folded monopole tri-band antenna array and its system level evaluation. *International Journal of RF and Microwave Computer-Aided Engineering, 28*(6), e21276.

[79] Gangwar, A., & Alam, M. S. (2018). A high FoM monopole antenna with asymmetrical L-slots for WiMAX and WLAN applications. *Microwave and Optical Technology Letters, 60*(1), 196–202.

[80] Gangwar, A. K., & Alam, M. S. (2020). Frequency reconfigurable dual-band filtenna. *AEU-International Journal of Electronics and Communications, 124*, 153239.

[81] Gangwar, A. K., & Alam, M. S. (2019). A miniaturized quad-band antenna with slotted patch for WiMAX/WLAN/GSM applications. *AEU-International Journal of Electronics and Communications, 112*, 152911.

[82] Anand, R., & Chawla, P. (2020). Optimization of inscribed hexagonal fractal slotted microstrip antenna using modified lightning attachment procedure optimization. *International Journal of Microwave and Wireless Technologies, 12*(6), 519–530.

[83] Anand, R., & Chawla, P. (2020). A novel dual-wideband inscribed hexagonal fractal slotted microstrip antenna for C- and X-band applications. *International Journal of RF and Microwave Computer-Aided Engineering, 30*(9), e22277.

[84] Anand, R., Shrivastava, G., Gupta, S., Peng, S. L., & Sindhwani, N. (2018). Audio Watermarking With Reduced Number of Random Samples. In *Handbook of Research on Network Forensics and Analysis Techniques*, eds. G. Shrivastava, P. Kumar, B.B. Gupta, S. Bala, N. Dey (pp. 372–394). IGI Global.

[85] Anand, R., & Chawla, P. (2016, March). A review on the optimization techniques for bio-inspired antenna design. In *2016 3rd International Conference on Computing for Sustainable Global Development (INDIACom)* (pp. 2228–2233). IEEE. N. Nikolova et al. (2011). Microwave imaging for breast cancer. *IEEE Microwave Magazine, 12*: 78–94.

[86] Chawla, P., & Anand, R. (2017). Micro-switch design and its optimization using pattern search algorithm for applications in reconfigurable antenna. *Modern Antenna Systems, 10*, 189–210.

[87] Dahiya, A., Anand, R., Sindhwani, N., & Deshwal, D. (2021). Design and construction of a low loss substrate integrated waveguide (SIW) for S band and C band applications. *MAPAN*, 1–9.

[88] Kaye, C., Jeffrey, I., & LoVetri, J. (2019). Improvement of multi-frequency microwave breast imaging through frequency cycling and tissue-dependent mapping. *IEEE Transactions on Antennas and Propagation, 67*(11), 7087–7096.

[89] Salucci, M., Oliveri, G., & Massa, A. (2015). GPR prospecting through an inverse-scattering frequency-hopping multifocusing approach. *IEEE Transactions on Geoscience and Remote Sensing, 53*(12), 6573–6592.

[90] Kohli, L., Saurabh, M., Bhatia, I., Shekhawat, U. S., Vijh, M., & Sindhwani, N. (2021). Design and Development of Modular and Multifunctional UAV with Amphibious Landing Module. In *Data Driven Approach Towards Disruptive Technologies: Proceedings of MIDAS 2020* (pp. 405–421). Springer Singapore.

[91] Kohli, L., Saurabh, M., Bhatia, I., Sindhwani, N., & Vijh, M. (2021). Design and Development of Modular and Multifunctional UAV with Amphibious Landing, Processing and Surround Sense Module. *Unmanned Aerial Vehicles for Internet of Things (IoT): Concepts, Techniques, and Applications*, 207. https://doi.org/10.1002/9781119769170.ch12

[92] Singh, P., "Vehicle Monitoring and Surveillance through Vehicular Sensor Network" IGI book series "Cloud-Based Big Data Analytics in Vehicular Ad-Hoc Networks" by the publisher, IGI Global.

[93] Kumar, S., & Raw, R. S. (2020). "Health Monitoring Planning for On-Board Ships Through Flying Ad Hoc Network. In *Advanced Computing and Intelligent Engineering* (pp. 391–402). Springer.

[94] Goyal, B., Dogra, A., Khoond, R., Gupta, A., & Anand, R. (2021, September). Infrared and Visible Image Fusion for Concealed Weapon Detection using Transform and Spatial Domain Filters. In *2021 9th International Conference on Reliability, Infocom Technologies and Optimization (Trends and Future Directions)(ICRITO)* (pp. 1–4). IEEE.

[95] Kaur, J., Sabharwal, S., Dogra, A., Goyal, B., & Anand, R. (2021, September). Single Image Dehazing with Dark Channel Prior. In *2021 9th International Conference on Reliability, Infocom Technologies and Optimization (Trends and Future Directions)(ICRITO)* (pp. 1–5). IEEE.

Chapter 10

# IoT implementation and challenges in healthcare industries

*Rahul and Sahithi Bommareddy*
Delhi Technological University, Delhi, India

*Monika*
Shaheed Rajguru College of Applied Sciences for Women,
University of Delhi, India

*Javed Ahmad Khan*
Govt. Girls Polytechnic Ballia, India

*Digvijay Pandey*
Department of Technical Education, Dr. A P.J Abdul Kalam Technical
University, UP, India

## CONTENTS

DOI: 10.1201/9781003239888-10

## 10.1 INTRODUCTION

The world of Internet of Things (IoT) [1, 2] is the most important computing process in the world. It has substantiated so many impossible things possible. If IoT meets medicine, it has been assisting in the enhancement of healthcare [3] in a more effective, healthier, and productive way. This new technology can be practiced from all parts of the country and can cause less time to deal with the diagnosis and the procedure of treatments [4]. IoT will speed up the process of delivering health amenities to individuals by making doctors access healthcare treatments through satellites and sensors. IoT has made so many miracles in the healthcare industry. Though there has been a drastic development, there has always been a gap in healthcare treatments all around the world. Many of the countries that have not yet developed are still picking up speed.

The opportunities that the industry receives will be talked upon. Telemedicine, preventive medicine, radio frequency identification (RFID), and trackers are something today's healthcare industry is being introduced to. With sufficient assistance from IoT, people will be able to get a diagnosis at any point of time, thereby being convenient for both the patients and the doctors. This also minimizes the long wait times for the appointments for the patients and also saves transportation time for the doctors as well.

Another aspect is the concept of wearable devices. Smart watches and bracelets to monitor necessary health information are a big aspect of today's healthcare industry. Without these, it is impossible to remain healthy in the cases of chronic patients. There are many IoT devices that monitor heart rate, blood pressure, and blood sugar, which also take Doppler and electrocardiogram (ECG) scans. During the COVID-19 pandemic, the importance of $SpO_2$ readings is also steepening the graph. Another IoT device is used for this purpose, which is now compatible with smartwatches.

There are numerous cases in which medicine was delivered late or where the diagnosis was not able to assist the patients within a reasonable time. Up to 1 million people died as a result of such untreated ailments. In a country like India, where the rural population is massive and there is minimal accessibility to healthcare centers, such devices can be used to establish telemedicine. Preventive medicine can also be practiced only with the help of IoT devices.

Though IoT has the capability to take healthcare to the next level, it also imposes a series of threats and challenges. In this chapter, we will talk about the challenges like data security and privacy, integration of such IoT devices, and the protocols that have to be followed. We will also tackle the problem of data overload and the difficulty in determining the accuracy of those IoT devices. Cost is also something that provides a great challenge in the healthcare sector as quality instruments have to be used. There are a wide variety of applications that should be explored as well. Many of the applications will be discussed in detail, like CV Technology [5], ingestible sensors, trackable inhalers, wearables to fight depression, medical alert systems, and many more.

In this particular article, we aim to give the details and a survey of the present situation of the healthcare industry in our country and analyze this existing information to facilitate further research. We will be able to find out the present working state of IoT in the healthcare industry in India as well as around the world. This will help us to compare both of them and use applications to solve many of the issues faced by today's healthcare industry.

## 10.2 RELATED WORK

There are numerous literatures available on IoT to improve quality, especially in the healthcare sector. There is a research article [4] that dealt with the risk management in the security aspect of the IoT devices in the healthcare industry. In this article, there was support from research that is focused on a hospital in Sudan. Therefore, a risk management system was developed to initiate the facilitation of the process in a better manner. This model was then evaluated by other experts and developed further. In the research article [6], on the challenges of IoT in healthcare, there was a point raised about data being an essential part of IoT devices. Therefore, the data collected will refer to more than 79.4 ZB of data. This large quantity of data will only result from the IoT devices hailing from the healthcare industrial equipment. Therefore, this challenge has been talked about. In another work [7, 8, 9], the authors talked about various such improvements and challenges in healthcare. Apart from this, they have also written about the opportunities provided by IoT devices and the advancements made in the IoT field of study. This leads to a breach in security as well. The authors in [10] have performed research on the future obstacles and research challenges imposed by the IoT. In this, they have stated that by the end of 2020 there will have been 212 billion products on IoT launched in the market for the individuals. Many such products will help in the contribution to the healthcare industry as well.

An Indian perspective was given on the IoT challenges by the authors in [11]. In this article, there has been a familiarization of the security issues ongoing in India and the hike in IoT growth in the present era. Excluding this, there was an issue of risk factors along with security challenges according to the Indian perspective. A book chapter [12] regarding IoT Service Utilization in Healthcare has talked about the IoT scenario in the healthcare industry along with the risk factors involved. Some of the healthcare challenges like teamwork were also explained in detail. Several models or frameworks used for IoT [13] in healthcare were defined and drawn attention upon. Apart from this, it was stated that healthcare has some limitations that are related to the identified factors in the healthcare sector as imposed by certain developing countries, especially India. Therefore, there have been certain frameworks that are designed for such countries to help safeguard security and threats.

According to the authors in [14, 15, 16], there must be a proper transition to a patient-centric treatment from a clinic-centric healthcare. Therefore, there has to be a multilayered architecture that supports this. Then they also emphasized the important drawbacks like regulation and interoperability issues. including security and privacy concerns. In [17], the authors have reviewed the IoT applications in high-risk industries like the environmental, health, and safety industries as these are the main ones where human life is at stake. Apart from this, there are IoT-based applications that are primed to offer a better solution at a granular level. The main purpose of this comprehensive and extensive review was to provide a better emergency response for the given high-risk environmental health (EH) industries. Therefore, more of the challenges were discussed and concluded with the proposed solutions. In addition to this, a novel architecture was introduced in [18], which supported a small mobile client module as well as an edge gateway supporting the local data process. In this way, many facilities can be made available through a private and public cloud by making sure that there is proper robustness and flexibility.

According to the authors in [19], there are many applications of IoT, ranging from basic wireless networks, cloud computing, and semantic technology to future internet. Through this, the devices are able to be connected all the time. They have compared the IoT to the "Internet of Everything," which emphazises that the IoT can connect all around the world and increase connectivity throughout devices. There has been a focus on how the capability of the IoT can be increased to ensure a better healthcare facility for each country. In a book chapter [20], there is a discussion about how network security can be enhanced through networking by connecting the devices through a remotely controlled atmosphere.

## 10.3  INTERNET OF THINGS IN THE HEALTHCARE INDUSTRY

IoT has many applications in the healthcare industry. Before the age of the internet of things devices, healthcare was mostly of doctors who are confined to hospital visits and prescriptions on paper. A more automated technique was made available for this purpose. IoT devices help to control remote monitoring [21, 22, 23]. This ensures that there is a higher potential for the physicians to deliver proper medical attention to the patients without having any concern about additional issues like remote access and patient monitoring. This has seen a significant change in the duration of admission at a hospital for a patient [24]. IoT in the prime of the healthcare industry has many applications for use by patients, elderly people, insurance companies, hospitals, and governments as well.

### 10.3.1  IoT for patients

Patients are mostly benefiting through IoT. They are able to access many wearable and internet-connected devices wirelessly to monitor heart rate and blood sugar and to take ECG and Doppler scans as well. This helps them to not only closely monitor the condition but also make sure that medical attention is given to the patients right away. There are many cases where a patient cannot be hospitalized at the correct time due to such delays. This ensures proper care is taken for the patient. According to surveys, diabetes is one of the few diseases that has to be closely monitored. Low or high glycemic indices can lead to life-threatening problems. These problems do not have any solutions and cannot be completely cured by medications. These medications have to be taken regularly, but still, glycemic values have to be properly managed. Therefore, IoT devices like glucometers provide proper checks to manage these symptoms. There are also IoT devices that send alerts to the healthcare provider when medical attention is needed in case of emergencies.

There is an example of photoplethysmography, which is a technique used to detect volume changes in blood circulation. This takes the measurements at the skin surface by passing an infrared light source. This infrared light source illuminates the skin and detects the observed light intensity through a photo sensor. The readings by the phtoplethysmography (PPG) sensor are then converted using a computer program, and the sensed data is transferred via Bluetooth, allowing us to check the readings in our smartphone.

### 10.3.2  IoT for doctors

Doctors are able to provide medical advice to people through IoT devices based on the data. The data collected through IoT devices provides a proper diagnosis to health care providers and physicians, which helps in the proper analysis of such treatments. A wearable monitor or an equipment embedded in IoT connects such devices and helps doctors to provide the most accurate diagnosis.

For example, a smart system is used to monitor sleep-deprived or sleep-walking patients. With the help of integrating IoT as well as using big data analytics, the patients' sleep cycles can be monitored by physicians [25]. The architecture of such sleep-operating IoT devices includes an IoT layer, a fog computing layer, and a cloud networking layer. In the IoT layer, all the devices using all the various elements that influence the parameters are considered. The data obtained is then computed through the fog computing layer [26]. This fog computing layer processes the data using the concept of fog nodes and stores the data in the cloud to centralize its processing. Then the data is stored in a database that includes analytical resources and accessibility through a graphical data interface.

### 10.3.3 IoT for hospitals

IoTs are used not only by patients at home but also in hospitals. They use the trackers for medical equipment and also defibrillators to know the location of the medical equipment. This can also be seen as a safety aspect during times of emergencies when a patient is in need of oxygen or a hospital bed. Infection spread and sanitation are aspects that are important for hospitals. There are IoT-enabled hygiene monitoring devices that help to prevent patients from getting infected [27].

For hygiene in hospitals, staff hygiene can be monitored by using Espressif System Programmable (ESP) modules as base stations connected to smartphones by a mobile node. The estimated Euclidean distance [28] is then calculated using Bluetooth Received Signal Strength Indicator (RSSI) values, which in turn measure the proximity-based solutions.

### 10.4 IOT IN INDIA

IoT is quite a hotspot in India. Many IoT devices are being used throughout the country, including in the capital city. India's first semi-high-speed train was launched with the safety feature of collision avoidance. This makes sure that accidents are avoided without human error. Almost one lakh people die every day due to train accidents. Every 30 minutes, one person dies in train accident. Thus, it is a very important strategy that needs to be devised to protect the passengers.

As India is a country that lags behind certain health indicators, IoT devices have made it possible in the healthcare industry. As India is the second most populated country, it accounts for 20% of the global diseases. Through IoT connection, there is enabled connectivity throughout the country, which enables it to access through all parts of the country for healthcare consultation. This is an advantage for the areas of poor healthcare services, which

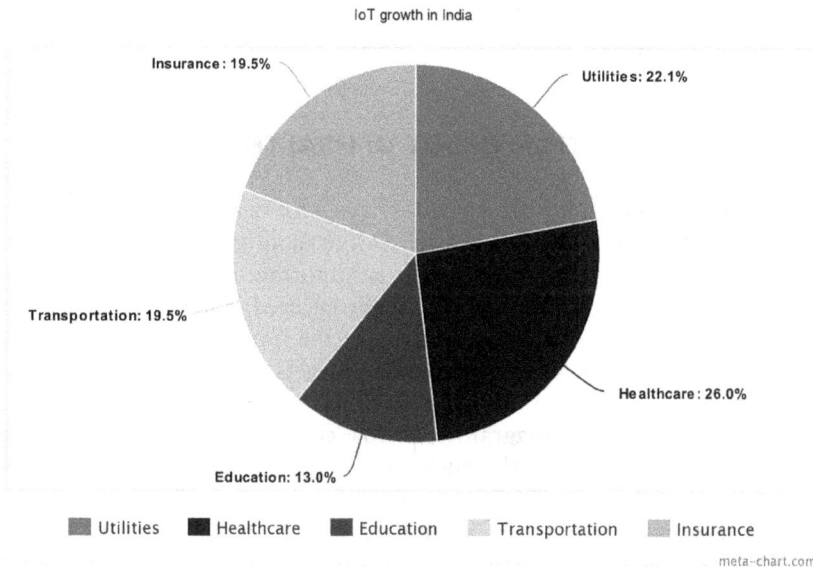

*Figure 10.1* Pie chart depicts the sectors in which IoT is influencing.

have inaccessibility to such quality healthcare. IoT devices make it possible for such problems to include a shortage of medical representatives due to the use of IoT devices. Through this, they are able to make sure that proper medical facilities are being ensured. The wait time for the diagnosis also decreases in such populated areas where the mortality rate decreases drastically. With the integration of such internet of things devices, IoT devices such as smart sensors [29, 30], health apps, and artificial intelligence (AI) are possible through the internet and clouds.

Figure 10.1 shows the chart that indicates the sectors in which IoT is influential.

In Indian healthcare, it is important to meet the demand of the patients receiving the healthcare.

Indian consumers are very demanding. They have a need for a well-developed healthcare facility. There is a demand for telemedicine and good healthcare insurance with government schemes. To make this possible, the revolutionizing technologies need to take a head start. Indian citizens need the right to proper healthcare necessities. Healthcare access will reduce the cost of treatment. It will limit the budgets that needto be allocated to healthcare. Without the complexity of the technology, it will be able to be deployed into the system. Through this, there will also be security and ease of access to healthcare for everyone. In India, because of the lack of standardization, there are more challenges involved in the deployment of IoT processes in the healthcare sector. The internet of medical things is based on predictive and preventive care [10]. It benefits patients, families, hospitals, doctors, nurses, and insurance companies.

## 10.5 IMPLEMENTATION OF IOT IN HEALTHCARE

IoT projects need high investments and have a lot of proof of concepts that will be suitable for many businesses. As the main goal for all businesses is a digital transformation initiative, it is important to recognize the project objectives for the technology to actually succeed. The various industries do have so many requirements. The aim of the implementation steps is to decrease operational costs. This, therefore, targets customer experience and can also increase the reach. To be able to understand the business analytics, we have to use case diagrams and IoT consulting companies to make sure that the IoT model has the business to understand that technology. IoT application-based companies make sure that the future of the company is ensured. For example, the IoT components must be aligned with the test cases. For any project, hardware and software selection are equally important. The components need to include sensors, edge gateways, communication protocols, IoT platforms, and cloud management software.

### 10.5.1 Sensors

Sensors are used to collect the data that is related to various factors like weight, volume, temperature, humidity, pressure, and many more. There are many sensors that help detect these aspects.

*Temperature sensor*: It is used to measure the temperature of the surroundings of an experiment. Temperature sensors often use resistance temperature detectors that are optimized [31–33] and easy to install. The resistance temperature detectors (RTDs) work on the principle of the expansion of the metals with respect to temperature. A DHT-11 sensor is a temperature sensor that is used in most of the projects in IoTs.

*Pressure sensors*: Pressure sensor works on the principle of the electromagnetic field. It constantly observes the changes in the field and returns the signal. This is a common feature used in the sensors of cars to detect objects. As there is no physical contact involved to detect the pressure, these proximity sensors are quite useful. Some examples of proximity sensors are Si114x and Si1102, which are mostly used in IoT devices.

*Smoke sensors*: Smoke sensor is one such IoT device that helps in detection. These are very common in our day-to-day life. The smoke detectors work on the principle of infrared radiation. The LED light pulses a beam of light into the sensor chamber, which checks for the smoke particles in the atmosphere. This is connected to Arduino and helps to build a circuit.

## 10.5.2 Edge gateways

Edge gateways are those which help in protocol translation, data processing, storage, filtering, and also for device security. Although edge computing is a relatively new approach for many companies, it is used to send the architecture to the cloud [34]. This is, therefore, used to process the source and send the data back to the cloud.

## 10.5.3 Cloud management software

This helps organizations to manage the cloud in private and public clouds and makes them aware of all the existing services and resources. This helps the system to administer and control the data received from the edge gateways. It helps to provide access control, data, applications, and services.

Software-as-a-Service (SaaS) application is used for cloud computing. In this, the data is distributed online and is used by the products through any browser. SaaS usually helps to improve IoT connectivity and also identifies the need for such universal usage of the data. Some of the softwares that provide support for IoT devices are Altair Smartworks, Watson studio by IBM, Salesforce IoT cloud, and Oracle IoT.

Figure 10.2 shows a graph of the number of billions of IoT devices over the last three decades.

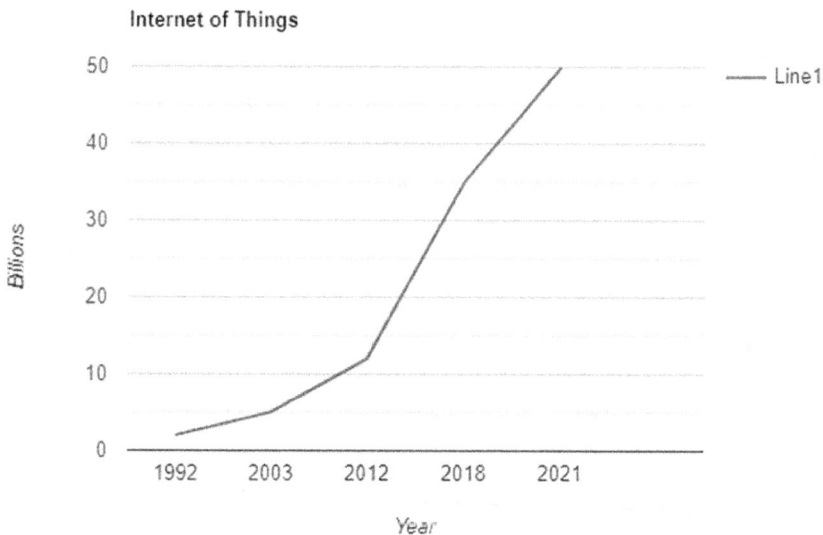

Figure 10.2 A line graph of the number of billions of IoT devices over three decades.

## 10.6 CHALLENGES IN THE HEALTHCARE SYSTEM IMPOSED BY IOT

IoT has flourished a lot, especially during pandemic times. There are many applications that have been published and are useful in every field. IoT has seen many investments coming its way in IoT app development.

According to Business Insider, the sales of IoT devices are growing exponentially. In 2015, over 46 million devices were shipped, and in 2020, over 161 million devices were shipped. Healthcare is always very costly and is increasing with the demands of the people [35]. There is a need for the automation of healthcare processes in the healthcare industry to offer better facilities to the patients.

With a proper diagnosis and treatment, healthcare-related IoT devices play a huge role in the minimization of hospital bills. It has been proved through research that a hospital bill using IoT to store and collect data saves up to 50% of what was being saved earlier.

### 10.6.1 Data security

Data security is one of the main issues with IoT devices. Data is the most important criterion for the functioning of IoT devices. The protection of patients' information and the data associated with it are important in the healthcare industry. Data security and insights always enhance our work structure and life. The trust built in these IoT devices helps to bring a better economy to the company providing them and also to the company investing in them. A study shows that 89% of the companies that provide IoT devices have customers who believe that there is a lack of security. In a 2019 survey that was conducted in prominent countries with respect to economic standards, 63% of people were unhappy with the way IoT security was being led. The first step for an IoT lifecycle to develop is to make sure there is a thorough examination of any vulnerability that may prevail. The user and customer back-end systems must also be checked for the same.

There are many IoT security issues, which include remote exposure, not being able to predict the industry's future, and constraints on resources.

IoTs have a large attack surface because of their internet connectivity. This makes them vulnerable to hackers interacting with the devices remotely. IoT security is also a similar thing to cloud security, which attracts users and is accountable for protecting the security of thousands of data privacy records.

IoTs have a concern to make sure that IoT security is the resource constraint. Tesla Model X was hacked in less than 90 seconds as it had a Bluetooth vulnerability. As Tesla works on Bluetooth and wireless key features to start and open the cars, this imposes a serious security concern.

## 10.6.2 Privacy

IoT devices are often available for public perception. This makes it important for IoT businesses to properly advertise their products to the local market. This advertising should also address most of the safety concerns the public might have. For example, to make a smart home, using Alexa is quite feasible, but 90% of Indians do not set up Amazon Alexa because of privacy concerns that the information might get stolen and hacked.

As there is a lot of data on the IoT devices, there are many entry points for hackers to steal the information. There is a lot of public profile as most of the IoT devices agree to use the collected data to make many decisions based on the product. For example, health insurance can gather your health statistics through a fitness tracker and can calculate the rate of insurance based on your vulnerability. Eavesdropping is something that everyone is scared of in today's world. Hackers are able to steal information from fitness trackers or listen to everyday conversations to either improve the quality of the fitness tracking or steal important information.

## 10.6.3 Integration to follow multiple protocols

IoT integration is important because each IoT device is designed through a set of applications. In order to get the desired results, they have to be integrated. IoT integration refers to the clubbing of IoT devices, IoT data, and IoT platforms with other businesses and cloud platforms. There are many different software to integrate such devices.

### 10.6.3.1 Mesh protocols

Zigbee is a type of mesh technology that extends coverage over a number of sensor nodes. Zigbee has a short range and has less power efficiency due to mesh configs.

Thread is also another low-power mesh protocol that is used in IoT devices. Mesh protocol is that which is able to network with the interconnected nodes so as to dynamically update the routing table. The goal of mesh IoT is to make connected devices over a local edge to route the data across this mesh network.

### 10.6.3.2 Bluetooth

Bluetooth is under the category of a wireless network. This is a short range of communication where the devices can be connected to a smartphone or smart home system within close proximity. This Bluetooth then helps to establish a connection for the transfer of data. Bluetooth devices these days have been widely integrated and are now seen in many fitness devices and medical wearables, such as pulse oximeters, glucometers, and blood pressure monitors.

### 10.6.3.3 WiFi

With the increase in technology, WiFi has been playing a crucial role. Without the involvement of additional smartphone devices and applications to process such obtained data, there is a limitation in coverage and scalability when it comes to IoT devices using WiFi.

### 10.6.3.4 LOW-POWER WIDE-AREA NETWORK (LPWAN)

LPWANs are the new technology observed in IoT devices. There is a longer range of communication. These devices also run on small, inexpensive batteries that last for many years and are very feasible. LPWAN can connect to the IoT sensors which help to monitor the data environmentally and check the occupancy. Though LPWAN is not an efficient way to send gigantic amounts of data, small blocks of code can be sent at a low rate if they are not time-sensitive. LPWAN provides quality service and has reached many goals of scalability [36].

## 10.6.4 Accuracy

Data and communication protocols help to keep the data policies and accuracy of those IoT devices in check. It is difficult to always calibrate the devices and check for proper functioning. IoT collects the data in bulk, so it needs to be checked for the proper analysis of the data in comparison to all the customers who are using it. Overloading of the data has the chance of affecting the decision-making process of hospitals and the healthcare sector in the future.

## 10.6.5 Increase in vulnerability

IoT devices are a big attraction to hackers. As IoT healthcare offers so much benefit, there are many ways the security spots are often vulnerable. It is important for the software developers to make sure that it is not vulnerable. Through IoT devices, hackers will be able to invade the personal space of such patients and also hospital details through a simple IoT breakout. The way the device works can be tampered with and is also life-threatening. That is why IoT devices are not fully automated. According to a source, Sentara Hospitals had a mailing error regarding the IoT medical devices, which caused the breach of over 577 patients. There have been statistics that show 82% of healthcare organizations have been attacked by IoT devices.

## 10.6.6 Regulation

The telecommunication framework does not always apply to all IoT devices. Only some IoT applications are compatible with the regulations. Communication with such IoT devices is restricted to machine-to-machine (M2m) with limited interaction. Telecommunication frameworks help to define those services and communicate between the networks of things. IoT sensors need the transmission of data and signals without involving humans. So sensors are also considered to be telecommunication services. Telecommunication frameworks regarding connectivity are not properly defined. Hence, the IoT providers are not responsible for any conveyance of connectivity issues. Spectrum is also a key enabler of IoT devices. It does not have any limitation to the technology that is used; hence, there can be satellite or terrestrial network connectivity across the IoT.

## 10.6.7 Compatibility

As IoT is one such technology where there are many technologies competing to become the standard, this makes connectivity even more difficult. It requires the deployment of extra software and hardware specifications. Generic computing devices do not have a longer lifespan, whereas IoT devices have a long lifespan, though it requires time-to-time calibration with the service. In general, IoT devices do not go out of service even though the manufacturing company does not sell that particular product.

There are some other compatibility issues which include bad standardization techniques of the M2M protocols as well as differences in firmware. In addition, the operating system software models also keep changing over the years, which do not make it compatible with the devices using the latest operating systems.

## 10.6.8 Bandwidth

IoT in the healthcare industry has resulted in the transformation of technology usage in the advances due to the COVID-19 pandemic. With the growth of technology in the healthcare industry, there has also been growth in the industry of IoT technology.

Figure 10.3 briefs about the challenges of the internet of things in the healthcare industry, and Figure 10.4 shows the percentage of IoT devices used in the healthcare industry for various sectors.

IoT Challenges in The Healthcare Industry

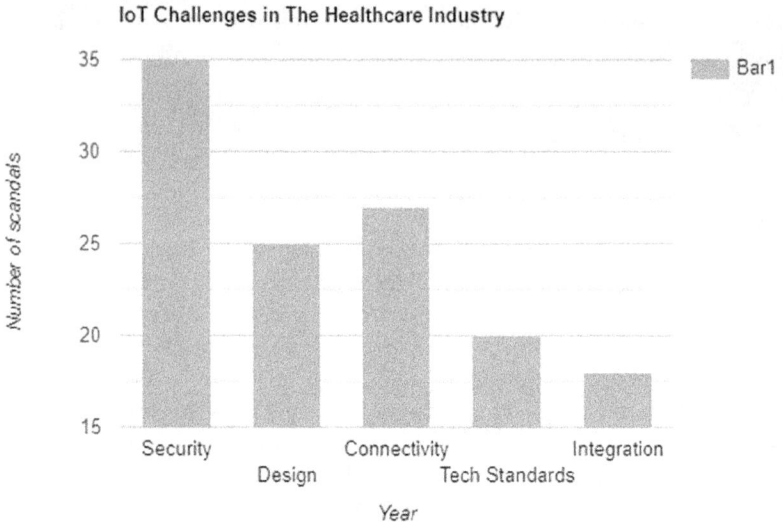

Figure 10.3 A bar graph depicting the challenges of the internet of things in the healthcare industry.

Divisions of IoT

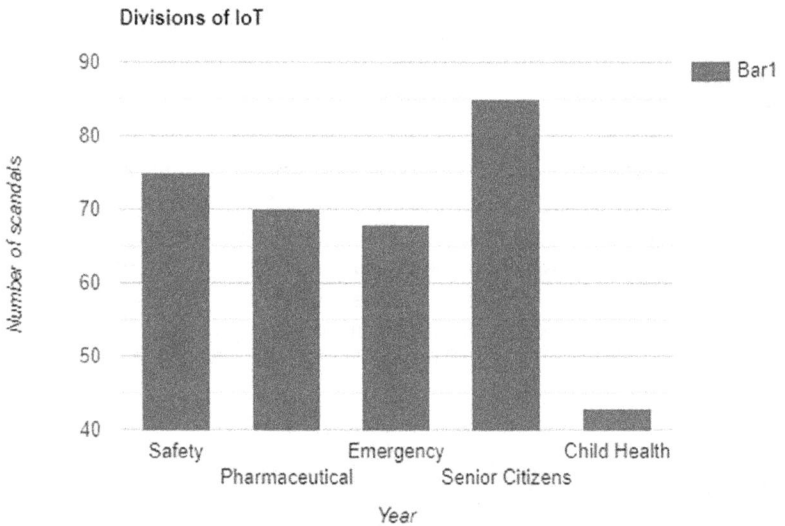

Figure 10.4 Percentage of IoT devices used in the healthcare industry for different sectors.

## 10.7 ADVANTAGES OF IOT

There are so many instances of healthcare redefining itself through the internet of things and many others. Similarly, there are many important aspects of IoT in the healthcare industry.

## 10.7.1  Less risk of error

As IoT is mostly handled by analyzing data and automated workflow, there is a very minimized error margin. It reduces the risk of error, thereby automating the procedure to make sure that it maintains accuracy. The data collected by the sensors is stored in the clouds. Therefore, human contact is not there by the tampering of data. Only the calibration and following protocols are the challenge. These errors are very crucial in the healthcare industry. The automation process reduces 55% of the medication errors. This makes sure that there is no risk factor involved for the person. A person in the healthcare industry needs to follow a certain role of diagnosis. He needs proper data to make sure that his diagnosis is correct and that there is no risk factor for the patient. When the data collection for the diagnosis is fully automated, there are less chances for the diagnosis to be incorrect.

## 10.7.2  Cost-effective

IoT makes sure that patient monitoring is effective. Through the network of IoT devices, it is easy to cut down on the need to visit the doctor's office. There is no need to travel all the way to see a doctor and get examined. All the tests required can be done remotely, and the test results can be faxed to the doctor respectively. An IoT facility of the connected homecare facility also reduces the risk of patients getting exposed to hospital stays.

The cost of whole treatment as supported by the health insurance company is very high for most of the middle-class people in India. Therefore, it is important to make healthcare available to all the citizens of the country. Internet of things implementation is possible by collecting the data and ensuring that particular data is used for the diagnosis.

## 10.8  AMBIENT-ASSISTED LIVING (AAL)

AAL is a branch that is associated with artificial intelligence. It is integrated with the internet of things. The purpose behind the introduction of AAL is to promote the independent lives of elderly people. Through this, a technique of real-time monitoring of these patients is done to see whether they receive the best medical facilities even in the time of medical fatalities [37]. This is made possible by using technologies like artificial intelligence, data analytics, and machine learning [38, 39]. The basic domains of AAL include activity recognition, data recognition, vitals recognition, and environmental recognition. These were experimented on and researched by many researchers in the field. There was the implementation of IPv6-based LPWAN used as a communication protocol. IoT-based healthcare systems are now able to track the quality of the air where the patients live. This makes sure that the patient can be transported to a different location if the environmental conditions are not favorable. IoT proposes a gateway that hopes to address many of the ongoing issues with advantages like data interoperability, accessibility, and security.

## 10.9 MOBILE IOT

Mobile IoT is the association of mobile computing with sensors and cloud computing techniques. This is used to ensure the proper tracking of the patient's information and makes it applicable to know the drastic changes in any physiological conditions. It works on the basic principle of the communication interface between the private network connection and the mobile networks. For example, there have been researches based on glucose systems that monitor through a mobile gateway. Based on such IoT devices, this locates the patient using an integrated global positioning system (GPS) module. IoT-based monitors have become so common that whenever there is a detection of any abnormal health condition like an irregular heartbeat, the primary contacts and technicians are informed. There are various methods in mobile IoT to safeguard the privacy and data security concerns of the parties involved. There are technical policies that require an app to collect the details on the basis of terms and conditions to the users in order to avoid legal proceedings in the future.

Mobile IoT or m-IoT is one such technology that is a part of the bigger IoT, which has changed the healthcare industry and the response stimuli of the entire sector.

## 10.10 WEARABLE DEVICES

These devices make sure that the professionals dealing with various patients have a maximum amount of data to work with for the proper diagnosis of the patient. These devices help to tackle various health issues and provide them at a low cost to healthcare seekers. These are usually completely non-invasive devices that safeguard the privacy concerns of the patient. Wearable devices are those which can be worn as a watch, bracelet, clip-on to a shirt, backpack, etc. The sensor is then placed at the site to make sure the data is collected. Wearable devices can also be connected to mobile applications through the network. They can be connected via Bluetooth as well. An IoT-enabled health monitoring device usually performs all the remote operations like checking body temperature, blood pressure, heartbeat, ECG, $SpO_2$ readings, and many more. Bio-signals like ECG and electromyography (EMG) are also analyzed through this. They can also be analyzed from time to time and be processed with the patient's vital information to check if the personalized normal goals are met. The interconnectivity of wearable devices extends its usage to another level. This computational power is used for easy processing and visualizing the collected data.

## 10.11 BLOCKCHAIN

Blockchain is one such technology that makes sure that data is shared between medical devices and medical healthcare providers from time to time. In the healthcare sector, the IoT network is a crucial step because data fragmentation is one of the major problems the sector is facing. Data fragmentation usually leads to gaps in data for healthcare providers, which results in insufficient data for the complete analysis. Blockchain technology helps to solve this data fragmentation. It helps to ensure the protective sharing of the data. Through this, sensitive medical information can be present in data repositories that can be safely accessed by authorized personnel. The transmission of the blockchain takes place due to three factors. This makes the process more secure. A ledger is present which is immutable and can be accessed by anyone. It can be operated from many different computers. It follows the data exchange policies that make it easier for data protection. An app called Healthcare Data Gateway uses blockchain technology, which allows patients to share their information securely. Patients can keep monitoring the sharing of their information and can control their information at any point of time without any violation of privacy policies.

## 10.12 CHILD HEALTH INFORMATION (CHI)

CHI deals with the program of creating awareness for a child's mental and health well-being. It is used to make sure that children are nurtured with the proper values both nutritionally and educationally. It makes sure their mental progress and behavior are tracked. Through this, the child's health can be regulated. This is easy for the patient's parents and guardians, especially as some special children require attention that might not be given adequately. If necessary, the doctors and parents can be prepared in case of an emergency. The IoT devices for children usually collect various readings like height, weight, heart rate, and $SpO_2$ readings based on which they will be able to think of a diagnosis in the case of emergencies without using up much time [40]. It can also track the nutritional values given to a child and can also make sure that the proper nutrients are being supplied by providing a tracker.

## 10.13 CONCLUSION

IoT is one of the many rapidly expanding fields in the technology sector. Day by day, people are getting benefits through remote access to healthcare without having to go anywhere in search of treatments. IoTs have also reduced the need for healthcare facilities in every location. It has reduced the need for humans to take tests and give a diagnosis on the basis of those tests. This reduces the use of machinery by humans, thereby reducing the human error involved. IoT in healthcare has solved many problems like data handling, security, privacy, interoperability, collaboration, and resource management. It has made the vast number of devices able to connect with the world today and serve a greater purpose. Interoperability between IoT devices makes sure of stakeholder collaboration. Security is a major problem IoT is facing today. The use of cloud computing and the upgradation of blockchain technology will definitely rule out the harm. IoT is an increasing industry, especially in the COVID-19 pandemic. It will affect the functioning and the role of healthcare in the future as well. This is the start of a new era of technology. Everything is being made possible up to the doorstep.

## REFERENCES

[1] Gupta, A., Srivastava, A., Anand, R., & Tomažič, T. (2020). Business Application Analytics and the Internet of Things: The Connecting Link. In *New Age Analytics* (pp. 249–273). Apple Academic Press.

[2] Gupta, R., Shrivastava, G., Anand, R., & Tomažič, T. (2018). IoT-based Privacy Control System through Android. In *Handbook of E-business Security* (pp. 341–363). Auerbach Publications.

[3] Juneja, S., Juneja, A., & Anand, R. (2020). Healthcare 4.0-digitizing healthcare using big data for performance improvisation. *Journal of Computational and Theoretical Nanoscience, 17*(9–10), 4408–4410.

[4] Zakaria, H., Bakar, N. A. A., Hassan, N. H., & Yaacob, S. (2019). IoT security risk management model for secured practice in healthcare environment. *Procedia Computer Science, 161*, 1241–1248. doi: 10.1016/j.procs.2019.11.238.

[5] Sindhwani, N., Verma, S., Bajaj, T., & Anand, R. (2021). Comparative analysis of intelligent driving and safety assistance systems using YOLO and SSD model of deep learning. *International Journal of Information System Modeling and Design (IJISMD), 12*(1), 131–146.

[6] Anmulwar, S., Gupta, A. K., & Derawi, M. (2020). Challenges of IoT in Healthcare. In *IoT and ICT for Healthcare Applications* (pp. 11–20). Springer, Cham.

[7] Rekha, H. S., Nayak, J., Sekhar, G. T., & Pelusi, D. (2020). Impact of IoT in Healthcare: Improvements and Challenges. *The Digitalization Conundrum in India: Applications, Access and Aberrations*, 73–107.

[8] Ahmed, A., Abdul Hanan, A., Omprakash, K., Lobiyal, D. K., & Raw, R. S. (2017). Cloud Computing in VANETs: Architecture, Taxonomy and Challenges. In *IETE Technical Review* (Vol. 35, pp. 523–547). India & USA: Taylor & Francis.

[9] Singh, P., Raw, R. S., & Khan, S. A. (2017). Link risk degree aided routing protocol based on weight gradient for health monitoring applications in vehicular ad-hoc networks. *Journal of Ambient Intelligence Humanized Computing.* https://doi.org/10.1007/s12652-021-03264-z.

[10] Joyia, G. J., Liaqat, R. M., Farooq, A., & Rehman, S. (2017). Internet of medical things (IoMT): Applications, benefits and future challenges in healthcare domain. *J. Commun., 12*(4), 240–247.

[11] Yadav, E. P., Mittal, E. A., & Yadav, H. (2018, February). IoT: Challenges and issues in Indian perspective. In *2018 3rd International Conference On Internet of Things: Smart Innovation and Usages (IoT-SIU)* (pp. 1–5). IEEE.

[12] Dauwed, M., & Meri, A. (2019). IOT service utilisation in healthcare. *Internet of Things (IoT) for Automated and Smart Applications*.

[13] Singh, P., "Vehicle Monitoring and Surveillance through Vehicular Sensor Network" IGI book series "Cloud-Based Big Data Analytics in Vehicular Ad-Hoc Networks" by the publisher, IGI Global.

[14] Farahani, B., Firouzi, F., Chang, V., Badaroglu, M., Constant, N., & Mankodiya, K. (2018). Towards fog-driven IoT eHealth: Promises and challenges of IoT in medicine and healthcare. *Future Generation Computer Systems, 78*, 659–676.

[15] Malsa, N., Singh, P. et al. (2020). Source of Treatment Selection for different States of India and Performance Analysis using Machine Learning Algorithms for Classification. *International Journal Series Book of Advances in Intelligent Systems and Computing*, Springer; volume: soft computing: theories and applications. 2020. ISSN: 2194–5357.

[16] Jain, S., Kumar, M., Sindhwani, N., & Singh, P. (2021). SARS-Cov-2 detection using Deep Learning Techniques on the basis of Clinical Reports. In *2021 9th International Conference on Reliability, Infocom Technologies and Optimization (Trends and Future Directions) (ICRITO)*, pp. 1–5, doi: 10.1109/ICRITO51393.2021.9596455.

[17] Thibaud, M., Chi, H., Zhou, W., & Piramuthu, S. (2018). Internet of Things (IoT) in high-risk Environment, Health and Safety (EHS) industries: A comprehensive review. *Decision Support Systems, 108*, 79–95.

[18] Bansal, R., & Monika, H. (2019, September). Classification Techniques Used in Sentiment Analysis & Prediction of Heart Disease using Data Mining Techniques. In *2019 International Conference on Issues and Challenges in Intelligent Computing Techniques (ICICT)* (Vol. 1, pp. 1–6). IEEE.

[19] Mathew, P. S., Pillai, A. S., & Palade, V. (2018). Applications of IoT in healthcare. In *Cognitive Computing for Big Data Systems Over IoT* (pp. 263–288). Springer, Cham.

[20] Anand, R., Sinha, A., Bhardwaj, A., & Sreeraj, A. (2018). Flawed Security of Social Network of Things. In *Handbook of Research on Network Forensics and Analysis Techniques* (pp. 65–86). IGI Global.

[21] Bishop, M. (2003). What is computer security? *IEEE Security & Privacy, 1*(1), 67–69.

[22] Saini, M. K., Nagal, R., Tripathi, S., Sindhwani, N., & Rudra, A. (2008). PC Interfaced Wireless Robotic Moving Arm. In *AICTE Sponsored National Seminar on Emerging Trends in Software Engineering* (Vol. 50).

[23] Singh, L., Saini, M. K., Tripathi, S., & Sindhwani, N. (2008). An Intelligent Control System For Real-Time Traffic Signal Using Genetic Algorithm. In *AICTE Sponsored National Seminar on Emerging Trends in Software Engineering* (Vol. 50).

[24] Qadri, Y. A., Nauman, A., Zikria, Y. B., Vasilakos, A. V., & Kim, S. W. (2020). The future of healthcare internet of things: A survey of emerging technologies. *IEEE Communications Surveys & Tutorials, 22*(2), 1121–1167.

[25] Yacchirema, D. C., Sarabia-Jácome, D., Palau, C. E., & Esteve, M. (2018). A smart system for sleep monitoring by integrating IoT with big data analytics. *IEEE Access, 6*, 35988–36001.

[26] Saheb, T., & Izadi, L. (2019). Paradigm of IoT big data analytics in the health-care industry: A review of scientific literature and mapping of research trends. *Telematics and Informatics*, *41*, 70–85.

[27] Karimpour, N., Karaduman, B., Ural, A., Challenger, M., & Dagdeviren, O. (2019, June). IoT based hand hygiene compliance monitoring. In *2019 International Symposium on Networks, Computers and Communications (ISNCC)* (pp. 1–6). IEEE.

[28] Anand, R., Singh, B. & Sindhwani, N. (2009). Speech perception & analysis of fluent digits' strings using level-by-level time alignment. *International Journal of Information Technology and Knowledge Management*, *2*(1), 65–68.

[29] Kohli, L., Saurabh, M., Bhatia, I., Shekhawat, U. S., Vijh, M., & Sindhwani, N. (2021). Design and Development of Modular and Multifunctional UAV with Amphibious Landing Module. In *Data Driven Approach Towards Disruptive Technologies: Proceedings of MIDAS 2020* (pp. 405–421). Springer Singapore.

[30] Kohli, L., Saurabh, M., Bhatia, I., Sindhwani, N., & Vijh, M. (2021). Design and Development of Modular and Multifunctional UAV with Amphibious Landing, Processing and Surround Sense Module. *Unmanned Aerial Vehicles for Internet of Things (IoT): Concepts, Techniques, and Applications*, 207.

[31] Chibber, A., Anand, R., & Arora, S. (2021, September). A Staircase Microstrip Patch Antenna for UWB Applications. In *2021 9th International Conference on Reliability, Infocom Technologies and Optimization (Trends and Future Directions)(ICRITO)* (pp. 1–5). IEEE.

[32] Dahiya, A., Anand, R., Sindhwani, N., & Kumar, D. (2021). A Novel Multi-band High-Gain Slotted Fractal Antenna using Various Substrates for X-band and Ku-band Applications. *MAPAN*, 1–9.

[33] Sindhwani, N., & Bhamrah, M. S. (2017). An optimal scheduling and routing under adaptive spectrum-matching framework for MIMO systems. *International Journal of Electronics*, *104*(7), 1238–1253.

[34] Pace, P., Aloi, G., Gravina, R., Caliciuri, G., Fortino, G., & Liotta, A. (2018). An edge-based architecture to support efficient applications for healthcare industry 4.0. *IEEE Transactions on Industrial Informatics*, *15*(1), 481–489.

[35] Somasundaram, R., & Thirugnanam, M. (2020). Review of security challenges in healthcare internet of things. *Wireless Networks*, 1–7.

[36] Rahul, Monika, Ray, P., Kharke, R. B., & Chauhan, S. S. (2021). Cardiovascular Disease Classification Using Different Algorithms. In *Inventive Communication and Computational Technologies* (pp. 189–201). Springer, Singapore.

[37] De Michele, R., & Furini, M. (2019, September). IoT healthcare: Benefits, issues and challenges. In *Proceedings of the 5th EAI international conference on smart objects and technologies for social good* (pp. 160–164).

[38] Kamalraj, R., Neelakandan, S., Kumar, M. R., Rao, V. C. S., Anand, R., & Singh, H. (2021). Interpretable filter based convolutional neural network (IF-CNN) for glucose prediction and classification using PD-SS algorithm. *Measurement*, *183*, 109804.

[39] Singh, H., Rehman, T. B., Gangadhar, C., Anand, R., Sindhwani, N., & Babu, M. (2021). Accuracy detection of coronary artery disease using machine learning algorithms. *Applied Nanoscience*, 1–7.

[40] Khamitkar, S.S., & Rafi, M.(2020). IoT based System for Heart Rate Monitoring. *International Journal of Engineering Research & Technology*, *9*(7). http://dx.doi.org/10.17577/IJERTV9IS070673.

Chapter 11

# Cloud-based artificial intelligence in healthcare systems

*Ghanshyam Raghuwanshi, Deepak Sinwar, and Vijaypal Singh Dhaka*
Manipal University, Jaipur, India

*Yogesh Gupta*
BML Munjal University, Gurgaon, India

## CONTENTS

DOI: 10.1201/9781003239888-11

## II.I INTRODUCTION

Initially, statistical approaches were widely used for extracting the information implicitly, and these approaches were not fruitful for data analysis as these are time-consuming because testing and formulation of hypothesis are the time taking tasks. Moreover, artificial intelligence (AI)/machine learning (ML) has replaced the traditional approaches and acts as a globally accepted approach for data analysis and scientific calculation purposes. ML plays a crucial role in different recent areas. However, there is always the greatest challenge to manage the effectiveness and accuracy of the method in corporation with the ML models. It is a growing field. Whenever it comes along with medical applications, it boosts the efficiency of the working system by providing a better prediction model. It is the process in which patterns are captured automatically from the existing data, and the reason is provided for the prediction of future events or in the diagnosis process. ML approaches change the medical domain with their richer and more advanced techniques. Currently, the Government of India is also promoting various startups [1] in the healthcare field by providing funds and other legal support. Some of the startups like SigTuple, Aindra, Niramai Health Analytix, Advenio Technosys, Ten3T, and QorQL, are employed in the area of medical fields. As per some of the leading reports, it is found that AI and ML [2, 3] will be involved everywhere for answering the queries of the patients related to medical issues, and these answers can be given by applying better and effective ML techniques on the existing data set. Currently, ML is working in the following areas of the medical field:

1. Disease Identification/Diagnosis;
2. Personalized Treatment/Behavioral Modification;
3. Drug Discovery/Manufacturing;
4. Clinical Trial Research;
5. Radiology and Radiotherapy;
6. Smart Electronic Health Records; and
7. Epidemic Outbreak Prediction;

The medical and healthcare system [4] has already been overloaded due to the large population in the countries like India. Developing countries are facing the problem of less-trained health workers and, also at the same time, exploding population. In India, 1:1700 is the proportion or ratio of doctor to patients, and it is very unrealistic as the rule, which is recommended by WHO, says that there must be the ratio of 1:1000. Worldwide many leading companies like Google, MedAware, and Enlitic have already launched their programs for achieving the better healthcare facilities, and these companies are continuously working on massive projects which include ML and AI as key technologies in healthcare. Instead of launching the spontaneous healthcare system, it is better to improvise the existing healthcare system with the

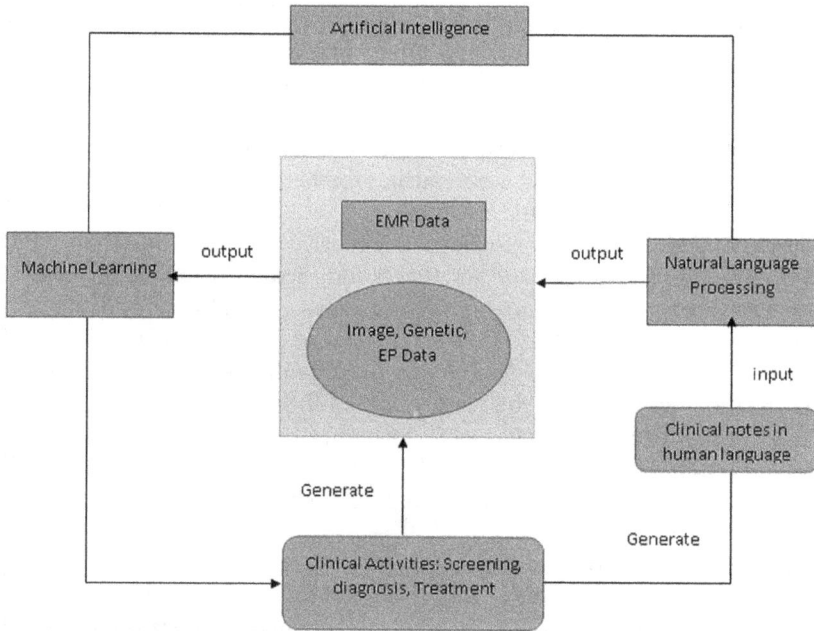

Figure 11.1  Machine learning, artificial intelligence, and natural language processing in healthcare.

latest ML technologies, and this can be helpful in enhancing productivity
along with precision. These technologies can save more lives in a lesser time,
and at the same time, expenses of healthcare systems can be reduced.

Machine Learning (ML) algorithms nowadays have influenced the healthcare system to a greater extent. Various tasks like detection and identification of body parts from medical images [5], lung disease classification [6],
detection of lungs [7], reconstruction of medical images [8, 9], and segmentation of brain tumor [10]. Nowadays, various applications of ML and AI
are working on analyzing clinical data and healthcare services. However,
analysis of the clinical data belongs to two categories: structured and
unstructured data. Meanwhile, genes, images, and biomarkers belong to the
unstructured data, whereas medical history, notes related to diseases, and
various medical journals come in the category of unstructured data.
Structured data can be better dealt with ML approaches, whereas unstructured data can be better dealt with by the specialized Natural Language
Processing (NLP) approaches as shown in Figure 11.1.

The advantages of AI have been discussed to the point where human physicians can be replaced by AI-based systems. AI can be used in the healthcare
system in different ways. It can be used for learning the attributes or features
from the huge data set of healthcare, and these features can be used for better assistance in the clinical process along with treatment, and this assistance

can be done by getting better insights into the system. Analysis of real-time data can be done by extracting useful information from the huge populated patient data set, and the patient can be instructed to be aware of the risk alert of a particular disease and also the health outcome prediction. The analysis of tests such as X-rays, computed tomography scans, and magnetic resonance images can also be done using the better AI tools and can reach any conclusion based on analysis.

Some of the clinical processes cannot be performed accurately, and there are some chances of diagnostic and therapeutic errors. However, the involvement of AI reduces the chances of these kinds of errors by introducing some specific error handling models. Better assistance to the patients can be provided by getting help from AI that can provide up-to-date medical knowledge to the physicians and thus results in better patient care. AI can manage medical records and analyze the performance of an individual institution and the whole healthcare system. AI can also be helpful in developing the model where digital consultations can be done by having digital nurses and doctors.

As far as the role of cloud computing in healthcare is concerned, it is the prime resource by which the cost of the healthcare system can be reduced to a greater extent, and at the same time, unbreakable service infrastructure can be provided at a minimum cost. It has been concluded by various researchers [11–13] that cloud computing can minimize the expanses in setting up Electronic Health Record (EHR) by providing the services of networking, hardware, software, and licensing fees at a minimum cost. However, it also ensures uninterruptable services to the customers.

Earlier attempts have been made toward improving healthcare services through the cloud computing infrastructure [12–19]. Rolim et. Al [20] introduced a new cloud-based system for collecting patient information from the network through a self-automated process, and hence, it eliminates the need for manual data collection, which may lead to typing errors and also relax the deployment process. Basically, the network is connected with the sensors [21–24] in the healthcare devices. This infrastructure also helps in distributing the required information on the cloud of medical centers, which facilitates the storage of data, processing, and distribution securely. The main advantages of the system are that it collects real-time data for local processing. However, there are some protocols proposed for cloud management. The method mentioned in [25] deals with the security-related issues in mobile devices while working in the cloud environment. It provides security as a service for mobile devices. This system relaxes the mobile devices from heavily loaded multimedia and security algorithms and facilitates the mobile devices to work effectively even with low memory and with lesser local resources. Another initiative came into existence that has been mentioned in Ref. [26]. This system provided anytime and anywhere services to doctors or physicians for accessing their patient's information. This system is leveraged with the power of wireless [27–29] along with cloud computing. The method in Ref. [30] proves its effectiveness for the emergency kinds of medical services which work for the Greek National Health Service by integrating the emergency system with the personal health record systems.

Further, cloud computing managed its presence in bio-informatics research also. Cloud-based system proposed in Ref. [31] works like a framework for colorectal cancer where medical images are analyzed for clinical and research use. Elastic Compute Cloud or EC2 is one of the services which is provided by amazon cloud, and this EC2 service is deployed by the method proposed in Ref. [32]. This approach uses 100 nodes for assembling or simulating the complete human genome, and a Sequence Search Alignment by Hashing algorithm is used for managing and aligning the 140 million reads. The authors in Ref. [33] also used the same Amazon's EC2 for calculating the relationship among 245,323 genome-to-genome. EC2 cloud service takes around 200 hours with an approximate cost of 8000 dollars. Although it seems higher in terms of cost, it is approximately 40% lesser than the system without cloud services. Harvard Medical School also avails the services of the cloud for developing genetic testing models which are used for managing a huge amount of information in very less time [34].

Apart from the academic research industry, some of the top-level software companies are also dealing in clouds for providing and offering better services for medical records. These companies are investing a huge amount in cloud infrastructures. World-class companies like Microsoft's HealthVault, Oracle's Exalogic Elastic Cloud and Amazon Web Services (AWS) are providing personal health-related data on their cloud servers. So, they can get the money in favor of their services to the clients. Also, the use of health cloud computing is reported worldwide [35].

We are living in the era of AI where a system can take over a large number of tasks. Moreover, as human beings and as a matter of fact, innovations are readily available to us. However, a combination of AI with the cloud can bring a major transformation in our healthcare systems. In the absence of the cloud, one can have better intelligence and classification techniques. If the data availability is too poor, then the technology and intelligence may not be able to make a proper justice with less data. A recent survey says that the worldwide market is totally captured by AI, and now, it will be reaching toward 89 billion dollars by 2025. This growth will further be fueled by the integration of AI with cloud infrastructure services.

Over the years, now, we have better healthcare systems with a richer cloud infrastructure along with ML techniques, which are basically the subset of AI-based approaches [36, 37]. Cloud provides a more cost-effective system for healthcare organizations by storing health-related data on cloud servers in a more cost-effective manner. Once we have a substantial availability of the data, ML [38] can play its role in better understanding and analysis of the medical data and in order to get better precision and accuracy of the data over a large period. However, the availability of a huge amount of medical data also makes the ML techniques more scalable, and these can be tested for different sizes and types of data sets at different points of time. The ML techniques after reaching any decision at one cloud site can also be sent over the network (i.e., over the different cloud servers) for testing and verification of the ML models on different datasets. Hence, it opens the door for more challenging and faster research opportunities. At this point, ML models can send their recommendations for treating individual patients suffering from chronic diseases, and as a result, it can minimize the unnecessary visits to emergency department.

Now, the time has come, when the researcher must seek the path where AI-based cloud computing and its implications must be used for improving the conditions and outcomes of the patients soon. This conjunction of the cloud with the AI facilitates us to do more insight research on a vast amount of healthcare data in this interconnected world of people. The future of the medical and healthcare system is depending on advancement, and new trends are occurring in cloud computing and AI.

## 11.2 HEALTH CLOUD COMPUTING OPPORTUNITIES AND CHALLENGES

Present research indicates that later or sooner within five years more than 75% of industries and small size organizations will require cloud services to fulfilling their needs. A large number of people, who are subscribing to cloud services, are increasing day by day, and this number can reach one billion in near future. Especially, in the health sector, most of the originations, experts, and managers believe that the inclusion of cloud services in healthcare will result in a better environment for research as well as medical facilities. Involvement of the cloud [39] in healthcare provides many opportunities as well as challenges in implementing and managing the services of the cloud. It requires the rigorous evaluation of the cloud before its widespread use and adoption through the network. There are some challenges and issues in the cloud when integrating it with healthcare from the perspective of legality, technology, management, and security.

## 11.3 MANAGEMENT ASPECTS OF CLOUD

As far as the management aspect of cloud computing is concerned, it is cost-effective to manage and avail the services of the cloud. Healthcare can manage the cost-effective and on-premises solution for different experiments and medical data with various facilities using the cloud computing services. IT services can be available for evaluation purposes in healthcare without purchasing the hardware and software resources. Due to this freedom, nowadays, healthcare systems can focus more on their operation part and critical tasks without worrying about the additional costs of IT staff and the training process.

At the same time, there might be challenges along with opportunities in the cloud system. The challenges may include privacy of the user, issues in data security, loss of governance, and sometimes undefined provider's agreement. Trust is the heart of any cloud system for its client, and it comes in concern when personal sensitive data move over the cloud computing model. In some challenging environments, service providers cannot guarantee the efficacy of the privacy controls and security concerns. Finally, if the provider does not meet the security and management requirement (e.g., applicable laws, regulations, standards, contracts, or policy changes), then the security, as well as the investment of the customer, may be at risk.

## 11.4 TECHNICAL ASPECTS OF CLOUD

As far as the technical aspect of cloud computing is concerned, there are a lot of opportunities and challenges. Hospitals, laboratories, and medical practices do not possess the in-house IT staff for maintaining the services and applications like EHRs. Cloud computing provides the opportunity to have IT services for medical staff and the whole healthcare system without worrying about the high cost of high maintenance, and EHRs adoption can be done efficiently [40, 41] at a low cost. Apart from opportunities, many technical challenges persist. These include the exhaustion of resources, data transfer bottlenecks, unpredictability in performance, bugs, and data lock-in issues. Most of the time, it has been observed that service providers over-commit to the healthcare systems due to the high competition in the market. However, they have failed in providing quality service and infrastructure. In order to gain a higher profit, cost cutting has also been introduced in the services of the cloud. However, healthcare organizations do not compromise on the quality and infrastructure services of the cloud because it requires a high level of accuracy and precision in medical trials and operations. Therefore, it is a great challenge for the cloud service providers to manage and assure quality services to the healthcare organization.

## 11.5 SECURITY ASPECTS OF CLOUD IN HEALTHCARE

Data lock-in is the greatest challenge for the healthcare system which is taking the services of the cloud. In most cases, healthcare systems may move the data from one service provider to another or to an in-house environment due to some personal reasons. For example, Google health services have been discontinued from January 2012, and in this case, users are supposed to download their personal health-related data. Unfortunately, most cloud service providers do not provide application and service interoperability.

Due to this reason, migration the data from one to another service provider gets difficult due to compatibility issues. So, if any healthcare system uses the services of some cloud provider, then in any case if the provider denies to continue its services, then migration of health data will be the greatest challenge. Biomedical laboratories for research may require need to repeatedly download and upload huge amounts of medical data from the cloud. Cloud application customers may feel the bottleneck in the data transfer due to the limited bandwidth, and this may suffer the clinical and medical operations and experiments. It is highly recommended for the cloud service provider to manage the bandwidth for the healthcare organizations to interrupt the services throughout the day.

Security is a very crucial aspect of the cloud in healthcare organizations. However, it is cheaper to manage the security issues at a larger scale on the cloud. For example, management of software, hardware, human resources, and management costs is lesser on the clouds. Due to the security and data availability reasons, data are replicated in multiple locations. This redundancy results in increasing data independence and, hence, manages the data recovery in the case of any failure. In addition to this, cloud service providers can relocate the resources and data dynamically to different locations for filtering, traffic management, and encryption in order to achieve a defensive security system against distributed denial-of-service attacks [42].

Apart from opportunities, it is a great matter of discussion regarding the security loopholes and challenges in the cloud environment such as attacks by hackers on sensitive medical data, breaks in the network, and poor management of encryption key. Generally, cloud servers are accessible to various customers. It is the responsibility of the provider to separate the resources. If the provider is unable to separate the resources of different clients, it may lead to a serious security risk. In some cases, the customers delete their unwanted data on virtual infrastructure, and it is the issue with various distributed operating systems that data will not be deleted immediacy, and meanwhile, that data can be accessed by other users. This results in a higher security risk to the cloud users than with dedicated hardware.

## 11.5.1 Legal aspects on cloud in healthcare

Besides the security threats in the cloud computing environment, there are also some legal issues like intellectual property rights, data privacy, and jurisdiction which are associated with the healthy cloud environment. Among all three, privacy and data jurisdiction are the major legal issue of concern and the most common issue of concern [42–45]. Different jurisdictions may impose different restrictions and rules on data security and usage and also on intellectual properties. Healthcare systems are very sensitive to jurisdiction and intellectual property rights. For example, the US Health Insurance Portability and Accountability Act (HIPAA) [46] denies cloud computing companies to share or restrict personal healthcare data with non-associated third parties. Moreover, the cloud service provider may replicate and transfer the data of its client in multiple jurisdictions without taking the concern of the client. Medical data in the cloud may have multiple legal places at the same time, with divergent legal significances.

## 11.6 BENEFITS OF CLOUD COMPUTING IN HEALTHCARE

Cloud computing offers numerous benefits to healthcare services. A few of them are highlighted as follows:

### 11.6.1 Intelligent visions

It is the beauty of cloud computing that all the stakeholders can be benefitted and empowered like patients, doctors, and management due to the more accurate processed data (information) for decision-making purposes.

### 11.6.2 Anticipative service

Better anticipation can be provided by better monitoring of the risks and threats which incorporate the better recommendation for dealing with abnormal situations in the future. This helps in managing the issues before they appear.

### 11.6.3 Higher transparency in system

It provides a huge system with great transparency where doctors and patients can utilize the services freely in a fearless environment. It provides great potential to the healthcare industry.

### 11.6.4 Complex picture

Cloud provides the data from the best possible sources and helps the healthcare teams in accessing the health-related data with more accuracy. Because the sources of the data will be multiple, greater role will be played by the cloud server along with the AI techniques in refining the data in a more accurate way.

### 11.6.5 Working with big data

It provides the input for the various industries where research is going on health-related big data [47] like medical images and prescription effectiveness on some set of diseases. In cloud computing, analytics can work with huge data sets, including active and extendable environments.

### 11.6.6 Accurate decision-making and treatment

The effectiveness of the medicines can be better calculated by AI-based techniques or by pro-data analysis. These pro-data can be found on various cloud servers which can help in making accurate decisions, and millions of lives can be saved and served in this way. There must be lesser errors in the medical area, and hence, better analytics and cloud data can also reduce the substantial medical errors.

### 11.6.7 Cost-effectiveness

It is always better to have services through the cloud on a rental basis instead of purchasing huge software which may lead to the overall high cost for the healthcare systems. That is why it is cheaper to avail of the services of the cloud instead of purchasing the complete infrastructure.

### 11.6.8 Great flexibility

Industry needs can be better adjusted in a fast and more accurate manner in the healthcare systems with the help of the cloud.

### 11.7 CLOUD COMPUTING ISSUES IN HEALTHCARE

In addition to providing several benefits to the healthcare industry, cloud computing suffers from various issues. Some of the issues are highlighted as follows:

### 11.7.1 Absence of good specialists

Although we have good healthcare workers and also a better healthcare infrastructure, still the main challenge of cloud computing in the healthcare systems is that despite having the raw data related to healthcare still, we are facing problems as we do not have good software specialists at all the places. This scarcity of software specialist may lead to serious consequences for the healthcare industry.

### 11.7.2 Limited functionality

Although cloud computing provides the base for huge data collection related to healthcare system, its functionalities are limited in analyzing the medical data. For better and effective analytical architecture, there will always be a need for AI approaches, data management techniques, and smart connected devices.

## 11.7.3 Security issues

The data are migrated from one cloud server to other cloud servers and from one network to another network. Sometimes, confidential data needs to be transmitted from one server to another for making it available to the nearby healthcare industry. This movement of confidential data throws a greater challenge to the researcher because there might be security issues, and handling these huge data might be a bigger challenge. In healthcare systems, medical practitioners may meet some privacy challenges in the cloud computing environment.

## 11.8 AI APPLICATION AREAS IN HEALTHCARE

Nowadays, AI is involved in almost all the areas of real-world applications and has replaced the traditional approaches of problem-solving with advanced computational techniques. The ability of AI-based techniques has proved that these are better than human abilities for performing specific tasks, for example, image [48, 49] and speech recognition [50]. Table 11.1 depicts a few applications of AI in the field of medical and healthcare as follows:

## 11.9 SOME REPRESENTATIVE HEALTHCARE SYSTEMS BASED ON CLOUD

Some representative systems are working in the healthcare industries such as the public cloud in Germany [51] and Sesam Vitale [52] in France. Netlink and Netcards developed a system that was focused on a huge trans-European network of health services for mobile citizens [53, 54], Palm vein-based health care [55–58]. Furthermore, new research was done for the card-based healthcare system for Slovenians which maintains the information of the patients and diseases on cards, and these cards were accepted for health-related operations and other activities. However, this was the newest invention ever which maintained the information of the patient at the national level [56, 59].

In the current era, dealing with healthcare issues for the developing as well as for developed countries is the biggest challenge. However, the inclusion of cloud services in the healthcare industry relaxes many managing authorities. As shown in Figure 11.2, if the record is managed on the cloud, then it is easier to maintain and at the same time services provided by healthcare can be improved both in time and quality.

Healthcare accreditation group released a report earlier which says that most of the time it has been observed that miscommunication among the healthcare representatives and patients leads the serious consequences for

*Table 11.1* Applications of AI in healthcare systems

| Technology | Application description | Application area |
|---|---|---|
| Robotics | It provides the best quality handling and cure by refining the precision and accuracy of the clinical procedures | Medical device, Health IT |
| Digital secretary | It monitors the condition of patients continuously and alerts the nursing staff and other doctors whenever necessary by raising alarming signals | Medical device, Health IT |
| Machine learning | Medical data analysis and prediction on healthcare data and patterns can be done which reduces the uncertainty issue in the medical treatment and decision-making process, and it takes a vast amount of diagnosed data of medical images for self-learning as an input | Diagnostic medical image, Health IT |
| Image processing | Medical images can be deeply analyzed, and judgment can be taken on the diseases regarding the disease types to obtain positive and negative results | Diagnostic medical image, Health IT |
| Natural language processing | Unstructured text data are converted into medical charts that can be easily understood and interrupted | Medical device, Health IT |
| Voice recognition | Can capture patient voice and language and store important information in electronic medical records | Medical device, Health IT |
| Natural language processing | Can convert long unstructured text data, such as medical charts, to be easily read and interpreted | Medical device, Health IT |
| Statistical analysis | Statistical approaches analyze the pre-existing health data of patients and predict the patient treatment results of health record data | Medical device, Health IT |

both patients and healthcare systems. In developing countries like India, due to illiteracy, there is a huge gap between patient saying and healthcare system perception. Mentally challenged, physically disabled, and dumb patients are not able to express their medical diseases and illness history to the medical practitioners. This is a major reason behind the higher death percentage in developed countries. However, with the increased growth in digitalization and multimedia devices, health-related data can possibly be gathered digitally and stored on the Cloud server. Countries like India will be more benefitted by the cloud-related services in the healthcare system because patient–to-doctor ratio in India is very high, and also, the number of hospitals is very less in order to fulfill the requirement of people.

Cloud will help us only in managing the medical data on the server and can be used for further research purposes. However, research on medical data can be more fruitful and beneficial by including more analysis using AI and ML approaches as shown in Figure 11.3.

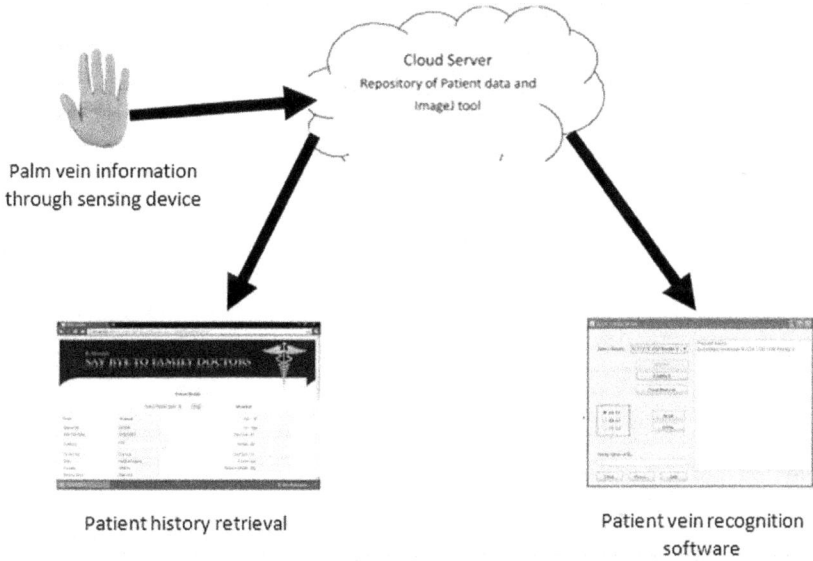

Palm vein information
through sensing device

Patient history retrieval

Patient vein recognition
software

*Figure 11.2* Cloud service for health care.

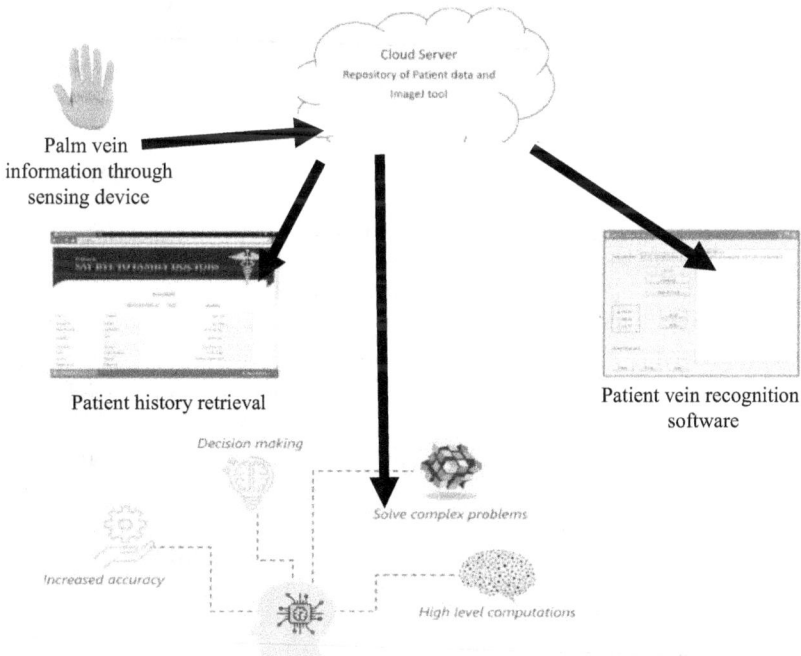

Palm vein
information through
sensing device

Patient history retrieval

Patient vein recognition
software

Decision making

Solve complex problems

Increased accuracy

High level computations

*Figure 11.3* Artificial intelligence and cloud server in healthcare system.

A method proposed Ref. [58] implements the palm vein pattern identification system which maintains the medical records of the patients on the cloud server and can be retrieved from the server by matching the pattern of the palm vein of patients. Somehow, this approach can reduce the burden at the places where patient registration and medical history management are the greatest issues. In this system, patients will put their palm on the sensor and medical records from the cloud server will be fetched based on the matched pattern. Distributed computing technology is coming in new forms such as Grid computing and Cloud computing. The introduction of Grid and Distributed Computing along with Information Technology (IT) led to a service concerned with developing software as a service (SaaS) using Cloud computing. This sets the goal for achieving better medical facilities in emergency medical situations also.

Apart from this, another system is also developed which helps the medical practitioners for getting better tools for processing and analyzing medical images. Further enhancement comes when mobile cloud computing is added to the healthcare systems as proposed in [60]. Mobile web servers and cloud computing work together to form a more promising architecture. Nowadays, due to the more revolution in handheld devices, it can be said that Mobile Cloud Computing is working like a heart or kernel for the transformation process of our traditional healthcare systems. This method took inspiration from Mobile Cloud Computing and proposed a system based on mobile medical web service for example, implementation of a Medical Cloud Multi-Agent Solution for polyclinic ESSALEMA Sfax—TUNISIA, using Google's Android operating system.

Nowadays, rich computing techniques have made their opportunities by accelerating the things related to medical and healthcare, and now, it is seeking its path in the hospitals, life sciences, and clinics. It makes sense to deal and analyze the large medical data of patients with greater accuracy, which is stored on cloud servers by availing the services of ML and AI services.

As per the survey done by Amazon Web Services (AWS), it is observed that around 94% healthcare persons feel that Artificial Intelligence and Cloud computing can better help the healthcare industry by minimizing unnecessary spending with great patient experience along with improved service quality.

It takes a very long time for the collection of healthcare data, and it also requires a lot of computing power in crunching the medical data for extracting meaningful information for the welfare of society, it is. Hence, it is a tedious task to transfer the data safely and securely from one server to another server. The development of efficient and adaptable ML models is also the biggest challenge to face for efficient healthcare systems. We use the power of cloud computing to automatically read documents and create data sets that can be used by data scientists to train and build models.

Computer vision in healthcare contributes to medical image analysis, cancer detection, lesion detection and classification, and measures blood lost

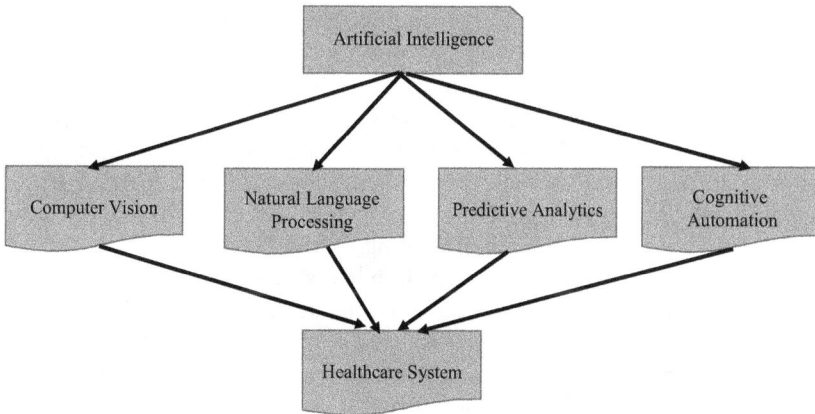

*Figure 11.4* Artificial Intelligence techniques in healthcare.

during surgeries, precise diagnosis. Computer vision can also support the medical system by saving the times of physicians and doctors with the automation of the report analysis process which results in fruitful and personalized advice.

On the other hand, NLP takes raw data as input such as summarizing clinical notes or academic journal articles, unstructured Electronic Health Record, question generation for the medical knowledge base, and self-configurable chatbots as shown in Figure 11.4. So, unstructured data can be transformed into meaningful information through NLP, and it makes sense for unstructured data. Generally, doctors and physicians record the patient's unstructured data in the notes section, and if these data are not mapped in the EMR, then they may be lost. These unstructured data will be processed with the NLP algorithms, and we can extract risk factors from these notes. In the end, risk scores and patient utilization patterns are calculated or predicted by predictive analytics. We can also predict the side effects and benefits of medicines on human bodies under different conditions such as countries, age groups, and temperature by doing the predictive analytics on the patient EHR data.

## 11.10 CONCLUSION

AI cloud technology is the most awaited innovation in the field of medical science. Limitation of data availability at low cost is now managed by the cloud computing infrastructure at low cost [61]. However, the integration of AI with cloud services does the proper justice to the AI models. This integration opens the path to the researchers as well as to the healthcare system for improving their research area to a greater extent. Nowadays, in the COVID-19 pandemic situation, AI plays a vital role in the identification of different versions of viruses [62]. It cannot be possible without the huge availability of COVID data sets [63] which is provided by the cloud infrastructure. The newly available AI- and cloud-based healthcare infrastructure [64] has proven outstanding results in precisely diagnosing and classifying patient circumstances and forecasting the sequence of diseases by using the gathered medical dataset. Eventually, better treatment and better learning for the medical staff can be expected with the hybrid AI- and cloud-based healthcare systems by providing the decision-making on the treatment process [65]. In order to maintain the safety, privacy, liability, and security of the data [66], still cloud computing infrastructures are facing a lot of challenges. Data integrity and security on cloud servers are the greatest challenges nowadays. Researchers are now working toward this area for establishing the faith of customers. There must be some set of rules and guidelines for the cloud services along with the systematic chances of improvement in the future, and this will guarantee a better, safe, and trusted healthcare system.

## REFERENCES

[1] Government Schemes, URL: https://www.startupindia.gov.in/content/sih/en/government-schemes.html [Available online, visited March 20, 2021].

[2] Anand, R., Shrivastava, G., Gupta, S., Peng, S. L., & Sindhwani, N. (2018). Audio Watermarking with Reduced Number of Random Samples. In *Handbook of Research on Network Forensics and Analysis Techniques* (pp. 372–394). IGI Global.

[3] Sindhwani, N., Verma, S., Bajaj, T., & Anand, R. (2021). Comparative analysis of intelligent driving and safety assistance systems using YOLO and SSD model of deep learning. *International Journal of Information System Modeling and Design (IJISMD)*, *12*(1), 131–146.

[4] Juneja, S., Juneja, A., & Anand, R. (2020). Healthcare 4.0-digitizing healthcare using big data for performance improvisation. *Journal of Computational and Theoretical Nanoscience*, *17*(9–10), 4408–4410.

[5] Yan, Z., Zhan, Y., Peng, Z., Liao, S., Shinagawa, Y., Zhang, S., ... & Zhou, X. S. (2016). Multi-instance deep learning: Discover discriminative local anatomies for bodypart recognition. *IEEE Transactions on Medical Imaging*, *35*(5), 1332–1343.

[6] Anthimopoulos, M., Christodoulidis, S., Ebner, L., Christe, A., & Mougiakakou, S. (2016). Lung pattern classification for interstitial lung diseases using a deep convolutional neural network. *IEEE Transactions on Medical Imaging*, *35*(5), 1207–1216.

[7] Shen, W., Zhou, M., Yang, F., Yang, C., & Tian, J. (2015, June). Multi-scale convolutional neural networks for lung nodule classification. In *International Conference on Information Processing in Medical Imaging* (pp. 588–599). Springer, Cham.

[8] Schlemper, J., Caballero, J., Hajnal, J. V., Price, A., & Rueckert, D. (2017, June). A deep cascade of convolutional neural networks for MR image reconstruction. In *International Conference on Information Processing in Medical Imaging* (pp. 647–658). Springer, Cham.

[9] Mehta, J., & Majumdar, A. (2017). Rodeo: Robust de-aliasing autoencoder for real-time medical image reconstruction. *Pattern Recognition, 63*, 499–510.

[10] Havaei, M., Davy, A., Warde-Farley, D., Biard, A., Courville, A., Bengio, Y., ... & Larochelle, H. (2017). Brain tumor segmentation with deep neural networks. *Medical Image Analysis, 35*, 18–31.

[11] Calabrese, B., & Cannataro, M. (2015). Cloud computing in healthcare and biomedicine. *Scalable Computing: Practice and Experience, 16*(1), 1–18.

[12] Sittig, D. F., & Singh, H. (2009). Eight rights of safe electronic health record use. *JAMA, 302*(10), 1111–1113.

[13] Wang, X., & Tan, Y. (2010, October). Application of cloud computing in the health information system. In *2010 International Conference on Computer Application and System Modeling (ICCASM 2010)* (Vol. 1, pp. V1–179). IEEE.

[14] He, C., Jin, X., Zhao, Z., & Xiang, T. (2010, October). A cloud computing solution for hospital information system. In *2010 IEEE International Conference on Intelligent Computing and Intelligent Systems* (Vol. 2, pp. 517–520). IEEE.

[15] Botts, N., Thoms, B., Noamani, A., & Horan, T. A. (2010, January). Cloud computing architectures for the underserved: Public health cyberinfrastructures through a network of healthatms. In *2010 43rd Hawaii International Conference on System Sciences* (pp. 1–10). IEEE.

[16] Yang, C. T., Chen, L. T., Chou, W. L., & Wang, K. C. (2010, December). Implementation of a medical image file accessing system on cloud computing. In *2010 13th IEEE International Conference on Computational Science and Engineering* (pp. 321–326). IEEE.

[17] Hoang, D. B., & Chen, L. (2010, December). Mobile cloud for assistive healthcare (MoCAsH). In *2010 IEEE Asia-Pacific Services Computing Conference* (pp. 325–332). IEEE.

[18] Guo, L., Chen, F., Chen, L., & Tang, X. (2010, April). The building of cloud computing environment for e-health. In *2010 International Conference on E-Health Networking Digital Ecosystems and Technologies (EDT)* (Vol. 1, pp. 89–92). IEEE.

[19] Alagöz, F., Valdez, A. C., Wilkowska, W., Ziefle, M., Dorner, S., & Holzinger, A. (2010, December). From cloud computing to mobile Internet, from user focus to culture and hedonism: The crucible of mobile health care and wellness applications. In *5th International Conference on Pervasive Computing and Applications* (pp. 38–45). IEEE.

[20] Rolim, C. O., Koch, F. L., Westphall, C. B., Werner, J., Fracalossi, A., & Salvador, G. S. (2010, February). A cloud computing solution for patient's data collection in health care institutions. In *2010 Second International Conference on eHealth, Telemedicine, and Social Medicine* (pp. 95–99). IEEE.

[21] Singh, L., Saini, M. K., Tripathi, S., & Sindhwani, N. (2008). An intelligent control system for real-time traffic signal using genetic algorithm. In *AICTE Sponsored National Seminar on Emerging Trends in Software Engineering* (Vol. 50).

[22] Saini, M. K., Nagal, R., Tripathi, S., Sindhwani, N., & Rudra, A. (2008). PC interfaced wireless robotic moving arm. In *AICTE Sponsored National Seminar on Emerging Trends in Software Engineering* (Vol. 50).

[23] Kohli, L., Saurabh, M., Bhatia, I., Shekhawat, U. S., Vijh, M., & Sindhwani, N. (2021). Design and development of modular and multifunctional UAV with amphibious landing module. In *Data Driven Approach Towards Disruptive Technologies: Proceedings of MIDAS 2020* (pp. 405–421). Springer, Singapore.

[24] Kohli, L., Saurabh, M., Bhatia, I., Sindhwani, N., & Vijh, M. (2021). Design and Development of Modular and Multifunctional UAV with Amphibious Landing, Processing and Surround Sense Module. In *Unmanned Aerial Vehicles for Internet of Things (IoT): Concepts, Techniques, and Applications* (p. 207).

[25] Nkosi, M. T., & Mekuria, F. (2010, November). Cloud computing for enhanced mobile health applications. In *2010 IEEE Second International Conference on Cloud Computing Technology and Science* (pp. 629–633). IEEE.

[26] Rao, G. S. V., Sundararaman, K., & Parthasarathi, J. (2010, October). Dhatri-A Pervasive Cloud initiative for primary healthcare services. In *2010 14th International Conference on Intelligence in Next Generation Networks* (pp. 1–6). IEEE.

[27] Meelu, R., & Anand, R. (2010 November), Energy efficiency of cluster based routing protocols used in wireless sensor networks. In *AIP Conference Proceedings* (Vol. 1324, No. 1, pp. 109–113). American Institute of Physics.

[28] Garg, P., & Anand, R. (2011). Energy efficient data collection in wireless sensor network. *Dronacharya Research Journal*, 3(1), 41–45.

[29] Paliwal, K. K., Anand, R., & Garg, P. Energy efficient data collection in wireless sensor network-a survey. In 2011 *International Conference on Advanced Computing, Communication and Networks*, 824–827.

[30] Koufi, V., Malamateniou, F., & Vassilacopoulos, G. (2010, November). Ubiquitous access to cloud emergency medical services. In *Proceedings of the 10th IEEE International Conference on Information Technology and Applications in Biomedicine* (pp. 1–4). IEEE.

[31] Avila-Garcia, M. S., Trefethen, A. E., Brady, M., Gleeson, F., & Goodman, D. (2008, December). Lowering the barriers to cancer imaging. In *2008 IEEE Fourth International Conference on eScience* (pp. 63–70). IEEE.

[32] Bateman, A., & Wood, M. (2009). *Cloud Computing*.

[33] Kudtarkar, P., DeLuca, T. F., Fusaro, V. A., Tonellato, P. J., & Wall, D. P. (2010). Cost-effective cloud computing: A case study using the comparative genomics tool, roundup. *Evolutionary Bioinformatics*, 6, EBO-S6259.

[34] Schmieding, M. L., Mörgeli, R., Schmieding, M. A., Feufel, M. A., & Balzer, F. (2021). Benchmarking triage capability of symptom checkers against that of medical laypersons: Survey study. *Journal of Medical Internet Research*, 23(3), e24475.

[35] Sharma, D. K., Chakravarthi, D. S., Shaikh, A. A., Ahmed, A. A. A., Jaiswal, S., & Naved, M. (2021). The aspect of vast data management problem in healthcare sector and implementation of cloud computing technique. *Materials Today: Proceedings*.

[36] Jiang, F., Jiang, Y., Zhi, H., Dong, Y., Li, H., Ma, S., ... & Wang, Y. (2017). Artificial intelligence in healthcare: Past, present and future. *Stroke and Vascular Neurology*, 2(4).

[37] Pesapane, F., Codari, M., & Sardanelli, F. (2018). Artificial intelligence in medical imaging: Threat or opportunity? Radiologists again at the forefront of innovation in medicine. *European Radiology Experimental*, 2(1), 1–10.

[38] Bakshi, G., Shukla, R., Yadav, V., Dahiya, A., Anand, R., Sindhwani, N., & Singh, H. (2021). An optimized approach for feature extraction in multi-relational statistical learning. *Journal of Scientific & Industrial Research*, 80, 537–542.

[39] Sajid, A., & Abbas, H. (2016). Data privacy in cloud-assisted healthcare systems: State of the art and future challenges. *Journal of Medical Systems*, *40*(6), 155.

[40] Sindhwani, N., Bhamrah, M. S., Garg, A., & Kumar, D. (2017, July). Performance analysis of particle swarm optimization and genetic algorithm in MIMO systems. In *2017 8th International Conference on Computing, Communication and Networking Technologies (ICCCNT)* (pp. 1–6). IEEE.

[41] Sindhwani, N., & Singh, M. (2016). FFOAS: Antenna selection for MIMO wireless communication system using firefly optimisation algorithm and scheduling. *International Journal of Wireless and Mobile Computing*, *10*(1), 48–55.

[42] Pearson, S. (2009, May). Taking account of privacy when designing cloud computing services. In *2009 ICSE Workshop on Software Engineering Challenges of Cloud Computing* (pp. 44–52). IEEE.

[43] Svantesson, D., & Clarke, R. (2010). Privacy and consumer risks in cloud computing. *Computer Law & Security Review*, *26*(4), 391–397.

[44] Mather, T., Kumaraswamy, S., & Latif, S. (2009). *Cloud Security and Privacy: An Enterprise Perspective on Risks and Compliance*. O'Reilly Media, Inc.

[45] Kuner, C. (2010). Data protection law and international jurisdiction on the Internet (part 1). *International Journal of Law and Information Technology*, *18*(2), 176–193.

[46] Act, A. (1996). Health insurance portability and accountability act of 1996. *Public Law*, *104*, 191.

[47] Sansanwal, K., Shrivastava, G., Anand, R., & Sharma, K. (2019). Big Data Analysis and Compression for Indoor Air Quality. In *Handbook of IoT and Big Data* (pp. 1–21). CRC Press.

[48] Gupta, M., & Anand, R. (2011). Color image compression using set of selected bit planes. *International Journal of Electronics & Communication Technology*, *2*(3), 243–248.

[49] Kumar, R., Anand, R., & Kaushik, G. (2011). Image compression using wavelet method & SPIHT algorithm. *Digital Image Processing*, *3*(2), 75–79.

[50] Anand, R., Singh, B. & Sindhwani, N. (2009). Speech perception & analysis of fluent digits' strings using level-by-level time alignment. *International Journal of Information Technology and Knowledge Management*, *2*(1), 65–68.

[51] Kardas, G., & Tunali, E. T. (2006). Design and implementation of a smart card based healthcare information system. *Computer Methods and Programs in Biomedicine*, *81*(1), 66–78.

[52] Bédère, P. (1997). The SESAM-Vitale system. In *Health Cards' 97* (pp. 123–125). IOS Press.

[53] Vikas, S., Gurudatt, K., Vishnu, M., & Prashant, K. (2013). Private vs public cloud. *International Journal of Computer Science & Communication Networks*, *3*(2), 79.

[54] Vossberg, M., Tolxdorff, T., & Krefting, D. (2008). DICOM image communication in globus-based medical grids. *IEEE Transactions on Information Technology in Biomedicine*, *12*(2), 145–153.

[55] Latha, N. A., Murthy, B. R., & Sunitha, U. (2012). Smart card based integrated electronic health record system for clinical practice. *International Journal of Advanced Computer Science and Applications*, *3*(10). http://dx.doi.org/10.14569/IJACSA.2012.031021.

[56] Heathfield, H. A., Peel, V., Hudson, P., Kay, S., Mackay, L., Marley, T., ... & Williams, J. (1997). Evaluating large scale health information systems: From practice towards theory. In *Proceedings of the AMIA Annual Fall Symposium* (p. 116). American Medical Informatics Association.

[57] Ferro Castro, B. J. (1969). Pattern-oriented software architecture: A system of patterns. *Computación y Sistemas, 1*(2), 1–4.

[58] Watanabe, M., Endoh, T., Shiohara, M., & Sasaki, S. (2005, September). Palm vein authentication technology and its applications. In *Proceedings of the Biometric Consortium Conference* (pp. 19–21).

[59] Kardas, G., & Tunali, E. T. (2006). Design and implementation of a smart card based healthcare information system. *Computer Methods and Programs in Biomedicine, 81*(1), 66–78.

[60] Hanen, J., Kechaou, Z., & Ayed, M. B. (2016). An enhanced healthcare system in mobile cloud computing environment. *Vietnam Journal of Computer Science, 3*(4), 267–277.

[61] Anand, R., Sindhwani, N., & Saini, A. (2021). Emerging Technologies for COVID-19. In *Enabling Healthcare 4.0 for Pandemics: A Roadmap Using AI, Machine Learning, IoT and Cognitive Technologies* (pp. 163–188).

[62] Ahmed, A., Abdul Hanan, A., Omprakash, K., Lobiyal, D. K., & Raw, R. S. (2018). Cloud computing in VANETs: Architecture, taxonomy and challenges. *IETE Technical Review, 35*, 523–547.

[63] Jain, S., Kumar, M., Sindhwani, N., & Singh, P. (2021). SARS-Cov-2 detection using deep learning techniques on the basis of clinical reports. In *2021 9th International Conference on Reliability, Infocom Technologies and Optimization (Trends and Future Directions) (ICRITO)* (pp. 1–5).

[64] Singh, P. (2021). Vehicle Monitoring and Surveillance through Vehicular Sensor Network. In *Cloud-Based Big Data Analytics in Vehicular Ad-Hoc Networks*. IGI Global.

[65] Malsa, N., Singh, P., Gautam, J., Srivastava, A., & Singh, S.P. (2020). Source of Treatment Selection for different States of India and Performance Analysis Using Machine Learning Algorithms for Classification. In *Soft Computing: Theories and Applications*. Springer, Singapore.

[66] Juneja, S., Juneja, A., & Anand, R. (2019, April). Reliability modeling for embedded system environment compared to available software reliability growth models. In *2019 International Conference on Automation, Computational and Technology Management (ICACTM)* (pp. 379–382). IEEE.

Chapter 12

# Nanomedicine in healthcare
## Impact and challenges for future generation

*K. Gunasekaran, N. Suthanthira Vanitha, K. Radhika, and P. Suresh*

Muthayammal Engineering College (Autonomous), Namakkal, India

## CONTENTS

## 12.1 INTRODUCTION

Currently, nanotechnology is one of the interesting emerging technologies. It occupies the golden period of nanotechnology with its new development, fabrication, and potential healthcare modalities. The impact of innovations in nanotechnology on healthcare [1] is quite furious. The nanoparticles play a profound role in the nanomedicine field and are proved to be effectively equipped in the healthcare scenario. On the other end, the negative impact

DOI: 10.1201/9781003239888-12

of nanotechnology can also be seen. In medicine, the new applied medical technology is nanomedicine. It is a specific medical subject that covers nano-medical science and nanomedical technology principle.

Nanotechnology alludes to the examination and deployment of little things estimated in a nanoscale. It can provide innovative provisions in an assorted scope of territories in the multidisciplinary field of Science like Physical Science, Electronic Sciences, and Material Science. The uses of nanotechnology in Biomedical and Medication affect the prosperity of people. The various modes of clinical utilization of nanotechnology are Nanomedicine, Nanoimplants, and Nanosensors.

The idea of nanotechnology was proposed in 1965 by Richard Feynman, a Physicist, and Nobel Laureate. The fundamental thought behind nano-technology is to benefit the scaling down of materials and inspect the eventual fate of making smaller devices [2]. Nanotechnology includes the investigation and utilization of issues on a Nuclear or Atomic-scale and regularly consolidates the information from different logical orders [3]. The standard working scope of nanotechnology is 1–100 nanometers (nm), referred to as nanoscale. Particles of this smaller size can handle singular molecules and atoms. The material shows better cell usefulness at the nanoscale when contrasted with a miniature or full scale [4]. The mat-ter changes the conduction based on its size decreased to nanoscale because of quantum size impacts [5], which express the particular conduct of the individual molecules or atoms. It gets conspicuous at the nanoscale sub-atomic conduct of the molecule [6]. Because of the capacity to work on sub-atomic scales, nanotechnology vows to create novel materials and components with extraordinary and improved substances [7]. For exam-ple, mass silver is nontoxic, while silver nanoparticles are fit for killing infections upon contact. The progression in nanotechnology is fetching nanomanufacturing which has a critical effect, particularly in medical ser-vices and clinical areas. Recently, nanomaterials have been generally applied in the field of diagnostics, imaging, and therapeutics. Nanomaterials are broadly acknowledged because of their size, shape, arrangement, structure, and other physical substances [8]. These properties are used to create the ideal materials with explicit absorptive, emissive, and light dispersion.

Nanomedicine has been characterized by the European Science Foundation. "Nanomedicine utilizes nano-sized devices for the finding, counteraction, treatment of sickness and to acquire expanded comprehen-sion of the complex fundamental pathophysiology illness." It consists of three nanotechnology spaces namely, findings, imaging specialists, and med-ication conveyance with nanoparticles in the 1–1000 nm range [9]. A signifi-cant word for "Theranostics" includes both diagnostics and treatment with the equivalent nanopharmaceuticals. Basic advancements have been made over the recent 15 years in the field of nanomedicine with more nanodrugs. The different sizes, calculations, materials, and focusing on moieties of nanoscale stages present the chance of focusing on organs, tissues, and individual cells. Thus, nanotechnology places its footprints in several fields of medicine and can support the practitioner in diagnostic, therapeutic, and preventive activities.

## 12.2 CLASSIFICATION OF NANOMATERIALS

The nanoparticles which are the category of nanomaterial place a significant role in medical care. Nanoparticles like proteins, infection, volcanic ejections, and so forth are normally found in the climate. These tiny particles are normally varied between 1 and 100 nm, having an encompassing interfacial layer. The half-life and circulation of the nanoparticles are dictated by their size. Hence, in biomedical applications specifically, the ideal nanoscale reach ought to be 10–100 nm with the goal that restorative nanoparticles can be disseminated all through the circulatory framework and enter through little vessels [10]. Nanoparticles have three key physical properties [11]:

(1) Highly mobile in the free state;
(2) Very large specific surface areas; and
(3) Capable of exhibiting quantum effects.

Based on the parameters, nanoparticles can be classified into various types. Figure 12.1 shows the classification of nanoparticles.

*Lipid-based Nanoparticles*: They contain lipid moieties, have various remedial applications with properties like enormous surface territory, high medication stacking limit, controlled delivery, and upgraded drug transportation [12]. They can be isolated into liposomes, solid lipid nanoparticles (SLNs), nanoemulsions, and nanosuspension. Normally, a lipid nanoparticle is circular with a breadth of 10–1000 nm, a strong center made of lipid, and a structure that contains dissolvable lipophilic atoms.

*Polymeric Nanoparticles*: They are natural particles that range from 1 to 1000 nm. Based on the morphological changes, nanocapsules and nanospheres are incorporated. Nanocapsules are made out of a slick center

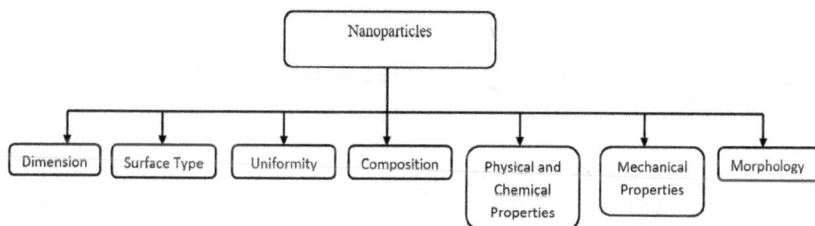

Figure 12.1 Classification of nanoparticles.

wherein the medication is normally broken down, encompassed by a polymeric shell that controls the delivery of the medication report from the center. Nanospheres depend on a consistent polymeric organization where the medication can be held inside or adsorbed onto their surface [13]. These nanoparticles are utilized as medication transporters for controlled delivery. The capacity to secure medication and different particles with the natural movement against the climate improves bioavailability.

*Metallic Nanoparticles*: They are in the size span of 10–100 nm. For illustration, Ag and gold. nanoparticles have expansive antiviral properties against flu, Herpes Simplex Virus (HSV), Human Immunodeficiency Virus-1(HIV-1), dengue infection type-2, hepatitis B virus (HBV), and vesicular stomatitis virus [14]. Additionally, gold nanoparticles discovered applications in natural imaging and materials science [15]. Likewise, silver nanoparticles can intrude the respiratory system and electron transport chain proteins are powerful in battling numerous infections [16]. Titanium nanoparticles (TiNPs) with properties, like high dissolvability and photocatalytic exercises, have wide antiviral properties for bacteriophages and H3N2 viruses. In addition to the above zinc oxide, nanoparticles, and superparamagnetic iron, nanoparticles are equally utilized for restorative applications.

*Semiconductor Materials*: They describe the wide clinical applications. The semiconductor nanocrystals like Quantum dots are in the range of 2–10 nm in size, utilized in detecting, imaging, and treatment of viral sickness because of their alluring optical and electronic properties [17, 18].

*Fullerenes and Carbon Nanotubes (CNTs)*: They address two significant classes of carbon-based nanoparticles. Fullerenes nanomaterial contains globular empty enclosure like allotropic types of carbon. Because of their electrical conductivity, high strength, structure, electron fondness, and adaptability, CNTs are generally utilized in the conveyance of chemotherapeutic medications with high pneumonic harmfulness. For moving antiviral medications, graphene is utilized attributable to its predominant mechanical strength and surface stacking properties [19].

*Ceramic Nanoparticles*: They are inorganic nonmetallic solids that are utilized for bone, teeth, and other clinical applications [20]. Calcium phosphate and tri-calcium phosphate, hydroxy-apatite, calcium sulfate, and carbonate, titania-based ceramics, zirconia, alumina are a few examples.

## 12.3 COMPONENTS OF NANOMEDICINE IN HEALTH SERVICE

Nanotechnology places its footprints in several fields of medicine and can support the practitioners in diagnostic, therapeutic, and preventive/monitoring of nanohealth services activities.

Figure 12.2 shows the various nanomedicine components.

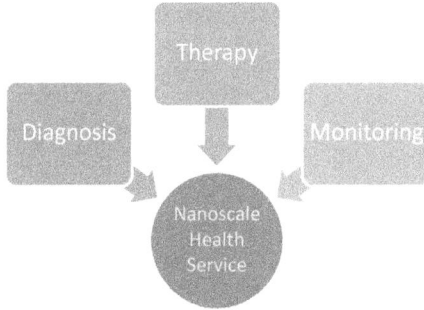

*Figure 12.2* Nanomedicine components.

## 12.3.1 Nanoparticles for diagnosis

The primary component of nanomedicine in healthcare is the Diagnostic system. Nanomedicine supports the development of new diagnostic tools. The measurement of substances such as vitamins and Hormones at nano-level seems to be a challenging one. On the other end, the use of nanomedicine in some substances is proven possible, for example, the measurement of substances at nanolevel like Electrochemiluminescence, Imaging/Cellular Imaging through nanoprobes due to its high volume to surface ratio, multifunctionality, and intrinsic characteristics. Normally, nanoprobes are Quantum Dots, Plasmonic Nanoparticles, Magnetic Nanoparticles, Nanotubes, Nanowires, and Multifunctional Nanomaterials. This nano-probe plays a vital role in Cancer and various infectious diseases. The integrated nanomedicine techniques namely Magnetic Relaxation, Plasma Spectroscopy, and Amperometry are the actual arrivals in diagnostic medicine [21]. Diagnostic applications of nanomaterials include pressure sensing by carbon nanotubes for blood pressure measurement, fullerenes for asthma and arthritis, and nanoshells for photonics-based imaging due to their wide optical scattering properties.

## 12.3.2 Nanoparticles for therapy

The secondary component of nanomedicine in healthcare is the Therapeutic system. Nanotechnology can help in improving drug plans and dispersion in the body. It assists in focusing on the particular therapeutic objective. Nanotechnology is additionally incorporated into the traditional operation for improved adequacy [21]. Therapeutic applications are directly involved with biological event. Nanomachines respond to the commands for specific drug delivery, replacement of tumors or restoration of blood glucose levels, etc. Therapeutic applications of nanoparticles include cancer therapy, gene therapy, drug delivery, and many more.

### 12.3.3 Nanoparticles for monitoring

The third component of nanomedicine in healthcare is Prevention/ Monitoring System. Nanotechnology can support in recovering the patients from diseases. Many new vaccines are ongoingly urbanized based on advancements in nanomedicine. In the case of hormone deficiency, aging is related to the levels of changes in menopause. Treating glands against aging at the cellular level would restore age hormone production. To maintain the desired hormone levels, artificial glands are inbuilt to bring the body to a younger state. With the support of the Heterostasis method, different hormone levels could be supplied to various organs something that the body could not perform itself.

## 12.4 ROLE OF BIOSENSORS IN NANOMEDICINE

Biosensors are the base of nanobiosensors. A biosensor is a diagnostic device capable of sensing the chemical and electrochemical actions happening at different biological extents tissues, cells, and molecules [22]. According to the International Union of Pure and Applied Chemistry definition, "a biosensor is an integrated device which provides specific quantitative analysis for the identification of biological element" [23].

### 12.4.1 Components of biosensors

- Bioelements
- Bioreceptors
- Transducer
- Electronic System

The main component in a biosensor is a bioreceptor or biologically derived sensing element which is coupled with a physiochemical transducer. The transducer converts the biochemical signal into an electrical signal. The signal generated by the transducer is of less magnitude; hence, it is amplified by an electronic system for further processes like displaying, analyzing, or transmitting. Generally, the purpose of a biosensor is to create an output signal that is directly proportional to the concentration of input biomolecules.

Figure 12.3 shows the flow diagram of biosensor.

### 12.4.2 Classification of biosensors

Biosensors are categorized into two groups:

(i) *Based on biological components*: DNA, enzymes, antibodies, microorganisms, tissues, and cell receptors are some of the examples.

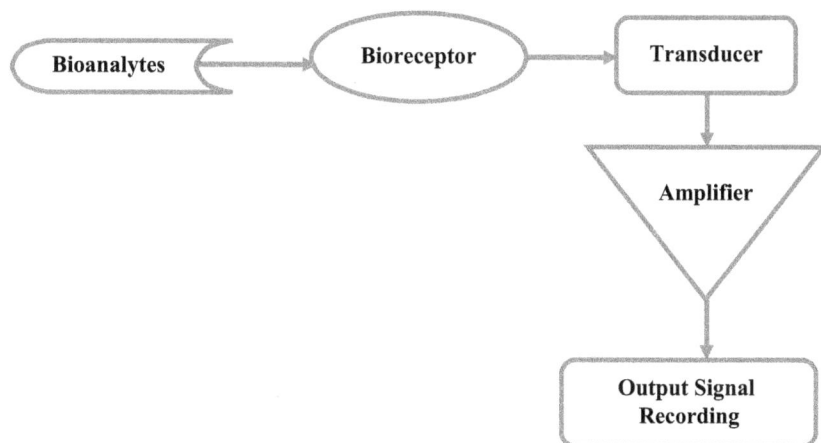

*Figure 12.3* Flow diagram of biosensor.

(ii)   *Based on the transduction method*: They are categorized as follows:
   - mass-based biosensors
   - optical based biosensors
   - electrochemical biosensors

*Optical Biosensors* use optical fiber to detect sensing elements based on absorption, scattering, and fluorescence properties. Refractive index of the contacting surface changes due to the above properties.

*Electrochemical Biosensors* use a noninterfering membrane over which this sensing molecule is placed. These molecules respond properly and produce an electrical signal proportional to the biological input.

*Mass Biosensors* are generally piezoelectric sensors also called acoustic biosensors since these are based on sound vibrations. Whenever a mechanical force is applied, they produce an electric signal.

Figure 12.4 shows the detailed classification of biosensors.

## 12.4.3 Characteristics of biosensors

(a)   *Linearity*: The ratio of the sensor output signal to the input signal that can be detected by a sensor. For biosensors, the linearity must be high.

(b)   *Sensitivity*: The number of outputs the sensor produces per unit substrate concentration is sensitivity.

(c)   *Selectivity*: The response of electrode in the presence of other external materials (or) chemical substances. Generally, for biosensors, selectivity should be minimum.

(d)   *Stability*: It represents how long the sensor produces output over some time.

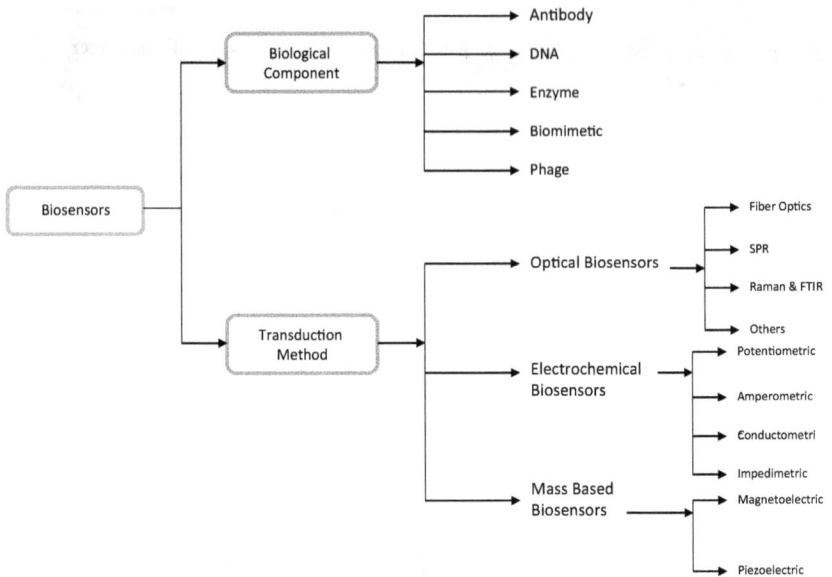

*Figure 12.4* Biosensor classification.

From the above discussion, it is clear that Biosensors are very important in the field of medicine, clinical analysis, and common health monitoring. Due to its user-friendly nature, properties like compactness, low cost, portability, and high speed of response made it very popular in nanomedicine.

## 12.4.4 Nanobiosensors

Nanobiosensor is a combination of nanotechnology and biosensor. It bridges the gap between advanced diagnostics and regular tests. It improves the sensitivity and other fundamental attributes for fabricating the sensor. With nanotechnology, nano biosensors become portable, wearable, and implantable in the human body or medical device. Nanobiosensors diagnose diseases like cancer in an early stage, and they also carry out detection with the aid of a biochemical and biophysical signal at the molecular level and single-cell level [24]. These sensors are becoming a modern instrumental in current diagnostic techniques by providing data access from the area which is not able to sense earlier [25, 26]. This allows for increasing new clinical information, discoveries, and better diagnosis of diseases. On the whole, this opens the entryway to the emerging clinical fields and improves general medical care.

## 12.4.5 Classification of nanobiosensors

Nanobiosensors are classified into five types. This classification is shown in Figure 12.5.

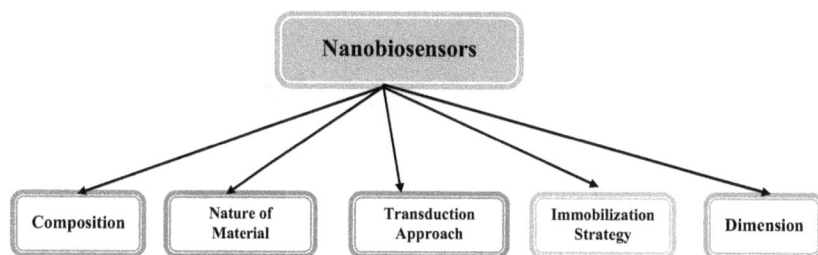

Figure 12.5 Classification of nanobiosensors.

## 12.4.6 Applications of nanobiosensors

Nanobiosensors are extensively used in wide fields of biomedical applications such as Tissue Engineering, 3D Printing, Biotechnology, Biomaterials, Sports, Medical Technology, and many more. They are employed for several purposes including diagnosing, preventing, clinical testing and treating, and monitoring diseases [27].

## 12.5 NANOMEDICINE DOMAINS

Nanomedicine is the application of nanotechnology in medicine that uses nanomaterials for diagnosis, monitoring, controlling, and prevention of diseases. Materials exhibit the best properties when they are in smaller sizes; i.e., nanomaterials have new physicochemical properties due to their size. These properties are utilized in nanomedicine for treating diseases. It involves implanting nanodevices in the human body for certain medical applications. Hence, nanomedicine acts as a boundary between biological systems and nanodevices. In addition, nanomedicine creates another element and efficient tool in the healthcare field for physicians to identify and heal traumatic diseases.

The major domain of nanomedicine is shown in Figure 12.6, which is discussed in the following sections.

## 12.5.1 Drug delivery

It refers to the transportation of pharmaceutical compounds into the desired area of the human body by conventional methods and technologies. In conventional techniques, oral pills and injections deliver the medicine to a specific part of the human body. Because traveling of medical compounds through potential cells has certain issues like weakening of immune system and taking a longer period to deliver the drug to the target area [28]. To overcome this, nanotechnology uses nanoparticles as a delivery vehicle to

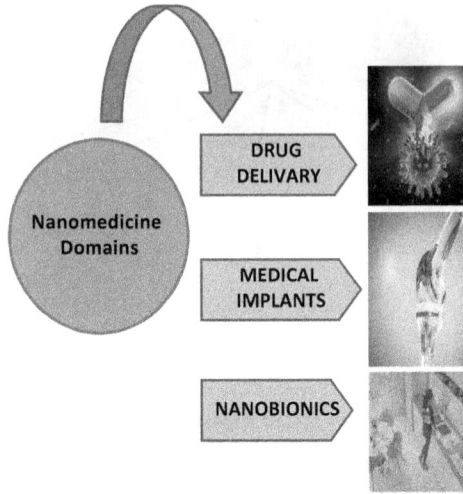

Figure 12.6 Domains of nanomedicine.

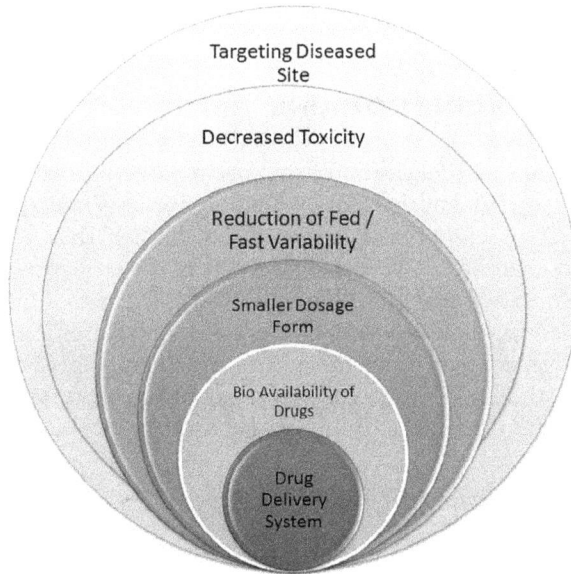

Figure 12.7 Merits of drug delivery.

transport the drugs to the target area as shown in Figure 12.7. Organic nanoparticles are nontoxic, easily biodegradable, and highly efficient. Due to these properties, a targeted drug delivery system is extensively used [29].

Normally drug delivery systems use submicron ranges from 3 nm to 2000 nm sized particles for the delivery of pharmaceutical compounds. In addition to organic nanoparticles, materials including lipids and polymers, for

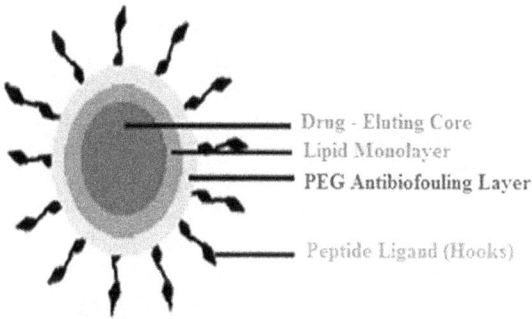

Figure 12.8 Nanoburrs.

example, polymeric nanoparticles, micelles, or dendrimers, are normally used for cancer treatment. In traditional cancer treatment, there are many side effects such as weakness, hair loss and so on that can be overcome with the help of nanoparticles in such treatments.

In addition, drug delivery is also utilized for supplying insulin to diabetic patients by the activated response. It has a sponge matrix usually 250 micrometers in diameter with nanocapsules, which consist of glucose oxidose injected into the patient's body. Whenever the sugar level of the patient gets increased, it reacts by activating nanocapsules to release insulin. Once the sugar level is decreased (or) attains normal, the sponge locks in the rest of the insulin.

Figure 12.8 shows nanoburrs that are tiny particles applied in drug delivery for affected arteries in the heart. These nanoburrs travel directly into the bloodstream and supply medicine to injured tissue [30].

### 12.5.1.1 Medical implants

Medical implants are positioned inside the surface of the human body. They may be either devices or tissues. These implants monitor body functions or provide support to organs and tissues. Recent researchers have developed implantable devices using nanoparticles such as Soft Tissue Implants, Bone substitute materials, Dental Implants, Hard Tissue Implants, and Orthopedic Implants.

Nanotechnology as nanorobotics and nanomaterials has shown incredible potential in the field of dentistry [31]. Other than dental fillers and dental remedial materials, nanomaterials are conceivably utilized in dental and prosthetic implants additionally [32]. Dental inserts are utilized as interfaces with the jaw bone and skull to help a dental prosthesis. The current dental implant is a biological interaction called Osseointegration where materials like titanium form a close link to the bone. The utilization of nanomaterials makes these materials solid, deformable, and erosion safe [33].

Nanofibers and nanoparticles are broadly used implants to increase the breast size (or) replacement of breast tissues. Generally used breast implants are of two types (i) saline-filled and (ii) silicone gel-filled. Both types have complications like breast pain, extrusion, infection, and inflammation. To overcome these side effects, nanofibre-coated implants are considered which enhance the quality and strength of implants. In nanotechnology, silicon rubber is enforced with $SiO_2$ and then utilized as the key component in a breast implant.

### 12.5.1.2 Nanobionics

Nanobionics is considered an innovation, a combination of science and electronics. Bionics, in the term nano bionics, implies the investigation of mechanical systems that are equipped for acting like a typical human body part. The recently utilized strategies for implants or body part substitution included embedding an artificial wooden leg or limb or a glass eyeball. These parts had no capacity which is embedded to help the patient. Nanobionics dive with a more effective and promising innovation of making of or designing artificial implants utilizing nanoscale devices that demonstrate actually like an ordinary human body part. The primary challenge looked at by the analyst in executing this idea into an electronic device correlates with the regular biological activities of the patient.

## 12.6 CHALLENGES OF NANOMEDICINE

Nanotechnology has created an infinitely attractive surge among researchers working in biomedical and healthcare modalities globally. Rapid progress in nanotechnology in the field of medicine has become evident to revolutionize Drug Delivery, Image-Based Therapy, Gene Therapy, Sustainable Drug Delivery, Diagnostics, Clinical Applications, and other related Thermostats [34]. Nanomedicine establishes nanotechnology concepts in medicine. It links two large cross-disciplinary fields with an extraordinary societal and economical perspective arising from the combination of specific accomplishments in the relevant fields. The incorporation of nanomaterials in medicine applies to the development of diagnostic devices, analytical tools, drug delivery, and therapeutic applications. The arrival of nanotechnology provides new opportunities in implants and the delivery of medications to specified areas. Even though the medical application of nanotechnology is steadily emerging, still there are challenges in the future of nanomedicine. Nanotechnology has got an adequate impact in the present medical research sector to extend the quality of the medical field. Though it solves many healthcare issues such as cancer diagnosis, implants, and delivery of medications without delay, still it is an apprehension for scientists and medical experts.

In drug delivery, the nanomaterials such as Silicon, Silver, and so on are used. The improved chemical reaction of nanoparticles causes to produce free radicals inside the cellular microenvironment. Exposing the human body to these materials for a longer period may change the functionality and create adverse effects such as oxidative stress, inflammation, and damage to biomolecules like DNA, proteins, and nucleic acids [35]. All human body reacts in a different way to the implanted nanodevices. The implanted electronic devices or materials can injure the soft tissues and organs. The particles gradually gather inside organs and block the blood flow. Therefore, nanodevices' compassion and their effect on the human body should be accurately analyzed before it is implanted.

Similarly, practical implementations of nano biosensors are very challenging since most people do not know how to use and when they are to be used. In addition, the moral, social, and lawful aspects of nanomedicine should be strategically focused on due to the potential risk factors whenever humans get exposed to it. Hence, it is basic to make the general public mindful of the advantages and dangers of nanomedicine.

## 12.7 CONCLUSION AND FUTURE PERSPECTIVES

The chapter discusses the impact and challenges of nanomedicine in healthcare. The opportunities for nanomedicine in healthcare are endless. The influence of nanotechnology in the development of nanomedicine supports the identification of the significant areas needed for technological innovation. The classification of nanoparticles and their applications in diagnosing treatment and prevention are also discussed. In addition to the components of nanomedicine, the role of biosensors in identifying the diseases, nanomedicine domains, and challenges is conferred.

The novel advances in nanomedicine act as an auspicious substitute technology over conventional cancer therapies that afford the opportunities for early detection, treatment, and diagnosis of cancer cells despite the cancer nanomedicines capable of delivering chemotherapeutic agents through lower toxicity. It is dominant to deliberate the cancer complication and dynamics for connecting the translational medical gap by conducting appropriate investigations for manipulating the tumor microenvironment. Furthermore, its role in achieving a more comprehensive kind of the fundamental biological process in cancer and modulating nanoparticle-protein interactions, blood circulation, and tumor penetration is discussed.

Nanotechnology deals with numerous potentials starting from detecting devices to energy transformation equipment and life-saving bio-implants. The success rate of graphene derivatives has proved an impressive search for other 2D materials which surpass the defects of graphene efficiently. The 2D materials have high potential in the medical field which comprises the transition metals such as transition metal dioxides, dichalcogenides, double hydroxides, laponite, graphitic carbon nitride, hexagonal boron nitride, silicene, and phosphorene. Through suitable surface modifications, the steady dispersions and wide-size tunable bandgap of 2D materials can be made possible. Hexagonal boron nitride is also known as a potent graphene analog having a completely inert characteristic nature and low fluorescence quenching property. Due to these properties, 2D materials beyond graphene are refined and diverse, which makes them impressive in biomedicine. Nanotechnology has grown to a spectacular status across the globe in various biomedical and engineering domains because of its significant characteristics.

Nanotechnology in nanomedicine is persistently growing, which creates opportunities in implantable delivery systems like injectable drug applications. It enhances the ability to deliver drugs less water-soluble and supports sites specific to reduce drug accumulation inside the healthy tissues that maintain the drug for a long term in the body for efficient treatment. It further protects the tissues through bioactivity from the biological environment. In addition, it permits the drugs to move around epithelial and endothelial barriers and then coalesces therapeutic and diagnostic tissues.

Future biomedicine covers tunable band gap-dependant characteristics, unique chemical composition and low cytotoxic potential and therapeutics. Currently, gold nanoparticles are used for enhancing the tumor-killing effect due to their ability to improve the apoptotic effect on tumors [35]. Hence, during combinatorial therapy of cancer disease, radiation dosages can be minimized. Apart from that, Quantum dots can be applied for locating tumors in patients and diagnostic tests in the future. Gold NPs can be assigned to proteins that support early-state detection of disease through lab samples. Similarly, various efforts to progress nanoparticle disease detection are in progress. In addition, early detection of blood-borne pathogens, peptide, and Aptamer-conjugated are several types of research worldwide and developed solutions for focused clinical challenges.

In today's healthcare [36, 37, 38], field drug discovery has become a potential market. It poses challenges to the researchers for the new findings. Nanomedicine lies in enhancing diagnostic methods, drug formulations, and drug disease therapy. In general, Pharmaceutical Industries follow the common process for drug discovery such as cloning, human receptors expression, and formats in enzymes. It has properties that allow high throughput, automated screening, combinatorial chemistries, speed, analysis, reliability, miniaturization, and automation [39]. The scarcity of nanomedicine has been considerably more with the increase and implementation of nanotechnology applications in medicine. This chapter focused on the nanomedicine applications, upcoming challenges, and opportunities in nanotechnology future perspectives.

## REFERENCES

[1] Juneja, S., Juneja, A., & Anand, R. (2020). Healthcare 4.0-digitizing healthcare using big data for performance improvisation. *Journal of Computational and Theoretical Nanoscience*, 17(9–10), 4408–4410.

[2] Toumey, C. P. (2008). Reading Feynman into nanotechnology: A text for a new science. *Techné: Research in Philosophy and Technology, 12*(3), 133–168.

[3] Silva, G. A. (2004). Introduction to nanotechnology and its applications to medicine. *Surgical Neurology, 61*(3), 216–220.

[4] Yi, H., Rehman, F. U., Zhao, C., Liu, B., & He, N. (2016). Recent advances in nano scaffolds for bone repair. *Bone Research, 4*(1), 1–11.

[5] Berger, M. (2009). *Nano-Society: Pushing the boundaries of technology* (Vol. 8). Royal Society of Chemistry.

[6] Vermae, S. R. D. A. (2018). Nanoscale modifications of dental implants: An emerging trend.

[7] Morganti, P. (2010). Use and potential of nanotechnology in cosmetic dermatology. *Clinical, Cosmetic and Investigational Dermatology: CCID, 3*, 5.

[8] Ealia, S. A. M., & Saravanakumar, M. P. (2017, November). A review on the classification, characterisation, synthesis of nanoparticles and their application. In *IOP Conference Series: Materials Science and Engineering* (Vol. 263, No. 3, p. 032019). IOP Publishing.

[9] Omanović-Mikličanin, E., Maksimović, M., & Vujović, V. (2015). The future of healthcare: Nanomedicine and internet of nano things. *Folia Medica Facultatis Medicinae Universitatis Saraeviensis, 50*(1), 23–28.

[10] Walmsley, G. G., McArdle, A., Tevlin, R., Momeni, A., Atashroo, D., Hu, M. S., ... & Wan, D. C. (2015). Nanotechnology in bone tissue engineering. *Nanomedicine: Nanotechnology, Biology and Medicine, 11*(5), 1253–1263.

[11] Dobson, P., Jarvie, H., & King, S. (2019, May 14). *Nanoparticle. Encyclopedia Britannica.* https://www.britannica.com/science/nanoparticle

[12] Mukherjee, S., Ray, S., & Thakur, R. S. (2009). Solid lipid nanoparticles: A modern formulation approach in drug delivery system. *Indian Journal of Pharmaceutical Sciences, 71*(4), 349.

[13] Ekladious, I., Colson, Y. L., & Grinstaff, M. W. (2019). Polymer–drug conjugate therapeutics: Advances, insights and prospects. *Nature Reviews Drug Discovery, 18*(4), 273–294.

[14] Gigliobianco, M. R., Casadidio, C., Censi, R., & Di Martino, P. (2018). Nanocrystals of poorly soluble drugs: Drug bioavailability and physicochemical stability. *Pharmaceutics, 10*(3), 134.

[15] De Jesus, M. B., & Zuhorn, I. S. (2015). Solid lipid nanoparticles as nucleic acid delivery system: Properties and molecular mechanisms. *Journal of Controlled Release, 201*, 1–13.

[16] Yu, M., Wu, J., Shi, J., & Farokhzad, O. C. (2016). Nanotechnology for protein delivery: Overview and perspectives. *Journal of Controlled Release, 240*, 24–37.

[17] Matea, C. T., Mocan, T., Tabaran, F., Pop, T., Mosteanu, O., Puia, C., ... & Mocan, L. (2017). Quantum dots in imaging, drug delivery and sensor applications. *International Journal of Nanomedicine, 12*, 5421.

[18] Probst, C. E., Zrazhevskiy, P., Bagalkot, V., & Gao, X. (2013). Quantum dots as a platform for nanoparticle drug delivery vehicle design. *Advanced Drug Delivery Reviews, 65*(5), 703–718.

[19] Bondavalli, P. (2018). Carbon and Its New Allotropes: Fullerene, Carbon Nanotubes and Graphene. In *Graphene and Related Nanomaterials: Properties and Applications* (pp. 1–40). Elsevier.

[20] Khan, I., Saeed, K., & Khan, I. (2017). Nanoparticles: Properties, applications and toxicities. *Arabian Journal of Chemistry, 12*: 908.

[21] Joob, B., & Wiwanitkit, V. (2017). Nanotechnology for health: A new useful technology in medicine. *Medical Journal of Dr. DY Patil University, 10*(5), 401.

[22] Alvarez, M. M., Aizenberg, J., Analoui, M., Andrews, A. M., Bisker, G., Boyden, E. S., ... & Khademhosseini, A. (2017). Emerging trends in micro-and nanoscale technologies in medicine: From basic discoveries to translation. *ACS Nano, 11*(6), 5195–5214.

[23] Thevenot, D. R., Toth, K., Durst, R. A., & Wilson, G. S. (1999). Electrochemical biosensors: Recommended definitions and classification. *Pure and Applied Chemistry, 71*(12), 2333–2348.

[24] Prasad, S. (2014). Nanobiosensors: The future for diagnosis of disease? *Nanobiosensors in Disease Diagnosis, 3*, 1–10.

[25] Saini, M. K., Nagal, R., Tripathi, S., Sindhwani, N., & Rudra, A. (2008). PC interfaced wireless robotic moving arm. In *AICTE Sponsored National Seminar on Emerging Trends in Software Engineering* (Vol. 50).

[26] Singh, L., Saini, M. K., Tripathi, S., & Sindhwani, N. (2008). An intelligent control system for real-time traffic signal using genetic algorithm. In *AICTE Sponsored National Seminar on Emerging Trends in Software Engineering* (Vol. 50).

[27] Banigo, A. T., Azeez, T. O., Ejeta, K. O., Lateef, A., & Ajuogu, E. (2020, March). Nanobiosensors: Applications in biomedical technology. In *IOP Conference Series: Materials Science and Engineering* (Vol. 805, No. 1, p. 012028). IOP Publishing.

[28] Mukherjee, S., Ray, S., & Thakur, R. S. (2009). Solid lipid nanoparticles: A modern formulation approach in drug delivery system. *Indian Journal of Pharmaceutical Sciences, 71*(4), 349.

[29] Naoum, G. E., Tawadros, F., Farooqi, A. A., Qureshi, M. Z., Tabassum, S., Buchsbaum, D. J., & Arafat, W. (2016). Role of nanotechnology and gene delivery systems in TRAIL-based therapies. *Ecancermedicalscience, 10*.

[30] Mariappan, N. (2019). Recent trends in nanotechnology applications in surgical specialties and orthopedic surgery. *Biomedical and Pharmacology Journal, 12*(3), 1095–1127.

[31] Bhardwaj, A., Bhardwaj, A., Misuriya, A., Maroli, S., Manjula, S., & Singh, A. K. (2014). Nanotechnology in dentistry: Present and future. *Journal of International Oral Health: JIOH, 6*(1), 121.

[32] Schmalz, G., Hickel, R., van Landuyt, K. L., & Reichl, F. X. (2017). Nanoparticles in dentistry. *Dental Materials, 33*(11), 1298–1314.

[33] Priyadarsini, S., Mukherjee, S., & Mishra, M. (2018). Nanoparticles used in dentistry: A review. *Journal of Oral Biology and Craniofacial Research, 8*(1), 58–67.

[34] Zhang, Y., Jin, Y., Cui, H., Yan, X., & Fan, K. (2020). Nanozyme-based catalytic theranostics. *RSC Advances, 10*(1), 10–20.

[35] Surendranath, A., & Valappil, M. P. (2020). Nanomedicine: Challenges and Future Perspectives. In *Functional Bionanomaterials* (pp. 451–476). Springer, Cham.

[36] Malsa, N., Singh, P., Gautam, J., Srivastava, A., & Singh, S.P. (2020). Source of Treatment Selection for different States of India and Performance Analysis using Machine Learning Algorithms for Classification. In *Soft Computing: Theories and Applications*.

[37] Ratnaparkhi, S. T., Singh, P., Tandasi, A., & Sindhwani, N. (2021). Comparative analysis of classifiers for criminal identification system using face recognition. In *2021 9th International Conference on Reliability, Infocom Technologies and Optimization (Trends and Future Directions) (ICRITO)* (pp. 1–6).

[38] Jain, S., Kumar, M., Sindhwani, N., & Singh, P. (2021). SARS-Cov-2 detection using deep learning techniques on the basis of clinical reports. In *2021 9th International Conference on Reliability, Infocom Technologies and Optimization (Trends and Future Directions) (ICRITO)* (pp. 1–5).

[39] Juneja, S., Juneja, A., & Anand, R. (2019, April). Reliability modeling for embedded system environment compared to available software reliability growth models. In *2019 International Conference on Automation, Computational and Technology Management (ICACTM)* (pp. 379–382). IEEE.

Chapter 13

# IoT for healthcare system
## Challenges and opportunities

*Jaspinder Kaur and Saarthak*

Chandigarh University, Mohali, India

**CONTENTS**

## 13.1 INTRODUCTION

We are living in that era of lifetime where almost everything is available on the internet from the answer of complex questions to movies for entertainment, same could be the thing with these day-to-day activities like controlling lights, fans, air conditioners, washing machines, etc. with the use of internet [1, 2]. Internet of things (IoT) have made these things possible, quite evidently it can be termed as the most important invention/development of generation. No doubt, it has come a long way and yet there is a long way to go. IoT [3–5] has impacted the day-to-day lives, professional living, and social circle as well [6, 7]. In numerous developed nations, IoT is well-known as the basic thing to have in homes, offices, shopping malls, etc. With this recognition, its cost is also decreasing drastically. For instance, today one can buy an Amazon Home for 4000 INR, which is as low a cost as that of a fancy dinner. One Amazon Home with all its accessory requirements can completely change the lifestyle of people to first-world standards.

After getting recognition in the personal and professional environments, and considering its success in these sectors, its worth in healthcare and medical sectors beholds a great chance of success in the same. As of the end of 2019, the whole world encountered a completely new era of living where people were either quarantined at homes or admitted to hospitals. This time of COVID-19 brought out the complete new need for IoT-based facilities in many ways. Hospitals are getting overcrowded, medical equipment is getting shorter on stock, manually taking patient's medical status is getting dangerous with every passing day. This is the place where IoT could outshine, like radio frequency identification (RFID) [8] patches for patient's details and wristwatch-based blood pressure monitor systems which can directly monitor and upload the information on the platform known as cloud and that information can be further analyzed by doctors to know patient's condition [7, 9].

IoT can mean a great deal not just in these times of coronavirus pandemic but also in maintaining overall health, as all have heard about wristwatch-based devices like "FitBit" and Apple watch which show the health status on all the owner devices in the environment where the information is stored on the cloud and can be retrieved at any moment from any source. With just a simple wristwatch design, these devices are capable enough to count your heart rate, blood pressure, oxygen saturation, steps walked, stairs climbed, and so much more. If there is an initiative for further improvement in these devices to a standard where they can assist in monitoring and foreseeing any future implications, then it will be possible to save the numerous lives which might become trouble in near future [2, 6].

The main goal of this chapter is to study the implementation and the numerous applications of IoT in healthcare industry [10]. With the incorporation of IoT, one can stay in regular touch with their doctors and fitness consultants as they do not need to visit them again and again. It can simply be made possible with the introduction of IoT. Patient's information can be regularly shared with the doctors as it is stored in the cloud itself. Talking about storing the information on the cloud, it does not just help with being up to date but also can save money. The various medical studies have proved that having long-term data of patients can help doctors realize the disease/problem faster and save a lot of time and money that would be wasted in random fishing around tests. A study on diabetic patients and high/low blood pressure patients has revealed that having the long-term-based data of the patients helps in identifying the problem and prescribing a better medicine [11, 12].

IoT is also a deal-breaker technology when it comes to keeping the records of patients. Hospitals had a hard time arranging those heavy binders filled with patient data which took forever to access whenever needed back in the 1950s. But with advancement in technology, there came yet another dust sitting technique of floppy disks followed by hard drives which are still a flop, but with IoT, all of these data can be made available securely online within seconds, which is even more secure than a bank guarded by several guards. These data can be accessed by the concerned personnel in any corner of the world, not like old times where accessing the patient's medical history was quite a big task. But now it is just as away as a push of a button or as easy as scanning a QR code [13, 14].

Complete implementation of IoT is already providing numerous benefits to its consumers. The inculcation of healthcare in this field will not just help doctors and patients but will also help in the administrative activities before and after the medical concerns and hence it might not be wrong to say that IoT can prove to be a firewall for the whole world against the pandemic that is going on [15, 16].

With its numerous advantages coming into the limelight on regular basis, there is no hidden fact that IoT platforms serve as a feast for hackers and phishers around the globe. Now that complete user data is available online, it has become an easy and more profitable target. Compromising these data have resulted in disclosure of personal things like transaction histories, credit card information etc. [17, 18]. Now that it is concerned with using these IoT platforms for healthcare purposes and so complications further increase because the medical background of a person is a concern between the doctor and that person himself. If these data leak and get into the hand of wrong people, it can have serious consequences as well. So, it might not be saying too much at this point that "With great power comes great responsibility", and hence, the organizations providing these facilities must stand out in this war against data phishers [19].

The rest of the chapter is organized as: The implementation of IoT in various sectors such as manufacturing and automobiles is discussed in Section 13.2. The five-level architecture of IoT is given in Section 13.3. In Section 13.4, directly implementable IoT applications in healthcare industry is presented. The IoT implementation in healthcare is discussed in Section 13.5. In Section 13.6, IoT advancements in India are well described. In Section 13.7, future scope of IoT advancements in healthcare is given. Advantages of IoT in healthcare are discussed in Section 13.7.3. Shortcomings of IoT in healthcare are defined in Section 13.8, and finally, in Section 13.9, conclusions are drawn.

## 13.2 IMPLEMENTATION OF IOT

Nowadays, IoT is implemented in the numerous sectors that include manufacturing, repairs, textile, research and development, and many other sectors around the globe. It has become an important asset for these sectors because IoT provides accuracy, time management, and quality that no human can provide irrespective of their experience and skills.

### 13.2.1 IoT in manufacturing sector

Over the years in transition from industry 3.0 to 4.0, a major portion of manufacturing units all over the world has adopted these IoT techniques to improve their manufacturing speed and quality, by using devices like programmable logical controller (PLC) which are not a part of IoT but are considered as the first step toward automating the manufacturing technologies.

PLCs can simply be programmed by using the graphical user interface (GUI) programming platforms and they use that programming logic to control the functioning of machines which do not have innate automation in them. Alongside PLCs, there are other advancements also where devices like "Arduino" and "Raspberry pi" are the development platforms being used to provide IoT support to the manufacturing industries.

### 13.2.2 IoT in automobile sector

The automobile sector deals with the most cumbersome and complex parts of machinery. So, implementation of IoT and automation was a great achievement. With the help of robotic arms [20] and automated assembly lines, automobile sector can achieve precision, quality, and speed of production that could never have been possible by human methods. These automated part assembly, welding, soldering, and cutting activities require ultimate precision. Robotic arms can work for as long as needed without needing any rest but human hands do not work like that. When people start getting tired, their precision decreases and the quality of the product also suffers [19].

Implementation of IoT in this sector is complicated yet simple. All of the controlled automation and robotic arms can be controlled from a safe environment with the use of microcontrollers using real-time cloud networks that make work rather simple for the operators. These automated devices can work with a very rare chance of mistake but the complicated thing here is that even if one of the assembly parts is damaged, whole line's working stops; if one assembly part is produced wrong, then again working of the entire line has to be stopped because it will keep producing the same defective product again and again, which could take hours before it can be resolved and hence is a complex asset.

Alongside these examples, there are infinite instances that it can see using these technologies and changing the world around them.

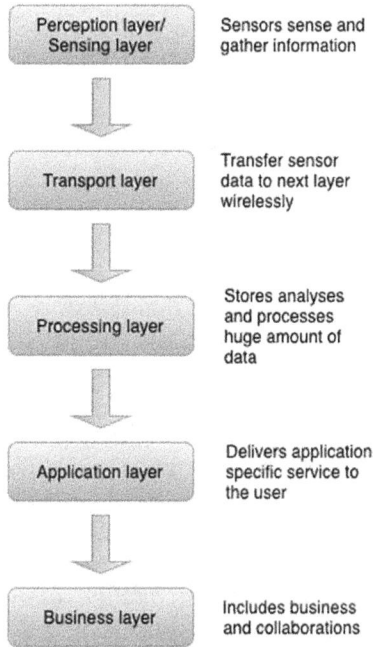

Figure 13.1 Five-level architecture of IoT.

## 13.3 ARCHITECTURE OF IOT

A common three-layer IoT architecture consists of the network, the perception, and the application layer. The first layer known as perception layer is the lowest layer in the IoT architecture in which the actuators, sensors, and other connected devices are present where they collect the information that are very necessary for the network. The network layer connects the devices in the network to other devices to handle the transmission of information. The third layer, i.e., application layer, provides some specific services to the user by providing data analytics, data reports, and control over the devices [21, 22]. The three-layered architecture is then upgraded to five layers with the addition of two more layers, namely the business layer and the processing layer. A five-layer IoT architecture (as shown in Figure 13.1) comprises of the perception layer, the network layer, the processing layer, the application layer, and the business layer [21].

A. Application layer

The application layer is the topmost layer of the five-layered IoT architecture. The application layer provides the global management of the applications. A few examples of the applications implemented through IoT can be listed as smart home, smart farming, smart health, smart city, intelligent transportation [21], etc. The functions of this layer range for designing applications for all types of businesses. It is also capable of performing some smart calculations [22].

B. Network layer

The second layer recognized as a network layer usually is a amalgamation of local area networks, access, and core networks. The main function of this layer is unique addressing and routing that makes sure that the integration of many devices is possible into a single application [23]. The network layer is also called the transmission layer because it transfers the data securely from the devices to the processing system. Thus, the network layer transfers the information from the perception layer to the middleware layer [24].

C. Perception layer

The perception layer, which is also known as the third layer, is the lowermost layer and most prone to various kinds of attacks. This layer includes various physical objects and sensor devices [25, 26] like an RFID, 2D barcode, infrared sensors, etc. This layer's basic functionality is to recognize the object and to help with the identification. The collected information is then passed to the network layer for its secure transmission to the information processing system [23].

D. Processing layer

This is the middleware layer in which the devices over the IoT implement different types of services. Each device connects and communicates with only those other devices that implement the same service type. This layer is responsible for the service management and has links to the database. It receives the information from the network layer. It performs information processing and ubiquitous computation and takes automatic decision based on the results [23, 24].

E. Business layer

The business layer is responsible for the management of the overall IoT system, including the applications and services. It builds business models, graphs, flowcharts, etc. based on the data received from the application layer. The real success of IoT technology also depends on good business models. Based on the analysis of results, this layer helps to determine the future actions and business strategies [23].

## 13.4 DIRECTLY IMPLEMENTABLE IOT APPLICATIONS IN HEALTHCARE INDUSTRY

Healthcare can be considered as one of the most important fields for implementation of IoT. Every year, there are a lot of accidents that happen in healthcare facilities such as fire, loss of oxygen supply, short circuits, and error in the medical equipment. With the help of IoT, all of these issues can be dealt with.

CAGR 20.2% (2016-2024)

2015    2016    2017    2018    2019    2020    2021    2022    2023    2024

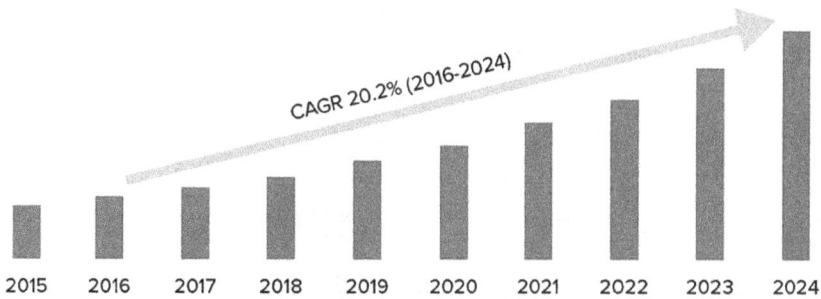

*Figure 13.2* Global IoT healthcare market size forecast, 2015–2024.

Like in the case of fire, WiFi-based smoke detectors can transmit the information to the concerned firefighters in the minimum time possible. Microcontroller devices can ring the alarms and inform all the patients in time to get out of the affected areas. In hospitals, it has all kinds of patients, so there might be some differently abled people also; for them, it can provide automated wheelchairs and high safety lifts to get them into a safe place. This application is not difficult at all as all the smoke detectors are connected to the internet, knowing the exact place of initiation of fire is possible and it can help to guide the people who are not able to escape the building in time, by telling them the relative safer position [27, 28].

Similarly, it can automate the oxygen supply systems with the use of basic IoT devices, where it can continuously monitor the level of availability, quality of the supply, locate blockages, monitor the usage, and forecast any future possibility of any disruption.

Figure 13.2 clearly shows how the implementation of IoT is being recognized by every country as healthcare is the key to keep the population healthy and working. Every year, there is a linear increase in the expenditure for research and implementation of the same in the healthcare sector. This implementation is although gaining speed, still there are a lot of challenges currently that had to be dealt with.

IoT projects need very high investments and have a lot of proof of concepts that will be suitable for many businesses. As the main goal for all businesses is a digital transformation initiative, it is important to recognize the project objectives for the technology to succeed. Various industries do have so many requirements. The implementation steps aim to decrease the operational costs. This hereby targets the customer experience and can also increase the reach. To be able to understand business analytics, we have to use case diagrams and IoT consulting companies to make sure that the IoT model has the business to understand that technology. IoT application-based companies make sure that the future of the company is ensured. For example, the IoT components must be aligned with the test cases. For any project, hardware and software selection is equally important. The components need to include sensors, edge gateways, communication protocols, IoT platforms, and cloud management software(s) [29].

### 13.4.1 Use of sensors

Sensors are used to collect the data related to various factors like weight, volume, temperature, humidity, pressure, and many more. Many sensors help to detect these aspects.

*Temperature Sensor*: It is used to measure the temperature of the experiment surroundings [1]. Temperature sensors often use resistance temperature detectors that are efficient and easy to install. The resistance temperature detectors (RTDs) work on the principle of expansion of the metals concerning temperature. A digital high technology (DHT) sensor is a temperature sensor that is used in most of the projects in IoTs. Similarly, uses of these sensors in the field are also mentioned below.

*Smoke detectors* – Smoke detectors work on the basic principle of completion of a circuit under normal circumstances. In a smoke detector, alpha rays are constantly flying off from one end of the sensor to another end which completes the circuit (flow of voltage is in microvolts) but when some smoke reaches the sensor, flow of electrons gets disrupted and circuits become inactive that triggers a microcontroller to ring the alarm, upload the effected coordinates on cloud, and perform all the activities needed by simply making use of IoT alongside this sensor.

*RFID tags* – RFID tag makes use of the electromagnetic fields to track and record the required data. After that, when it is contacted by another RFID receiver device, it transmits the data digitally. This technology can be used to provide all the information of patients and concerned personally in the form of these smart tags that can track and record all the needed activities and can help monitor the patients better.

*Motion detectors* – Motion detectors are rather a complex piece of technology that makes use of multiple phenomena like Doppler's effect, inertial navigation, or sensors to identify a relative position of the target. These sensors can be used in hospitals that have memory loss patients, mentally disabled, or differently abled people. These sensors can help in monitoring the activities of those people and locating them whenever needed.

## 13.5 IMPLEMENTATION OF IOT IN HEALTHCARE INDUSTRY

IoT has changed the entire healthcare industry. Now, there is no need to visit the doctor every time you face an issue, it can be done straight with the internet. All of the essential data of the patient can be stored online and can be accessed by the doctor. A lot of countries are spending heavily to bring these techniques into practice and with every coming year, this budget is increasing.

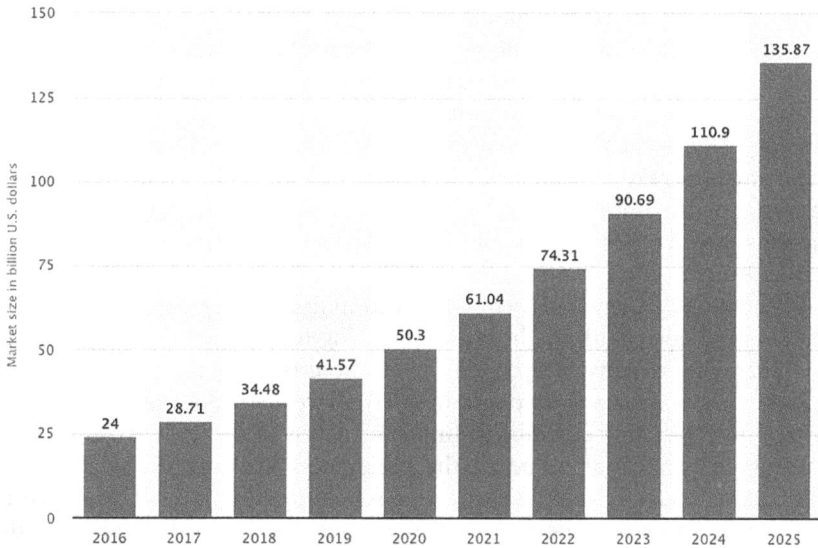

*Figure 13.3* Expenditure in the IoT healthcare sector.

Figure 13.3. clearly shows how expenditure in the IoT healthcare sector is increasing exponentially in international markets. The countries are identifying the advantages and needs of IoT in the healthcare sector, and this development brings out different advantages for doctors, patients, hospitals, and governments.

## 13.5.1 Implementation advantages for patients

With the implementation of IoT and cloud computing in the healthcare sector, patients are at a great advantage as they can access the concerned medical doctors as per their needs from anywhere in the world without actually stepping into the hospital. By using the devices like Fitbit and Apple watch, they can keep a record of their health, and these data can further be stored on clouds for it to be accessed by doctors who can help them prescribe in a better way.

According to the research, patients with diseases like diabetes, high/low blood pressure, and Alzheimer's need constant monitoring and hence IoT devices can be used to constantly monitor these patients and optimize their data [30–32] as per the need. This can help to prescribe medicines as well as to inform the concerned person if there are some unusual readings [33].

## 13.5.2 Implementation advantages for doctors

Analyzing data and storing it on cloud platforms is not just useful for patients only, it is more useful for doctors as they can virtually meet the doctors and get the proper guidance especially in times of global pandemics like the one going on right now. This helps in the protection of doctors as well whenever there are some patients with acute infectious diseases who are at high risk of spreading if not quarantined.

Every year, some patients consult doctors in very late phases of diseases, which makes treatment impossible or very difficult. This is one of the major reasons for the importance of IoT devices, where it will help doctors and patients, predict these diseases in time and prevent any serious repercussions in the future.

For example, a smart system is used to monitor sleep-deprived or sleep-walking patients. With the help of integrating IoT as well as using big data analytics, the patients' sleep cycle can be monitored by the physicians. The architecture of such a sleep operating IoT devices includes the IoT layer, fog computing layer, and cloud layer. In the IoT layer, all the devices using all the various elements that influence the parameters are considered. The data obtained is then computed through the fog computing layer. This fog computing layer processes the data using the concept of fog nodes and stores the data into the cloud to centralize its processing. Then, the data are stored in a database which includes analytical resources and accessibility through a graphical data interface.

### 13.5.3 Implementation advantages for hospitals

Hospitals have to store a large amount of data about the patients and with conventional methods of storing the data, it is a cumbersome process to retrieve the data and use it for further processes. With the implementation of IoT, this process consumes no time at all. Be it storing the data on cloud or programming RFIDs for individual patients, all of these tasks take no time at all.

IoT-based platforms also help the hospitals in keeping a track of the order, cleanliness, and patient hygiene as well in real-time, that can help them in providing first-class facilities to their patients and improve the overall quality of healthcare [28].

### 13.5.4 Implementation advantages for government

Governments around the world are spending a huge amount every year on research and development for the same as it improves the living and healthcare standards of the country and it brings out a healthy population that is ready to work for the country and every worker brings ultimately more money which is important for the country.

Having a better healthcare system attracts people from all over the world for getting good healthcare facilities and ultimately attracts money and revenue. Therefore, the implementation of IoT is very important from the government's perspective [34].

## 13.6  IOT ADVANCEMENTS IN INDIA

Because of cheap labor forces and vast land availability, India offers a great deal of international development and that is the reason India is becoming a major hub for the IoT applications. Indian government has been vigilant in understanding the opportunities this field of IoT has to provide in the development of the country.

If these projections follow the same increment every year, the cost for an IoT commodity will reduce significantly and its application will be more robust and it will no longer be a first-world commodity [19].

People in India might not realize it, but in the next 5 years, India will need these IoT products more than any other country in the world. Because of the increasing population and overcrowding of cities, it will be a better deal to have everything available with the people with the help of internet only.

Despite having one of the biggest pharma sectors in the world, India still lacks behind in the overall medical and healthcare facilities which it has to offer. India lacks in providing sustainable state-owned medical facilities at a reasonable cost, that is where the integration of IoT sector comes in to play a huge role. It will not just reduce its long-term cost in the development of its healthcare facilities, but also increase its standards that are held together by the weak strings right now.

## 13.7  FUTURE SCOPE OF IOT ADVANCEMENTS IN HEALTHCARE

Despite providing healthcare sector as a drastic change from the previous generations, the advancement of IoT does not stop there. As mentioned earlier, IoT is a very vast field of science and so it can combine technologies from the various fields and can improve the quality of healthcare furthermore. Some of those future ideas are explained below.

### 13.7.1  Hologram-based patient interaction

Once the objective of advancement in technology is achieved, there are a million ways to make it better. For example, in this particular approach, a hologram-based doctor–patient meeting can improve the standard of meeting and understanding rather than just being on a video call. Scientific studies have proved this factor that people's mentality and way of expression changes drastically when people actually look at each other. Along with this, there are numerous psychological factors also that affect the overall behavior and thought process of the people. That is why, psychological factors can be handled better using this approach. It is true that this technology exists currently to an extent but it is not completely operable from a commercial perspective and that is where the role of IoT strikes in as it can make that thing possible [16].

## 13.7.2 Remote robotic surgeries

IoT alongside robotic arms is already proving its worth in the manufacturing sector, where it stands out because of its precision and accuracy and that is one of the most important things while performing surgeries [35, 36]. The scope of this particular area is a way more than people might realize as there are a lot of instances where the required surgeons are unavailable or are currently not available in those cases. These robotic surgeries outshine because there is no need for the actual presence of that doctor at that place and he can perform the surgery from any location just because of IoT. One another factor that affects value is that if this technology is ever made possible, surgeons who have lost their ability to keep their hand still, or have met an accident or have grown old or who cannot perform surgery by their hands but have unmatched experience in those cases, this development can outshine and prove its worth [37].

## 13.7.3 Advantages of IoT in healthcare

IoT not only makes human life easier but also helps many businesses to revolutionize themselves in being established worldwide. It can be deployed in many fields such as healthcare when combined with high technology. Because it can automate any object, it helps in improving machine to human interactions. The application of IoT is diverse and embedded in every activity of life. There are numerous applications such as smart transportation, smart home, smart agriculture, animal tracking, smart industry, smart living, smart health, smart city, and smart energy. Some of the advantages are explained as:

1. Low cost of treatment in the future.
2. Better quality of healthcare facilities.
3. Good for the citizens depending on the government to provide basic healthcare facilities.
4. Improves living standard of people.
5. Beneficial for the country as better living and healthcare standards attract immigration of people.
6. Improves net healthy to unhealthy people ratio which is of major concern in an overcrowded country like INDIA.
7. Attracts foreign investment and revenue for technology transfer.
8. Increases the need for skilled labor forces and helps in the development of people with weak financial background [19, 38].

## 13.8 SHORTCOMINGS OF IOT IN HEALTHCARE INDUSTRY

As discussed above, IoT undoubtedly delivers some amazing benefits such as better healthcare facilities, low cost of treatment, and improves living standard of people. However, it surely has its own set of shortcomings. Some of the disadvantages of IoT are discussed below. In addition to this, there are many challenges because of which the need of security in IoT arises.

A. Risk of data security

While talking about IoT advancements in the field of healthcare, storing and uploading of data on to cloud platforms is one of the most important task as it enables the entire functioning of IoT healthcare system and it serves the sole purpose of providing a base to act upon. But these cloud platforms are not the most secured places in the world. Time and often, these cloud platforms remain on the top priority list of hackers and phishers. Their activities to first extract that data and leaking it online can be very harmful for everyone related with that data. Constant measures are being taken by every country's cyber laws and cloud providing platforms that user data must be kept a secret and protected from attackers [39].

Various big players in the market of IoT have drastically failed in keeping their data secured from these hackers. According to a report, Tesla's model X was hacked and quite often we hear about data servers being hacked. Be it of Dominos or Facebook or any other company, data security is one of the biggest concern when it comes to IoT applications.

B. Privacy

IoT devices are often available for public perception. This makes it important for IoT businesses to properly advertise their products to the local market. This advertising should also address most of the safety concerns the public might have. For example, to make a smart home using Alexa is quite feasible, but 90% of Indians do not set up Amazon Alexa because of the privacy concerns that the information might get stolen and hacked. As there is a lot of data on IoT devices, there are many entry points for hackers to steal information. There is a lot of public profile as most of the IoT devices agree to use the collected data to make many decisions based on the product. For example, health insurance can gather your health statistics through a fitness tracker and can calculate the rate of insurance based on your vulnerability. Eavesdropping is something that everyone is scared of in today's world. Hackers can steal the information from fitness trackers or able to listen to everyday conversations to either improve the quality of the fitness tracking or to steal important information [2, 15].

C. Short range

Most of the IoT devices work on either Bluetooth or WiFi-based systems which are very effective for short-range applications but suffer when a long-distance constraint arrives. IoT devices also support Ethernet-based communication support which makes them very well suited in confined system applications, but not for long distances.

D. Vulnerability

IoT devices are a big attraction to hackers. As IoT healthcare offers so much benefits, there are so many ways in which the security [40] is often vulnerable. The software developers need to make software and developers need to make sure that it is not vulnerable. Through IoT devices, hackers will be able to invade the personal space of such patients and also the hospital details through a simple IoT breakout. The way the device works can also be tampered with, which is also life-threatening. That is why IoT devices are not fully automated. According to a source, Sentara Hospitals had a mailing error regarding the IoT medical devices, which made the breach of over 577 patients. There have been statistics that 82% of healthcare organizations have been attacked by hackers targeting IoT devices [41, 42].

E. Regulation

The telecommunication framework does not always apply to all IoT devices. Only some IoT applications are compatible with the regulations. Communication with such IoT devices restricts from machine to machine (M2M) with limited interaction. Telecommunication frameworks help define those services and communication between the network of things. IoT sensors need the transmission of data and signals without involving humans. So sensors are also considered as telecommunication services. Telecommunication frameworks regarding connectivity are not properly defined. Hence, the IoT providers are not responsible for any conveyance of connectivity issues. Spectrum is also a key enabler of IoT devices. It does not have any limitation to the technology that is used; hence, there can be satellite or terrestrial network connectivity across the IoT.

F. Acceptance as standard

There are a lot of people who still have the thinking that IoT and other technological advancements should not be made as a standard level of healthcare but consider conventional methods to be a better way to deal with healthcare, which is slowing down the growth of IoT and is also hindering it from becoming a standard practice.

G. Compatibility

As IoT is one such technology where many technologies are competing to become the standards, this makes connectivity even more difficult. It requires the deployment of extra software and hardware specifications. Generic computing devices do not have a larger lifespan, whereas IoT devices have a long lifespan, although it requires time to time calibration with the service. Generally, IoT devices do not go out of service even though the manufacturing company does not sell that particular product. There are some other compatibility issues which include bad standardization techniques of the M2M protocols as well as differences in firmware. The operating system software models also keep changing over the years, which do not make it compatible with the devices using the latest operating systems [35].

## 13.9 CONCLUSION

Considering all the possible ways in which IoT can be implemented in everyday healthcare facilities of people, it can be concluded that no doubt it can change the lives of people drastically for good. It is going to have its effect on the medical standards of the people. IoT might be able to bring many of the futuristic technologies that felt impossible out of movies to reality but some things cannot be ignored for sure. IoT brings some great advantages to people by giving them employability not just in the medical sector but in the manufacturing and research sectors as well, still some security risks and high vulnerability cannot be ignored. Cloud facilities that hold the user data when left vulnerable to these hackers make the person's whole data available on the internet in simplest terms. It makes their life open book to the world but the only difference is that these data also consist of their credit card info, bank info, their location details and everything they do every day, which is neither safe nor legal. So, IoT might bring an ultimate number of advantages but there are some serious drawbacks to look toward also [43]. Despite providing healthcare sector a drastic change from previous generations, the advancements of IoT does not stop there. As mentioned earlier, IoT is a very vast field of science and so it can combine technologies from various fields and improve the quality of healthcare [44]. The future scope of IoT in healthcare industries has already been discussed above.

In addition, IoT is very well accepted for some of the future applications such as robot taxi, gaming room, and agriculture. Robot taxis are made to understand to avoid the traffic areas in a city and to take alternative ways, thereby helping in traffic management. They can be called from the side of the road by showing hand motions. The client's area is obviously trailed by GPS and authorizes clients to request a taxi to be at a specific area at a specific time by simply calling attention to it on an itemized map [45, 46, 47, 48]. When the robot taxi is not being used, it will end up taking refuelling breaks. Another important future application is handling the information of the city by means of IoT [49, 50, 51, 52, 53]. For instance, all the structures, constructions, sewers, rails, cycle ways, and any other framework can be checked by the government with publicly available information (APIs). Another fun application is the use of game rooms with the help of gadgets to detect, cause the temperature of the game room to increase and decrease. The room utilizes these data to quantify energy and vitality levels so as to control the game movement as indicated by status of the player.

## REFERENCES

[1] Al-Fuqaha, A., Guizani, M., Mohammadi, M., Aledhari, M., & Ayyash, M. (2015). Internet of things: A survey on enabling technologies, protocols, and applications. *IEEE Communications Surveys & Tutorials*, 17(4), 2347–2376.

[2] Ara, T., Shah, P. G., & Prabhakar, M. (2016). Internet of things architecture and applications: a survey. *Indian Journal of Science and Technology*, 9(45), 1–7.

[3] Anand, R., Sinha, A., Bhardwaj, A., & Sreeraj, A. (2018). Flawed Security of Social Network of Things. In *Handbook of Research on Network Forensics and Analysis Techniques* (pp. 65–86). IGI Global.

[4] Gupta, A., Srivastava, A., Anand, R., & Tomažič, T. (2020). Business Application Analytics and the Internet of Things: The Connecting Link. In *New Age Analytics* (pp. 249–273). Apple Academic Press.

[5] Gupta, R., Shrivastava, G., Anand, R., & Tomažič, T. (2018). IoT-Based Privacy Control System through Android. In *Handbook of E-Business Security* (pp. 341–363). Auerbach Publications.

[6] Guin, U., Singh, A., Alam, M., Canedo, J., & Skjellum, A. (2018, January). A secure low-cost edge device authentication scheme for the internet of things. In *2018 31st International Conference on VLSI Design and 2018 17th International Conference on Embedded Systems (VLSID)* (pp. 85–90). IEEE.

[7] Dhanvijay, M. M., & Patil, S. C. (2019). Internet of things: A survey of enabling technologies in healthcare and its applications. *Computer Networks*, 153, 113–131.

[8] Gupta, A., Srivastava, A., Anand, R., & Chawla, P. (2019). Smart vehicle parking monitoring system using RFID. *International Journal of Innovative Technology and Exploring Engineering*, 8(9S), 225–229.

[9] Pace, P., Aloi, G., Gravina, R., Caliciuri, G., Fortino, G., & Liotta, A. (2018). An edge-based architecture to support efficient applications for healthcare industry 4.0. *IEEE Transactions on Industrial Informatics*, 15(1), 481–489.

[10] Juneja, S., Juneja, A., & Anand, R. (2020). "Healthcare 4.0-Digitizing Healthcare Using Big Data for Performance Improvisation". *Journal of Computational and Theoretical Nanoscience*, 17(9–10), 4408–4410.

[11] Suo, H., Wan, J., Zou, C., & Liu, J. (2012, March). Security in the internet of things: a review. In *2012 International Conference on Computer Science and Electronics Engineering* (Vol. 3, pp. 648–651). IEEE.

[12] Jing, Q., Vasilakos, A. V., Wan, J., Lu, J., & Qiu, D. (2014). Security of the internet of things: perspectives and challenges. *Wireless Networks*, 20(8), 2481–2501.

[13] Shouran, Z., Ashari, A., & Priyambodo, T. (2019). Internet of things (IoT) of smart home: privacy and security. *International Journal of Computer Applications*, 182(39), 3–8.

[14] Kalmeshwar, M., & Prasad, N. (2017). Internet of Things: architecture, issues and applications. *International Journal of Engineering Research and Application*, 7(06), 85–88.

[15] Sengupta, J., Ruj, S., & Bit, S. D. (2020). A comprehensive survey on attacks, security issues and blockchain solutions for IoT and IIoT. *Journal of Network and Computer Applications*, 149, 102481.

[16] Oh, S. R., & Kim, Y. G. (2017). Security requirements analysis for the IoT. In *2017 International Conference on Platform Technology and Service (PlatCon)*.

[17] Farahani, B., Firouzi, F., Chang, V., Badaroglu, M., Constant, N., & Mankodiya, K. (2018). Towards fog-driven IoT eHealth: Promises and challenges of IoT in medicine and healthcare. *Future Generation Computer Systems*, 78, 659–676.

[18] Zhang, Z. K., Cho, M. C. Y., Wang, C. W., Hsu, C. W., Chen, C. K., & Shieh, S. (2014, November). IoT security: ongoing challenges and research opportunities. In *2014 IEEE 7th International Conference on Service-Oriented Computing and Applications* (pp. 230–234). IEEE.

[19] Yacchirema, D. C., Sarabia-Jácome, D., Palau, C. E., & Esteve, M. (2018). A smart system for sleep monitoring by integrating IoT with big data analytics. *IEEE Access*, 6, 35988–36001.

[20] Saini, M. K., Nagal, R., Tripathi, S., Sindhwani, N., & Rudra, A. (2008). PC interfaced wireless robotic moving arm. In *AICTE Sponsored National Seminar on Emerging Trends in Software Engineering* (Vol. 50).

[21] Islam, S. R., Kwak, D., Kabir, M. H., Hossain, M., & Kwak, K. S. (2015). The internet of things for health care: A comprehensive survey. *IEEE Access*, 3, 678–708.

[22] Bhatia, H., Panda, S. N., & Nagpal, D. (2020, June). Internet of things and its applications in healthcare—A survey. In *2020 8th International Conference on Reliability, Infocom Technologies and Optimization (Trends and Future Directions)(ICRITO)* (pp. 305–310). IEEE.

[23] Baker, S. B., Xiang, W., & Atkinson, I. (2017). Internet of things for smart healthcare: Technologies, challenges, and opportunities. *IEEE Access*, 5, 26521–26544.

[24] Nazir, S., Ali, Y., Ullah, N., & García-Magariño, I. (2019). Internet of things for healthcare using effects of mobile computing: A systematic literature review. *Wireless Communications and Mobile Computing*, 2019.

[25] Kohli, L., Saurabh, M., Bhatia, I., Sindhwani, N., & Vijh, M. (2021). Design and Development of Modular and Multifunctional UAV with Amphibious Landing, Processing and Surround Sense Module. In *Unmanned Aerial Vehicles for Internet of Things (IoT): Concepts, Techniques, and Applications* (p. 207).

[26] Kohli, L., Saurabh, M., Bhatia, I., Shekhawat, U. S., Vijh, M., & Sindhwani, N. (2021). Design and development of modular and multifunctional UAV with amphibious landing module. In *Data Driven Approach Towards Disruptive Technologies: Proceedings of MIDAS 2020* (pp. 405–421). Springer, Singapore.

[27] Tiburski, R. T., Amaral, L. A., De Matos, E., & Hessel, F. (2015). The importance of a standard securit y archit ecture for SOA-based iot middleware. *IEEE Communications Magazine*, 53(12), 20–26.

[28] De Michele, R., & Furini, M. (2019, September). Iot healthcare: Benefits, issues and challenges. In *Proceedings of the 5th EAI International Conference on Smart Objects and Technologies for Social Good* (pp. 160–164).

[29] Karimpour, N., Karaduman, B., Ural, A., Challenger, M., & Dagdeviren, O. (2019, June). Iot based hand hygiene compliance monitoring. In *2019 International Symposium on Networks, Computers and Communications (ISNCC)* (pp. 1–6). IEEE.

[30] Sindhwani, N., Bhamrah, M. S., Garg, A., & Kumar, D. (2017, July). Performance analysis of particle swarm optimization and genetic algorithm in MIMO systems. In *2017 8th International Conference on Computing, Communication and Networking Technologies (ICCCNT)* (pp. 1–6). IEEE.

[31] Bakshi, G., Shukla, R., Yadav, V., Dahiya, A., Anand, R., Sindhwani, N., & Singh, H. (2021). An optimized approach for feature extraction in multi-relational statistical learning. *Journal of Scientific and Industrial Research (JSIR)*, *80*(6), 537–542.

[32] Sindhwani, N., & Singh, M. (2016). FFOAS: antenna selection for MIMO wireless communication system using firefly optimisation algorithm and scheduling. *International Journal of Wireless and Mobile Computing*, 10(1), 48–55.

[33] Silva, B. N., Khan, M., & Han, K. (2018). Internet of things: A comprehensive review of enabling technologies, architecture, and challenges. *IETE Technical Review*, 35(2), 205–220.

[34] Zakaria, H., Bakar, N. A. A., Hassan, N. H., & Yaacob, S. (2019). IoT security risk management model for secured practice in healthcare environment. *Procedia Computer Science*, 161, 1241–1248.

[35] Geng, H. (Ed.). (2017). *Internet of Things and Data Analytics Handbook*. John Wiley & Sons.

[36] Yu, Y., Li, Y., Tian, J., & Liu, J. (2018). Blockchain-based solutions to security and privacy issues in the internet of things. *IEEE Wireless Communications*, 25(6), 12–18.

[37] Thibaud, M., Chi, H., Zhou, W., & Piramuthu, S. (2018). Internet of things (IoT) in high-risk environment, health and safety (EHS) industries: A comprehensive review. *Decision Support Systems*, 108, 79–95.

[38] Saheb, T., & Izadi, L. (2019). Paradigm of IoT big data analytics in the healthcare industry: A review of scientific literature and mapping of research trends. *Telematics and Informatics*, 41, 70–85.

[39] Ahemd, M. M., Shah, M. A., & Wahid, A. (2017, April). IoT security: A layered approach for attacks & defenses. In *2017 international conference on Communication Technologies (ComTech)* (pp. 104–110). IEEE.

[40] Anand, R., Shrivastava, G., Gupta, S., Peng, S. L., & Sindhwani, N. (2018). Audio Watermarking with Reduced Number of Random Samples. In *Handbook of Research on Network Forensics and Analysis Techniques* (pp. 372–394). IGI Global.

[41] Somasundaram, R., & Thirugnanam, M. (2020). Review of security challenges in healthcare internet of things. *Wireless Networks*, 1–7.

[42] Ngu, A. H., Gutierrez, M., Metsis, V., Nepal, S., & Sheng, Q. Z. (2016). IoT middleware: A survey on issues and enabling technologies. *IEEE Internet of Things Journal*, 4(1), 1–20.

[43] Aman, M. N., Chua, K. C., & Sikdar, B. (2017, December). A light-weight mutual authentication protocol for IOT systems. In *GLOBECOM 2017-2017 IEEE Global Communications Conference* (pp. 1–6). IEEE.

[44] Anand, R., Sindhwani, N., & Saini, A. (2021). Emerging Technologies for COVID-19. In *Enabling Healthcare 4.0 for Pandemics: A Roadmap Using AI, Machine Learning, IoT and Cognitive Technologies* (pp. 163–188).

[45] Singh, P., Pareek, V., & Ahlawat, A. K. (2017). Designing an energy efficient network using integration of KSOM, ANN and data fusion techniques. *International Journal of Communication Networks and Information Security (IJCNIS)*, 9(3), pp. 466–474.

[46] Singh, P., Nayak, P., Datta, A., Sani, D., Raghav, G., & Tejpal, R. (2019). Voice control device using raspberry Pi. In *SOUVENIR, IEEE Conference, Amity International Conference on Artificial Intelligence (AICAI'19), Amity University Dubai, Dubai International Academic City, IEEE, UAE Section.* February 4–6.

[47] Singh, P. (2021). Vehicle Monitoring and Surveillance Through Vehicular Sensor Network. In *Cloud-Based Big Data Analytics in Vehicular Ad-Hoc Networks.* IGI Global.

[48] Singh, P., Raw, R. S., Khan, S. A., Mohammed, M. A., Aly, A. A., & Le, D.-N. (2021). W-GeoR: Weighted geographical routing for VANET's health monitoring applications in urban traffic networks. *IEEE Access.* https://doi.org/10.1109/ACCESS.2021.3092426.

[49] Singh, P., Raw, R. S., & Khan, S. A. (2021). Link risk degree aided routing protocol based on weight gradient for health monitoring applications in vehicular ad-hoc networks. *Journal of Ambient Intelligence Humanized Computing.* https://doi.org/10.1007/s12652-021-03264-z.

[50] Rana, K., Tripathi, S., & Raw, R. S. (2019). Fuzzy logic-based directional location routing in vehicular ad-hoc network. In *Proceedings of the National Academy of Sciences, India Section A: Physical Sciences Springer, (SCI, SCOPUS, DBLP) (IF = 1.544, Q-3R).*

[51] Ahmed, A., Abdul Hanan, A., Omprakash, K., Lobiyal, D. K., & Raw, R. S. (2017). Cloud Computing in VANETs: Architecture, Taxonomy and Challenges. In *IETE Technical Review* (Vol. 35, pp. 523–547). Taylor & Francis, India & USA.

[52] Kumar, S., & Raw, R. S. (2020). Health Monitoring Planning for On-Board Ships through Flying Ad Hoc Network. In *Advanced Computing and Intelligent Engineering*, Springer, ISBN: 978-981-15-1483-8 (pp. 391–402).

[53] Kumar, A., Tripathi, S., & Raw, R. S. (2016). Bringing healthcare to doorstep using VANETs. In *3rd IEEE International Conference as INDIACom-2016*, Delhi, India (pp. 4747–4750).

Chapter 14

# Automatic heart-rate measurement using facial video

*Geetanjali Sharma, Neelam Nehra, and Aman Dahiya*
Maharaja Surajmal Institute of Technology, New Delhi, India

*Nidhi Sindhwani*
Amity University, Noida, India

*Pooja Singh*
University Institute of Engineering (UIE)- Computer Science and
Engineering (CSE), Chandigarh University, Gharuan, Mohali, Punjab, India

## CONTENTS

## 14.1 INTRODUCTION

The number of heart beats per minute is measured by a person's heart rate (HR). It is a significant biological parameter that offers information about the whole of cardiovascular system and is important in the diagnosis and

DOI: 10.1201/9781003239888-14

| Age | 18 - 25 | 26 - 35 | 36 - 45 | 46 - 55 | 56 - 65 | 65 + |
|---|---|---|---|---|---|---|
| Athlete | 54 - 60 | 54 - 59 | 54 - 59 | 54 - 60 | 54 - 59 | 54 - 59 |
| Excellent | 61 - 65 | 60 - 64 | 60 - 64 | 61 - 65 | 60 - 64 | 60 - 64 |
| Great | 66 - 69 | 65 - 68 | 65 - 69 | 66 - 69 | 65 - 68 | 65 - 68 |
| Good | 70 - 73 | 69 - 72 | 70 - 73 | 70 - 73 | 69 - 73 | 69 - 72 |
| Average | 74 - 78 | 73 - 76 | 74 - 78 | 74 - 77 | 74 - 77 | 73 - 76 |
| Below Average | 79 - 84 | 77 - 82 | 79 - 84 | 78 - 83 | 78 - 83 | 77 - 84 |
| Poor | 85 + | 83 + | 85 + | 84 + | 84 + | 85 + |

(a)

| Age | 18 - 25 | 26 - 35 | 36 - 45 | 46 - 55 | 56 - 65 | 65 + |
|---|---|---|---|---|---|---|
| Athlete | 49 - 55 | 49 - 54 | 50 - 56 | 51 - 56 | 51 - 56 | 50 - 55 |
| Excellent | 56 - 61 | 55 - 61 | 57 - 62 | 58 - 63 | 57 - 61 | 56 - 61 |
| Great | 62 - 65 | 62 - 65 | 63 - 66 | 64 - 67 | 62 - 67 | 62 - 65 |
| Good | 66 - 69 | 66 - 70 | 67 - 70 | 68 - 71 | 68 - 71 | 66 - 69 |
| Average | 70 - 73 | 71 - 74 | 71 - 75 | 72 - 76 | 72 - 75 | 70 - 73 |
| Below Average | 74 - 81 | 75 - 81 | 76 - 82 | 77 - 83 | 76 - 81 | 74 - 79 |
| Poor | 82 + | 82 + | 83 + | 84 + | 82 + | 80 + |

(b)

*Figure 14.1*  Heart-rate chart: (a) men and (b) women.

evaluation of a person's stress levels [1]. Normal heart rate values vary by age, medical history, and level of physical activity as shown in Figure 14.1. For decades, this is widely recognized that any irregular changes in the cardiac pulse should be examined and diagnosed further. As people become more fitness and health conscious, several tele-health monitoring platform concepts are being created. These include, among other items, assisting vulnerable people or seriously ill individuals in residential settings. Furthermore, any communication system can only track one patient at a time, which is inconvenient when a quick or ongoing inspection of individual from a particular place – such as an office or a metro station – is needed [2–4]. The heart rate monitoring using facial video has become a popular method because of its convenience and easy access. Facial data collection and processing do not require any complex hardware or software architecture. Through video processing, this chapter presents a novel automatic method of measuring heart rate remotely. The subject must be comfortable and close to a webcam for this technique to work.

Photoplethysmography (PPG) detects the variations of light transmission or reflectance during cardiovascular pulse cycle to determine blood volume.

As is the case with pulse oximetry sensors [5, 6], PPG is normally conducted with specific light infrared or red wavelength light sources [7–13]. Similar to Ref. [8], we investigate a method for detecting heart rate using RGB change in color of faces in video. We also look at some ways to enhance the pixel range used to measure heart rate, such as separating out the pixels that make up a person's face.

Using a reimplementation of GrabCut, for example, we can segment out the facial pixels. We can compare how these algorithm variants perform in stationary videos and videos with movement or noise. The remainder of this chapter explains how to calculate a person's heart rate from a video of their face. The technical approach is defined in Section 14.2, and the experimental setup is discussed in Section 14.4. Section 14.5 discusses results, and Section 14.6 gives some conclusions.

## 14.2 TECHNICAL APPROACH

### 14.2.1 Introduction to Haar-like features

Digital image features called Haar-like features are used in object recognition. They were used in the first real-time face detector and acquired their name from their intuitive resemblance to Haar wavelets. Working with only image intensities (i.e., RGB pixel values at each and each pixel of an image) made efficient feature calculation computationally costly in the past. Working with an alternative feature set centered on Haar wavelets instead of the normal picture intensities was explored in an article by Werner et al. [9].

A Haar-like function considers neighboring rectangular regions in a detection window at a particular spot, sums the pixel intensities in each region, and calculates the difference between the sums [14], as shown in Figure 14.2. This distinction is then used to break an image into sub-sections [4]. For example, it is a well-known fact that the region of the eyes is darker than the region of the cheeks. A group of two parallel rectangles appears above the eye and on the cheeks, region is a typical Haar function for face detection (FD). These rectangles are identified with the help of a detection window that acts as a bounding box for the targeted object (e.g., the face in this case).

A window of the target size is moved over the input image in the Viola–Jones object detection framework's detection process, and the Haar-like feature is calculated for each subsection of the image. The difference is then compared to a threshold for separating nonobjects from objects that has been learned. A large number of Haar-like features are needed to accurately describe an object because a single Haar-like feature is a poor classifier (its detection efficiency is only a bit better than random guessing).

In the Viola–Jones object detection system, the Haar-like features are grouped in a classifier cascade to form an efficient learner or classifier. A Haar-like feature has a significant speed advantage over most of the other features. A Haar-like function can be computed in a fixed time with the help of integral images (approximately 60 microprocessor instructions for a two-rectangle feature) [15].

#### 14.2.1.1 Rectangular Haar-like feature

The variation between the number of pixels in a rectangle that can be anywhere in the original image and at any size can be described as a simple

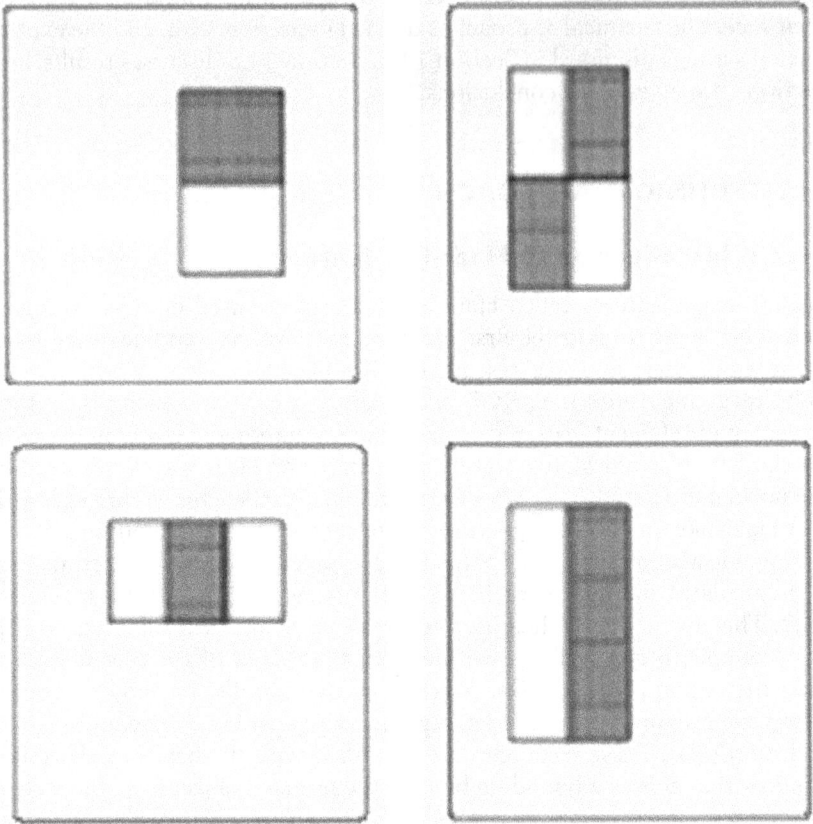

*Figure 14.2* Face classifier with Haar-like features.

rectangular Haar-like function. Two-rectangle function is the name given to this updated feature collection. Viola and Jones also distinguished between three-rectangle and four- rectangle functions.

The output represents certain aspects for a specific image field. These feature type may represent the presence (or absence) of specific image properties like edges or texture changes [16–20].

A two-rectangle function, for example, will show where the dark-light border is placed as shown in Figure 14.3.

## 14.2.2 Software used

### 14.2.2.1 Python (programming language)

Python is a high-level, interpreted programming language that can be used for a variety of tasks. Python was designed by Guido van Rossum in 1991. Its design methodology prioritizes the feasibility of code and makes liberal

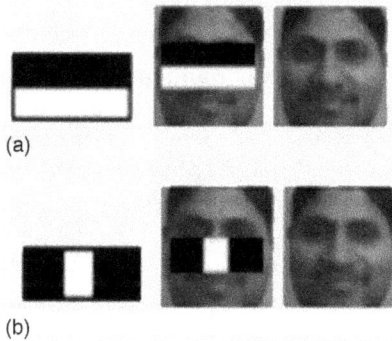

*Figure 14.3* Haar like features map (a) highlighting the eyes and (b) highlighting the nose.

use of whitespace [14, 16]. Its object-oriented approach and language constructs were created to help researchers write quick and conceptual code for both large and small projects.

It is a dynamically typed language. Structured (especially procedural) programming, object-oriented programming, and functional programming are all supported. Because of its large standard library, Python is sometimes referred to as a "batteries included" language. Python was created in the late 1980s as a replacement for the ABC programming language. Python 3.0, published in 2008, is a big revision of the language that is not fully backward compatible, and most of the Python 2 codes will not run on Python 3. Python 2 was officially discontinued in 2020 (it was originally scheduled for 2015), and "Python 2.7.18 is the last Python 2.7 update and hence the last Python 2 release." It will no longer receive security updates or other changes.

Python 2 is no longer available, so only Python 3.5.x and later are supported. For a wide range of operating systems, Python interpreters are available. CPython, an open-source reference implementation, is developed and maintained by a global group of programmers. The Python Software Foundation is a nonprofit organization that manages and directs resources for Python and CPython development.

### 14.2.2.2 PyCharm

PyCharm is a computer programming integrated development environment (IDE) that primarily focuses on Python programming language. JetBrains, a Czech company, built it. It includes code implementation, a graphical debugger, and unit tester, web creation and VCS integration with Django and Data Science with Anaconda. The Apache License applies to the Community Version, and a proprietary license applies to the Advanced Edition, which has additional features.

Features of PyCharm:

1. Fast fixes for coding assistance and review.
2. Mapping of projects and code: It refers to file structure views, advanced project views, and quick jumps among usages, methods, files, and classes.
3. Python refactoring: It extracts process, rename, add vector, introduce constant, push down, pull up, and other refactoring techniques.
4. Installed Python emulator.
5. Line-by-line application inspection for installed units.

### 14.2.2.3 OpenCV

Stanley, the vehicle that won the 2005 DARPA Grand Challenge, used OpenCV in 2005. OpenCV is available on Linux, Windows, OS X, iOS, Android, and other platforms, and supports a number of programming languages. Interfaces based on CUDA and OpenCL for high-speed GPU operations are also under research.

OpenCV (Open-Source Computer Vision Library) is a programming library oriented primarily toward artificial intelligence. This was created by Intel and then sponsored by Willow Garage and Itseez (that was then acquired by Intel). Under the open-source BSD license, the library is cross-platform and free to use.

The OpenCV-Python library is a compilation of Python bindings for solving computer vision problems. Python is a general-purpose programming language created by Guido van Rossum that quickly gained popularity due to its simplicity and readability of code. It allows the programmers to communicate their ideas in fewer lines of code while maintaining readability. A tracking example for same is shown in Figure 14.4. Python is slower than the languages such as C/C++. Python, on the other hand, can be easily extended with C/C++, allowing us to write computationally intensive code in C/C++ and then wrap it in Python to use as a module. This has two benefits: first, the code is as quick as the original C/C++ code (because it is the real C++ code running in the background), Second, Python is easier to code than C/C++. The Python wrapper for the original OpenCV C++ implementation is called OpenCV-Python.

OpenCV's application areas are given below:

1. Toolkits for 2D and 3D applications
2. Face-detection framework
3. Sign-language recognition
4. Brain–computer interface
5. Motion recognition
6. Object recognition
7. Optimization and identification

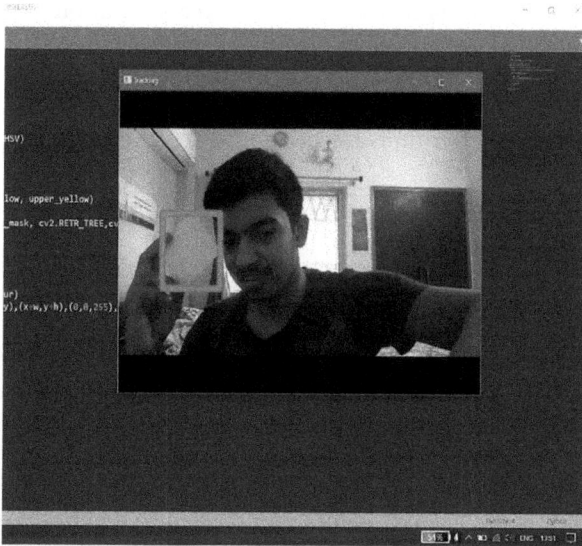

*Figure 14.4* Tracking using OpenCV.

8. Stereopsis stereo vision: depth by two cameras
9. Structure from motion (SFM) application
10. Motion detection
11. Virtual and augmented reality
12. Understanding of gesture

## 14.3 BRIEF LITERATURE SURVEY

In some recent years, experts have explored several remote-based detection techniques based on computer vision [21–28]. The authors in Ref. [29] proposed physiological measurement using human faces as a biomarker. As per this article, a thin layer of tissue has been observed using face area. Then, in the year 2007, detection of heart rate has been done with the help of facial thermal imaging based on bio-heat architectures [30]. Thereafter, a different method based on a specific light source (infrared light or red lights) has been implemented, which is called photoplethysmography (PPG) method. PPG is an optical and noninvasive method, which has been proved very effective in heart rate detection [31, 32]. Later, Verkruysse et al. [33] proposed a possibility of detection of heart rate from video data using face as a marker and this has been done using PPG with light signal.

In 2010, the authors in Ref. [34] proposed a new method for automatic heart rate detection, wherein a standard camera has been used for colorful recording of human face. Later, the previous method was also explored and improved by several other researchers [35–37]. The primary concept behind all the previous studies is to use a blind source separation method on the basis of variation of face color to classify heart rate [38, 39]. Thereafter, a different method of heart detection was proposed using subtle head motion in the years 2013 [40–42]. Some researchers also explored optical modeling and noise reduction algorithms for heart rate detection.

## 14.4 EXPERIMENTAL SETUP

### 14.4.1 Methods of detection of heart rate

There are three key steps for detecting heart rate in video. These are explained later in the chapter. First, face is identified as it is the only identified part of the frame that contains the information of heart rate. Second, inside the face-bounding box, the required region of interest (ROI) is picked. Ultimately, the plethysmography signal must be extracted from the ROI's time-dependent shifts in pixel colors and studied to identify the prominent frequency inside the heart rate range.

### 14.4.2 Face detection and tracking

We use the OpenCV Cascade Classifier that has been educated on both negative and positive frontal face pictures. A face detector is made up of a series of increasingly complex classifiers, each of which employs one or more Haar-like features. The features are made up of two, three, or four rectangular pixels. Easy vertical, horizontal, and diagonal edges and blobs can be detected using these features. Because each sub-window has over 180,000 possible features, only a small subset of these is used for the same. The AdaBoost learning algorithm with one to some hundred features is utilized to train the classifiers. The FD is demonstrated in Figure 14.5. The associated features with the minimum error and classifier associated are selected for that stage, the weights are changed, and the entire process is then repeated till the required number of classifiers has been reached. This method generates a unit-heavy classifier from a weighted combination of several fewer complex classifiers. The cascade starts with a simple classifier (based on a single feature) that has a low threshold and is built with a low false negative rate (or with high false positive rate). Even if a window receives a positive outcome from this classifier, it is passed on to the later classifier. The sub-window is rejected if the classifier returns a negative result as it must separate out sub-windows that all pass through the preceding stage.

Every successive stage of the cascade uses a more complex classifier based on an increasing number of features. However, each round has fewer windows and hence the processing time is reduced than if all of the image's windows were subjected to the complex classifiers. To obtain invariance with respect to lighting and volume, sub-windows are normalized, and the

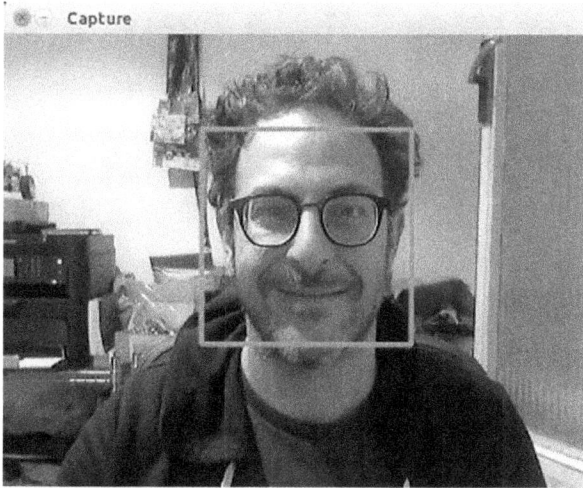

*Figure 14.5* Face detection using OpenCV.

final detector is slid over the image [43–45] at various window sizes. To build a single facial bounding box, any overlapping positive-classification windows are averaged. Each frame in the video is subjected to this FD algorithm and the bounding box is established for each face that it sensed. If no face is found in a frame, the previous frame's face is used; if several faces are detected, the nearest face to the preceding frame's face is used.

Haar cascades were used to introduce FD. Paul Viola and Michael Jones presented it in their research article [13], and it is a simple but very effective procedure. It is all about machine learning [46–48] and it has been evaluated on a range of both negative (photos of things without people) and positive (photos of people) images as shown in Figure 14.6. Following are some of the main features of the Viola-Jones detector:

1. Haar features: These are the various rectangular shape images.
2. Converting an Integral Image from the pixel intensity values.

From a large number of choices, the most efficient AdaBoost learning algorithm is used to choose the most effective features. The Cascades Filter eliminates negative windows to concentrate the computational complex process as much as possible on the positive ones.

## 14.4.3 Region of interest selection

The part of the image that has been chosen based on certain parameters will be used throughout the computational process. The most suitable place to observe skin color variation is the person's forehead, because this offers

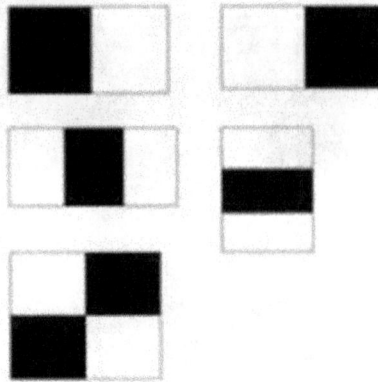

Figure 14.6 Haar features.

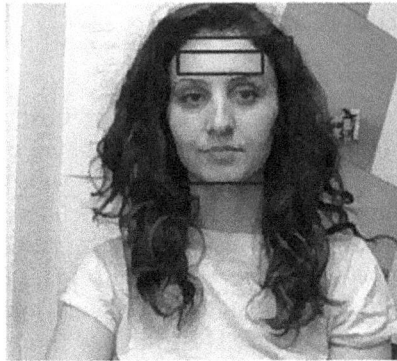

Figure 14.7 ROI selective area.

extensive changes featured. Although the size of the facial detection frame depends greatly on the subject's distance from the camera [49], the rectangle put on this area is measured in relation to it. Inside the area of interest, the median or mean of the vectors is then calculated for each frame used. The ROI is shown in Figure 14.7.

As the face-bounding box created by face recognition includes both background and facial pixels, an ROI must be selected inside the bounding box. As per the authors in Ref. [10], the simplest ROI is to use the entire height and the middle 60% of the bounding box width. Because the bounding box is normally within the face area in terms of height but outside the face in terms of width, this technique effectively changes the bounding box to eliminate the background pixels to the sides of the face. Any background pixels are typically still visible on the box's corners while using this process.

We also look at the other options for determining the ROI. The results of eliminating the eye region that contains nonskin pixels varying between

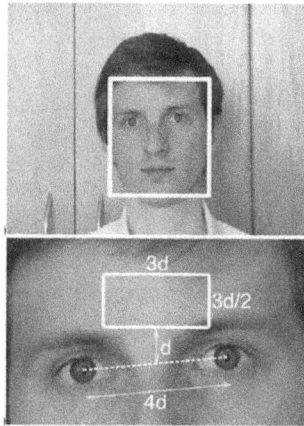

*Figure 14.8* ROI selection for whole face and forehead.

frames as a result of blinking or eye movement are studied. The eyes were successfully removed by eliminating the pixels from between 25% and 50% of the height of bounding box. We also consider keeping the pixels that are above the eye area, as the authors in Ref. [20] found that the plethysmography signal is strongest on the forehead. Finally, we look at the distinguishing facial pixels from background pixels as shown in Figure 14.8.

## 14.4.4 Object tracking

There are two approaches that can be used to classify the subject's face. For each frame, the FD algorithm is used in first approach. In the second approach, using the face recognition algorithm for the specific frames, only face monitoring is applied to them. The second approach is chosen because it is faster. This is due to the fact that when tracking an object seen in the previous photo, information about its existence is also given as shown in Figure 14.9. Multiple instance learning (MIL) tracker and boosting tracker are the best tracking algorithms, according to this research. We selected MIL for testing because its average processing time per face is around 9 milliseconds compared with around 15 milliseconds for boosting tracker.

## 14.4.5 System model for heart rate measurement

The signal from the previous stage is transformed into a 200-frame window using Fast Fourier Transform (FFT). Frequency filtering can be used to correct the incorrect readings because natural pulse rates are between 37 and 192 beats per minute. A heart rate of 0.5 to 3 Hz corresponds to a frequency of 0.5 to 3 Hz. Because the frequency range is too different

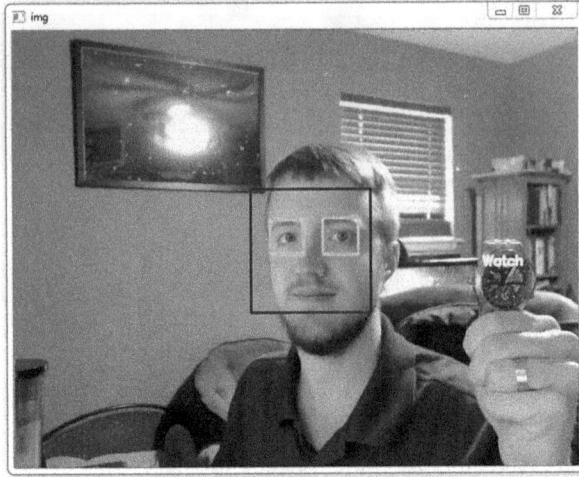

*Figure 14.9* Object tracking using OpenCV.

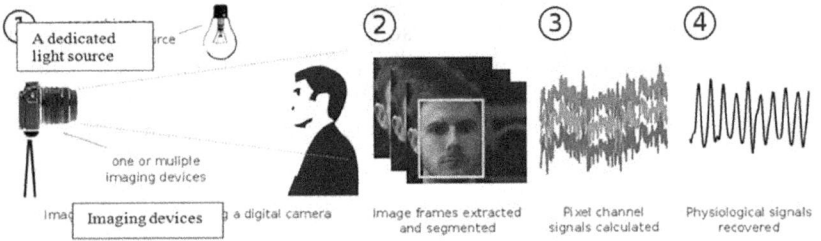

*Figure 14.10* Heart-rate detection.

from the frequency of the power line, which is 50 Hz to 60 Hz, this introduces a very little risk of power interference.

Because this algorithm runs with the frequency of the web camera, the sampling frequency only affects the spectral density during the operation [2, 3]. The limit is first found while avoiding the 0 Hz portion. An aspect ratio is determined between the median and maximum of the continuum to ensure that the maximum represents an HR frequency. We found that a 3:1 ratio is a strong discriminant for this case. Heart-rate detection system is shown in Figure 14.10.

## 14.4.6 Implementation

To make the final process, the previous steps are combined. As shown in Figure 14.11, these are represented as a series of blocks. The first block runs FD on each frame until it finds a face (or many faces). Following the frame, an object tracker is used to control each face separately and FD is no longer used on each frame. Every 10 seconds for up to ten consecutive frames, a

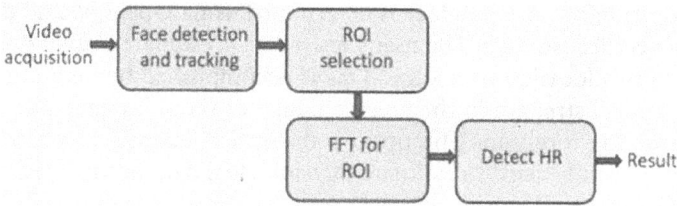

*Figure 14.11* Diagram of a heart rate measuring algorithm.

novel FD is used to see whether the tracked object is a face or if new faces had also emerged to the image.

## 14.5 RESULTS

### 14.5.1 Testing environment

Tests were carried out on the following hardware during development:

- Processor: Intel(R) Core (TM) i5-7200U CPU @ 2.50 GHz.
- RAM: 8.00 GB.
- 720p HD webcam.

In this study, the results evaluated for people were compared with a noticeable difference in skin tone, after measuring the average of the pixels from the ROI space. For each of the 20 people involved, the experiments were conducted under the same conditions. None of the participants wore any kind of makeup, and none had any sort of skin disorder. HR experiments were also carried out then in parallel with other two heart-rate control systems [50, 51] to make sure that the measurements were correct.

There were 3% errors found, but the true error rate is difficult to ascertain because monitors have inherent errors. In the experiments, different skin tones representing people from European origin and two people from the Indian subcontinent are used as shown in Figure 14.12. There were no significant differences in HR accuracy discovered.

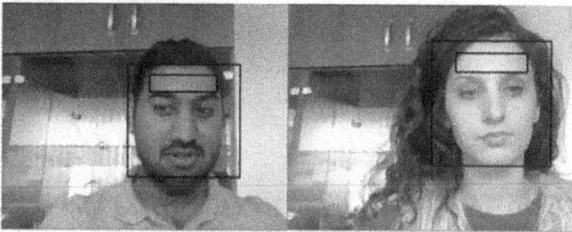

*Figure 14.12* Running test on different skin tones.

The location of the user's face is determined using OpenCV, and the forehead area is then isolated. The user's heart rate is estimated using data gathered from this location over time. This is accomplished by determining the average optical strength in the green channel of the sub-image alone at the position of the forehead. The optical absorption characteristics of (oxy-)hemoglobin can be used to estimate physiological data in this way. A stable

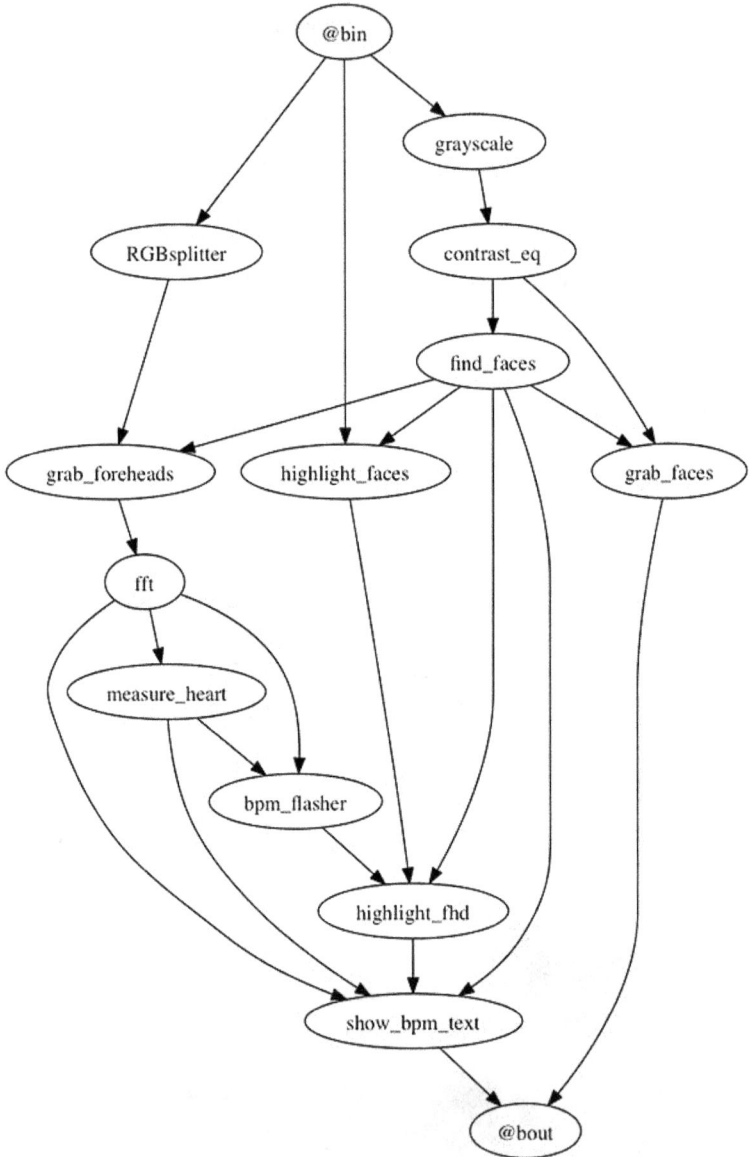

Figure 14.13 Execution order.

heartbeat can be isolated in around 15 seconds with good lighting and minimal motion noise. In the raw data stream, other physiological waveforms (such as Mayer waves) should also be available.

After estimating the individual heart rate, the value of real-time phase variance associated with this frequency is calculated. After that, in post-process frame rendering, the heartbeat can be exaggerated, causing the highlighted forehead position to pulse in time with the user's actual heartbeat. Multiple simultaneous individual identifications in a single camera's image stream are definitely possible, yet only one face's information is currently collected for analysis. Execution order is given in Figure 14.13. As per the execution order, initially the image is divided into grayscale and RGB. Then, forehead has been detected from both types of images that can be used for the detection of heart rate and bpm.

## 14.6 CONCLUSION

Heart rate monitoring is necessary because irregular changes in the cardiovascular system are obtained in diagnosis. The noncontact pulse monitoring methods are believed to be the most effective in everyday life and internet of things (IoT) applications are used among the several pulse monitoring techniques. The approach we have proposed here solves the issue of multiple-subject–based heart-rate monitoring process while still allowing for a smart phone implementation. Although a quite low-quality camera of laptop was used here, up to four people's HR could be tracked using a single webcam. Because it has used face recognition and object tracking altogether, the algorithm takes less time to compute. In the future, we plan to look into the effect of image quality [52–57] with the number of several faces that can be recognized and that too with the maximum distance between the subject and the camera [58, 59]. Some extra features can also be included such as temperature detection. The HR calculation algorithm will also be implemented on a number of platforms, including Raspberry-Pi and Android. In this way, multiple-camera monitoring of multiple people and their HR can be established.

## REFERENCES

[1] Hart, J. (2015). Normal resting pulse rate ranges. *Journal of Nursing Education and Practice*, 5(8), 95–98.

[2] Evans, J., Papadopoulos, A., Silvers, C. T., Charness, N., Boot, W. R., Schlachta-Fairchild, L., … & Ent, C. B. (2016). Remote health monitoring for older adults and those with heart failure: Adherence and system usability. *Telemedicine and e-Health*, 22(6), 480–488.

[3] Hassan, M. A., Malik, A. S., Fofi, D., Saad, N., Karasfi, B., Ali, Y. S., & Meriaudeau, F. (2017). Heart rate estimation using facial video: A review. *Biomedical Signal Processing and Control*, 38, 346–360.

[4] Stanković, R. S., & Falkowski, B. J. (2003). The Haar wavelet transform: Its status and achievements. *Computers & Electrical Engineering, 29*(1), 25–44.

[5] Kohli, L., Saurabh, M., Bhatia, I., Shekhawat, U. S., Vijh, M., & Sindhwani, N. (2021). Design and development of modular and multifunctional uav with amphibious landing module. In *Data Driven Approach Towards Disruptive Technologies: Proceedings of MIDAS 2020* (pp. 405–421). Springer, Singapore.

[6] Kohli, L., Saurabh, M., Bhatia, I., Sindhwani, N., & Vijh, M. (2021). Design and Development of Modular and Multifunctional UAV with Amphibious Landing, Processing and Surround Sense Module. In *Unmanned Aerial Vehicles for Internet of Things (IoT): Concepts, Techniques, and Applications* (p. 207).

[7] Talukder, K. H., & Harada, K. (2010). Haar wavelet based approach for image compression and quality assessment of compressed image. *arXiv preprint arXiv:1010.4084.*

[8] Datcu, D., Cidota, M., Lukosch, S., & Rothkrantz, L. (2013, June). Noncontact automatic heart rate analysis in visible spectrum by specific face regions. In *Proceedings of the 14th International Conference on Computer Systems and Technologies* (pp. 120–127).

[9] Werner, P., Al-Hamadi, A., Walter, S., Gruss, S., & Traue, H. C. (2014, October). Automatic heart rate estimation from painful faces. In *2014 IEEE International Conference on Image Processing (ICIP)* (pp. 1947–1951). IEEE.

[10] Li, J., Chen, Z. Z., Huang, L., Fang, M., Li, B., Fu, X., ... & Zhao, Q. (2018). Automatic classification of fetal heart rate based on convolutional neural network. *IEEE Internet of Things Journal, 6*(2), 1394–1401.

[11] Laukkanen, R. M., & Virtanen, P. K. (1998). Heart rate monitors: State of the art. *Journal of Sports Sciences, 16*(sup1), 3–7.

[12] Monkaresi, H., Calvo, R. A., & Yan, H. (2013). A machine learning approach to improve contactless heart rate monitoring using a webcam. *IEEE Journal of Biomedical and Health Informatics, 18*(4), 1153–1160.

[13] Otoom, A. F., Abdallah, E. E., Kilani, Y., Kefaye, A., & Ashour, M. (2015). Effective diagnosis and monitoring of heart disease. *International Journal of Software Engineering and Its Applications, 9*(1), 143–156.

[14] Van Rossum, G. (2007, June). Python programming language. In *USENIX Annual Technical Conference* (Vol. 41, p. 36).

[15] Chawla, P., Sindhwani, N. & Anand, R. (2020). Smart coal payload delivery system using pic microcontroller. *International Journal of Advanced Science and Technology, 29*(10s), 1485–1490.

[16] Sanner, M. F. (1999). Python: A programming language for software integration and development. *J Mol Graph Model, 17*(1), 57–61.

[17] Hasan Talukder, K., & Harada, K. (2010). Haar wavelet based approach for image compression and quality assessment of compressed image. *arXiv e-prints, arXiv-1010.*

[18] Tamboli, S. S., & Udupi, V. (2013). Image compression using Haar wavelet transform. *International Journal of Advanced Research in Computer and Communication Engineering, 2*(8).

[19] Nadrag, C., Poenaru, V., & Suciu, G. (2018, June). Heart rate measurement using face detection in video. In *2018 International Conference on Communications (COMM)* (pp. 131–134). IEEE.

[20] Viola, P., & Jones, M. (2001). Robust real-time object detection. *International Journal of Computer Vision, 4*(34–47), 4.

[21] Nosrati, M., & Tavassolian, N. (2017). High-accuracy heart rate variability monitoring using Doppler radar based on Gaussian pulse train modeling and FTPR algorithm. *IEEE Transactions on Microwave Theory and Techniques*, 66(1), 556–567.

[22] Grigulo, J., & Becker, L. B. (2018, September). Experimenting sensor nodes localization in WSN with UAV acting as mobile agent. In *2018 IEEE 23rd International Conference on Emerging Technologies and Factory Automation (ETFA)* (Vol. 1, pp. 808–815). IEEE.

[23] Gupta, A., Srivastava, A., Anand, R., & Tomažič, T. (2020). Business Application Analytics and the Internet of Things: The Connecting Link. In *New Age Analytics: Transforming the Internet through Machine Learning, IoT, and Trust Modeling* (p. 249).

[24] Anand, R., Sinha, A., Bhardwaj, A., & Sreeraj, A. (2018). Flawed Security of Social Network of Things. In *Handbook of Research on Network Forensics and Analysis Techniques* (pp. 65–86). IGI Global.

[25] Juneja, S., Juneja, A., & Anand, R. (2020). Healthcare 4.0-digitizing healthcare using big data for performance improvisation. *Journal of Computational and Theoretical Nanoscience*, 17(9–10), 4408–4410.

[26] Sansanwal, K., Shrivastava, G., Anand, R., & Sharma, K. (2019). Big Data Analysis and Compression for Indoor Air Quality. In *Handbook of IoT and Big Data* (Vol. 1).

[27] Hwang, S., Seo, J., Jebelli, H., & Lee, S. (2016). Feasibility analysis of heart rate monitoring of construction workers using a photoplethysmography (PPG) sensor embedded in a wristband-type activity tracker. *Automation in Construction*, 71, 372–381.

[28] Xiuping, Y., Jia-Nan, L., & Zuhua, F. (2015, June). hardware design of fall detection system based on ADXL345 sensor. In *2015 8th International Conference on Intelligent Computation Technology and Automation (ICICTA)* (pp. 446–449). IEEE.

[29] Pavlidis, I., Dowdall, J., Sun, N., Puri, C., Fei, J., & Garbey, M. (2007). Interacting with human physiology. *Computer Vision and Image Understanding*, 108(1–2), 150–170.

[30] Garbey, M., Sun, N., Merla, A., & Pavlidis, I. (2007). Contact-free measurement of cardiac pulse based on the analysis of thermal imagery. *IEEE Transactions on Biomedical Engineering*, 54(8), 1418–1426.

[31] Hyvärinen, A., & Oja, E. (2000). Independent component analysis: Algorithms and applications. *Neural Networks*, 13(4–5), 411–430.

[32] Jeanne, V., Asselman, M., den Brinker, B., & Bulut, M. (2013, December). Camera-based heart rate monitoring in highly dynamic light conditions. In *2013 International Conference on Connected Vehicles and Expo (ICCVE)* (pp. 798–799). IEEE.

[33] Verkruysse, W., Svaasand, L. O., & Nelson, J. S. (2008). Remote plethysmographic imaging using ambient light. *Optics Express*, 16(26), 21434–21445.

[34] Poh, M. Z., McDuff, D. J., & Picard, R. W. (2010). Non-contact, automated cardiac pulse measurements using video imaging and blind source separation. *Optics Express*, 18(10), 10762–10774.

[35] Poh, M. Z., McDuff, D. J., & Picard, R. W. (2010). Advancements in non-contact, multiparameter physiological measurements using a webcam. *IEEE Transactions on Biomedical Engineering*, 58(1), 7–11.

[36] Pursche, T., Krajewski, J., & Moeller, R. (2012, January). Video-based heart rate measurement from human faces. In *2012 IEEE International Conference on Consumer Electronics (ICCE)* (pp. 544–545). IEEE.

[37] Kwon, S., Kim, H., & Park, K. S. (2012, August). Validation of heart rate extraction using video imaging on a built-in camera system of a smartphone. In *2012 Annual International Conference of the IEEE Engineering in Medicine and Biology Society* (pp. 2174–2177). IEEE.

[38] Balakrishnan, G., Durand, F., & Guttag, J. (2013). Detecting pulse from head motions in video. In *Proceedings of the IEEE Conference on Computer Vision and Pattern Recognition* (pp. 3430–3437).

[39] Rubinstein, M. (2014). *Analysis and visualization of temporal variations in video* (Doctoral dissertation, Massachusetts Institute of Technology).

[40] Li, X., Chen, J., Zhao, G., & Pietikainen, M. (2014). Remote heart rate measurement from face videos under realistic situations. In *Proceedings of the IEEE Conference on Computer Vision and Pattern Recognition* (pp. 4264–4271).

[41] Stricker, R., Müller, S., & Gross, H. M. (2014, August). Non-contact video-based pulse rate measurement on a mobile service robot. In *The 23rd IEEE International Symposium on Robot and Human Interactive Communication* (pp. 1056–1062). IEEE.

[42] Xu, S., Sun, L., & Rohde, G. K. (2014). Robust efficient estimation of heart rate pulse from video. *Biomedical Optics Express*, 5(4), 1124–1135.

[43] Kumar, R., Anand, R., & Kaushik, G. (2011). Image compression using wavelet method & SPIHT algorithm. *Digital Image Processing*, 3(2), 75–79.

[44] Vyas, G., Anand, R., & Holê, K. E. Implementation of advanced image compression using wavelet transform and SPHIT algorithm. *International Journal of Electronic and Electrical Engineering*.

[45] Saini, P., & Anand, M. R. (2014). Identification of defects in plastic gears using image processing and computer vision: A review. *International Journal of Engineering Research*, 3(2), 94–99.

[46] Kamalraj, R., Neelakandan, S., Kumar, M. R., Rao, V. C. S., Anand, R., & Singh, H. (2021). Interpretable filter based convolutional neural network (IF-CNN) for glucose prediction and classification using PD-SS algorithm. *Measurement*, 183, 109804.

[47] Singh, H., Rehman, T. B., Gangadhar, C., Anand, R., Sindhwani, N., & Babu, M. (2021). Accuracy detection of coronary artery disease using machine learning algorithms. *Applied Nanoscience*, 1–7.

[48] Bakshi, G., Shukla, R., Yadav, V., Dahiya, A., Anand, R., Sindhwani, N., & Singh, H. (2021). An optimized approach for feature extraction in multi-relational statistical learning. *Journal of Scientific & Industrial Research*, 80, 537–542.

[49] Anand, R., Singh, B. & Sindhwani, N. (2009). Speech perception & analysis of fluent digits' strings using level-by-level time alignment. *International Journal of Information Technology and Knowledge Management*, 2(1), 65–68.

[50] Singh, L., Saini, M. K., Tripathi, S., & Sindhwani, N. (2008). An intelligent control system for real-time traffic signal using genetic algorithm. In *AICTE Sponsored National Seminar on Emerging Trends in Software Engineering* (Vol. 50).

[51] Saini, M. K., Nagal, R., Tripathi, S., Sindhwani, N., & Rudra, A. (2008). PC interfaced wireless robotic moving arm. In *AICTE Sponsored National Seminar on Emerging Trends in Software Engineering* (Vol. 50).

[52] Choudhary, P., & Anand, M. R. (2015). Determination of rate of degradation of iron plates due to rust using image processing. *International Journal of Engineering Research*, 4(2), 76–84.

[53] Juneja, S., & Anand, R. (2018). Contrast Enhancement of an Image by DWT-SVD and DCT-SVD. In *Data Engineering and Intelligent Computing* (pp. 595–603). Springer, Singapore.

[54] Gupta, M., & Anand, R. (2011). Color image compression using set of selected bit planes. *International Journal of Electronics & Communication Technology*, 2(3), 243–248.

[55] Ratnaparkhi, S. T., Singh, P., Tandasi, A., & Sindhwani, N. (2021). Comparative analysis of classifiers for criminal identification system using face recognition. In *2021 9th International Conference on Reliability, Infocom Technologies and Optimization (Trends and Future Directions) (ICRITO)* (pp. 1–6).

[56] Jain, S., Kumar, M., Sindhwani, N., & Singh, P. (2021). SARS-Cov-2 detection using Deep Learning Techniques on the basis of Clinical Reports. In *2021 9th International Conference on Reliability, Infocom Technologies and Optimization (Trends and Future Directions) (ICRITO)* (pp. 1–5).

[57] Malsa, N., Singh, P., Gautam, J., Srivastava, A., & Singh, S. P. (2020). Source of treatment selection for different states of india and performance analysis using machine learning algorithms for classification. In *Soft Computing: Theories and Applications*. Springer, Singapore.

[58] Goyal, B., Dogra, A., Khoond, R., Gupta, A., & Anand, R. (2021, September). Infrared and visible image fusion for concealed weapon detection using transform and spatial domain filters. In *2021 9th International Conference on Reliability, Infocom Technologies and Optimization (Trends and Future Directions)(ICRITO)* (pp. 1–4). IEEE.

[59] Kaur, J., Sabharwal, S., Dogra, A., Goyal, B., & Anand, R. (2021, September). Single image dehazing with dark channel prior. In *2021 9th International Conference on Reliability, Infocom Technologies and Optimization (Trends and Future Directions)(ICRITO)* (pp. 1–5). IEEE.

Chapter 15

# An intelligent model for coronary heart disease diagnosis

*T. K. Revathi, B. Sathiyabhama, and S. Sankar*
Sona College of Technology, Salem, India

*Digvijay Pandey*
IET Lucknow, Department of Technical Education Kanpur, India

*Binay Kumar Pandey*
Govind Ballabh Pant University of Agriculture and Technology, Uttarakhand, India

*Pankaj Dadeech*
Swami Keshvanand Institute of Technology, Management & Gramothan, Jaipur, India

## CONTENTS

## 15.1 INTRODUCTION

Heart attack is the primary cause for the mortality rate in the world. Recently, one in every four people dies due to heart failure worldwide. Lancet (medical journal) reported that, in India, Tamil Nadu is the second highest state in the prevalence rate of heart disease. People are affected as they do not get timely treatment and diagnosis of the disease. Usually, heart disease happens because of the disorders in the heart rhythm called arrhythmias [1]. Among many arrhythmias, myocardial infarction (MI) commonly known as heart attack is the main reason for mortality rate [2]. It happens due to the stopping of blood flow in a particular portion of the heart which directs to the complete blockage in coronary arteries causing heart attack. Thin fat plaque formation inside the coronary artery disrupts the blood flow in and out to the heart. But complete blockage in coronary arteries causes MI [3]. The proposed work uses a novel imaging biomarker fat attenuation index (FAI) that is able to detect fatty tissue formation in and around the arteries using computed tomography (CT) image. The significance of FAI is to diagnose the fatal heart attack many years before it happens [4, 5]. It acquires the details about the type of heart attack and the place of arteries where it exactly occurs [6].

The amount of fat in and around the artery wall is taken from online Visual Lab repository. A deep learning approach with convolutional neural network (CNN) [7] is used to predict the heart attack with this cardiac fat database. There are two classes being obtained from CNN, one is normal class, i.e., no blockage in artery, another is abnormal class, i.e., cardiac mortality. CNN implements data augmentation to train the model with huge volume of data and hence it reduces computational burden of the testing phase [8, 9]. It is vital to fit the learning model with a suitable trained structure of the data. Thus, the proposed system is competent enough that it eliminates the need for pre-processing and manual feature extraction for the identification of disease. Typically, the bootstrap aggregation strategy is used to train and validate the diagnostic performance of the proposed system [10, 11]. FAI renders many significant features such as once patients are detected with the high risk of FAI, they are treated as having a higher risk of adverse heart attack for the next five years. With this new technology, clinicians may find the patients who have greater risk of deadly heart attack and give aggressive medical treatment to prevent them from heart attack.

## 15.2 RELATED WORK

CHD is identified as one of the primary deadly diseases. It occurs due to plaque build-up inside the artery tube. This results in narrowing of the coronary artery lumen that restricts the flow of blood to the heart [12, 13]. Narrowing of arteries is called as stenosis. The whole blockage in the artery leads to MI, generally recognized as a heart attack [14]. There are various types of diagnosis that do exist for predicting the disease [15]. These plaques diffuse the fat content to the proximal side wall to the tube and they cause the inflammation in the artery. This kind of inflammation is the cause of heart attack.

Current tools are suitable for diagnosing the heart disease only after it happens [16, 17]. It is a tough task to diagnose a heart attack as early as it happens. Recently, a new biomarker, FAI, was introduced by the Centre of Research Excellence, British Heart Foundation for predicting future adverse heart attack many years before it happens [18]. It is difficult to notice and categorize the coronary artery inflammation to prevent MI as early as possible. FAI is an imaging biomarker that computes the inflamed coronary artery and is medically obtained using noninvasive coronary CT angiography (CCTA) test [19, 20]. To prevent patients from heart attack, they are recommended to take up further noninvasive tests. The artery plaque can be classified into three categories. They are calcified plaque, noncalcified plaque, and mixed plaque based on its composition [21, 22]. The formation of these plaques and their breakage leads to the severe coronary syndrome and it causes MI [23]. Coronary artery stenosis is narrowing of the arteries. Severe blockage of arteries may cause a heart attack [24]. Coronary artery calcium score (CACS) is a tool that plays a vital role in diagnosing artery stenosis disease. It does not correctly predict all types of causes of the CHD [25]. The prognostic value of CACS is used to discover the existence and severity of CHD in patients.

Artery inflammation enables the timely exploitation of events to prevent future MI. FAI around coronary artery is used to diagnose coronary inflammation and it also identifies the individuals at risk of cardiac mortality. It captures fat attenuation of perivascular and detects vascular inflammation at an early stage with routine CCTA [26]. There are both invasive and noninvasive procedures offered to detect heart disease. CCTA is a well-established heart imaging tool that gives the information on the plaque present in the coronary arteries [27]. It is a sensitive and commonly used diagnostic tool for diagnosing CHD [28]. The width of luminal plaque and the plaque composition is found by CCTA. The vessels can also be diagnosed like retinal images, because both CCTA and retinal images are vessel-based structures [29, 30]. Analysis of coronary arterial vessel provides needs details about conditions of the blood flow and systemic level of the blood voltage [31]. Cardiologists can detect the sign of systemic vessel burden much earlier before it happens. Speed of blood flow helps in assessing the cardiac threatening diseases such as CHD and MI. It is done from the structure of abnormality in the coronary artery structures [32]. The noises have been eliminated using 3D artifacts removal technique [33] so that the arteries look clear in viewing the vessels. An adaptive block-matching 3D algorithm is applied for treating low-dose CT images [34].

CHD can also be predicted using another diagnosing tool called retinal fundus risk factors [35]. Researchers can gather the retinal image based on which they can validate their model. To support the examination, automatic artery segmentation method, mainly from CCTA images, has been used extensively for doing research study. In ancient days, several computer visions-based methods were deals about this problem from the perception of signal processing [36–39]. In this type of assumption, the scientists have been followed to denoise the CCTA images from specific patterns for segmenting the vessels [40]. Singular value decomposition (SVD)–based algorithm has also been proposed for the sparse representation of an image dataset [41]. Long-term recurrent CNN is being used for the visual recognition of image data and semantic approaches also give better outcome to the image visualization [42]. Various heuristic methods such as line detection [43] and feature extraction–based handcrafted methods were used in determining the disease [44]. However, much more improved results are obtained, with the advance techniques of machine learning and from feature learning automation technique [45]. For instance, the features of vessel may be automatically extracted using gradient boosting [46], and scientists need to anticipate to introduce conditional random field (CRF). Their parameters are qualified from curvilinear structure segmentation of the data with the structured support vector machine (SVM) [47].

In the modern times, CNN [48] has remarkable outcomes for several computer vision problems. Several literature surveys portray that CNN has better performance in doing the segmentation process of vessels in any body organs and it even outstands to the ability of human specialists in multiple datasets [49]. Nevertheless, the segmented vessels of all the methods mentioned are rather unclear and they suffer from tiny and faint tubes of the arteries. This happens because of the kernel function applied in the CNNs. The existing methodologies only depend on the pixel-wise kernel functions and they also compare the model generated images with the standard images.

This is not providing the desirable outcome because it cannot aggressively accommodate natural vessel structure that exists in CCTA images. In fact, the segmentation of coronary arteries can be measured as an image conversion problem. From an input image, a segmented artery vessel map is generated. If the output images are inhibited to look like the doctors' annotation, then clear and sharp artery vessel maps can be attained from the proposed method of generative adversarial network (GAN).

GAN is a special kind of system that allows the creation of a rational output [50, 51]. GAN contains two different networks, namely discriminator and generator. The discriminator tries to differentiate the regular images from the outputs generated through generator. The generator is responsible in producing realistic outputs. This cannot be done by the discriminator, whereas the generator cannot differentiate the standard image from model-generated image.

Clinical database contains patients' heart-related information that is used to recognize the factors that support heart attack prediction [52]. The knowledge discovery is used to identify the influence that helps in improving the quality and provides better patient care. Differential diagnostic procedure [53] is a systematic diagnostic method. In this method, condition-based identification is used to find the presence of a disease entity where multiple alternatives are possible. The major complaint is examined with respect to the causal factors [54]. According to various theoretical paradigms, the presence of the disease is identified and compared to known categories of any disease which the researcher encounters for diagnosis. This method may establish several algorithms to the process of elimination and also it is used to obtain the information that minimizes the probabilities of candidate conditions. This is an insignificant level for the scientists who are working with the evidence such as symptoms, patient history, and medical knowledge.

Retinal images are one of the most significant tools to predict the various cardiovascular risk factors. It is stated that rather than numerical and electrocardiogram (ECG) signals, the image data could be correlated directly with cardiovascular events [55, 56]. Recently, the use of deep learning helps in getting the outcome for detecting age, patient's gender information, systolic blood pressure (BP), diastolic BP, and smoke practice from the fundus images. The artificial intelligence (AI)–based system [57] had equivalent area under curve (AuC) to the traditional risk calculators in predicting severe cardiovascular risks. The model developed seems to be actual imaging modality to assess the CHD events.

In most developing countries, CHD is the principal cause of mortality. By 2020, in India, the estimated prevalence rate of CHDs would be 54.5 million. Due to CHDs, one in four deaths happens. Cardiovascular diseases (CVDs) have not been addressed properly under specific control programs as like existing communicable diseases. Hypertension accounted for 80% of the CHDs. It is designated that risk factors like systolic BP and plasma cholesterol contribute to the surplus risk of CHD [58].

Indian Council of Medical Research (ICMR) estimates that the count of hypertensive is expected to rise up to 214 million in 2025. So, this chapter wants to address these hypertensive risk factors appropriately. The retinal fundus is the potential biomarker to find the hypertensive periodically based on its microstructural changes. Also, India needs priority action to highlight the knowledge of physicians, individuals, and communities about the risk factors and make them adhere to the proper treatment of patients. This article produces the evidence-based recommendation to emphasize the physicians' knowledge on treating patients. The improper follow up of bedside patients can cause the patients to revisit hospital infinitely.

## 15.3 PROBLEM FINDINGS

Heart disease causes death to people. Heart is the main part of a human body which circulates blood in and out of the heart muscle. Coronary artery is a kind of tube that plays a vital role in passing the blood circulation to the heart. If the tube is clear, then there is no problem in passing the blood. If it is thin plaque, then disruption happens in blood flow that sometimes causes chest pain or angina. Sometimes, the complete blockage blocks the coronary artery which is not able to pass the blood into the heart, which causes MI. The risk of heart attack is evaluated based on the plaque formation. The fatty tissue formation in and around the blood vessel is called as perivascular fat. To diagnose the fatty tissue inflammation, a new imaging biomarker FAI is used. FAI is measured using CT scan image. The CT scan image of heart along with ECG signal is given to CNN model to classify the test data into normal or heart attack based on the trained data. The only classifier to deal with the image datasets is CNN. There is no need to filter the noise. It is robust classifier that swallows overall burden in training phase and takes less computational time to test the data.

### 15.3.1  Objective of the proposed CNN model

- To develop a neural network for the patients suffering from heart disease and heart beat disorders.
- To detect the present cases of heart attack analyzed so as to generate a knowledge base of potential occurrence to strengthen preventive treatment to the patients.
- To apply big data–based prognostic analytics and image processing procedures [59–62] to learn the essential knowledge and valuable insights accessible in the clinical databases.
- To assess an exclusive instructive interference on heart attack and risk reduction for the patients.

### 15.3.2  Data acquisition

The dataset is taken from the online visual lab Cardiac Fat Database – CT. These data describe about the fat content backgrounds of the heart corresponding to the risk factors of carotid stiffness, coronary artery calcification, atherosclerosis, atrial fibrillation (AFib) cancer incidence, and others. The image is already segmented and denoted with red color representing the epicardial fat, the green color representing the mediastinal fat, and the blue color indicating the gap among the epicardial and mediastinal fats. In total, there are about 20 patients' data available and the relevant extracted features are kept separately in the database. The data are further tuned with feature extraction such as pixel level and weighted vicinity based on Gaussian method.

### 15.4  PROPOSED METHODOLOGY

### 15.4.1  Design of neural network

Neural networks form a significant role to find a transformation of data for making a decision. Neural network plays a vital role to obtain significance from complex data. Its remarkable ability can be applied to segment patterns and identify features that are too complex to be noticed by either humans or other computer techniques. There are several neural networks available in present for meeting different applications dealing with different data. The proposed system is to develop a CNN for heart attack prediction and control. CNN is the most commonly used neural network applied to analyze the visual imaginary. Building of big data, cloud-centred CNN, and scientific interference for heart attack control and prevention is a challenging task. It involves the sharing of prompt accessible health details [63] and domain-oriented insights to the medical practitioners for quality prediction.

CNN is capable of handling the clinical images and it explicitly represents the medical insights executed through software packages. The clinical insights are strides into the various layers of CNN; in each layer, the low- and high-level features are to be extracted for efficient decision making.

CNN consists of input, output, and multiple hidden layers. The hidden layer comprises of convolutional, pooling, and fully connected layers. Every layer is made up of neurons with learnable weights and biases. Every time, a series of layer gets activated. In the input layer, the image data are given as an input to train the model. The given image is represented in three-dimensional matrix (WxHxD) of pixel values. Part of an input image pixel is given to convolutional layer (ConV) used to extract the features of the input volume. The convolution layer comprises of a set of independent filters that take a weighted sum over every image pixel used for feature detection. Figure 15.1 illustrates the CNN structure in classifying CT image.

Striding is calculated with dot product between the kernel and pixel of an input for feature map. Low-level layer will identify a set of features such as line or edges of a given image. The high-level layers will find the more complex features of the original image. The process is repeated until all the pixels of the entire input image are visited. The outcome of convolution layer is a simple integer such as positive number or negative number that

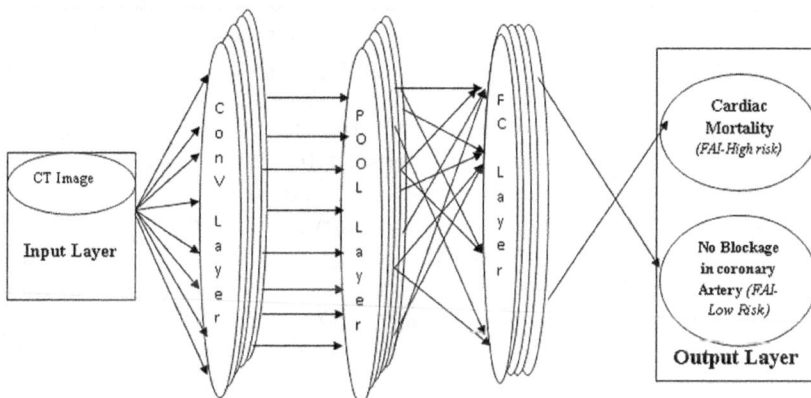

*Figure 15.1* CNN layer for classifying CT image.

will be given as input to the next layer rectifier linear unit (ReLU). This applies activation function max() on every element, which turns all negative values into zeros. The size of the image remains the same. The next layer is pooling layer (POOL layer) that performs reduction of spatial magnitudes of the input. The last unit is fully connected unit layer that applies the softmax function for the classification of generated features into different classes based on the trained data. This system is useful in diagnosing the future heart attack in a short time and effective via identifying FAI and irregular heartbeat of ECG.

## 15.4.2 Work plan

### 15.4.2.1 Knowledge acquisition

The details are collected from domain-specific researchers like medical practitioners and cardiologists about the heart attack to create a knowledge base. Knowledge base also meets the clinical documentation, review consultation of details, clinical diagnosis, treatment process and guidelines of best practice with the help of doctors. The data required to build the network model is taken from the online visual lab Cardiac Fat Database – CT.

### 15.4.2.2 Image pre-processing

Deep learning has the ability to deal with medical imaging, including object recognition and image segmentation. Clinical images portray only the human structure and no background image is present other than human body. In this proposed system, CT scan image depicts only the structure of heart and not more than that. The images have to pre-processed for the feature extraction. Pre-processing technique is better for improving the visualization of CT image in contrast enhancement. In this work, no pre-processing is needed, because the available data itself is denoised with Gaussian filters. All the images are enhanced and contrasted to the level of better recognition. The purpose of contrast enhancement is to increase the effectiveness of the low contrast CT image. The contrast-enhanced images are better for the model to extract the desired features.

The original CCTA image has cardiac motion artifacts due to several reasons. The first and foremost step is to perform the removal of cardiac motion artifacts in the right coronary artery (RCA). It is done by doing image reconstruction process to the CCTA. Image reconstruction refers to recovering the original clean CCTA image from the corruption arising from the motion blur and low resolution. The image noise refers to the variations in color, brightness, or imperfect camera sensor [64–67].

The fundamental impact of image reconstruction is image quality. The main purpose of doing reconstructions is to improve image quality [68]. Sometimes, the low radiation dose degrades the original image quality.

Deep CNN considers the low-dose CT scan image for noise reduction and produces normal-dose CT scan image patch by patch. It is very tough to remove all noises fully with the conventional denoising methods [69].

The block-matching 3D (BM3D) algorithm is suggested as a fine method for image restoration. It has been enhanced with performing denoising in a local noise level estimation. Non local means (NLM) low-dose CT image restoration with similar means is considered for image noise reduction process. Sparse representation technique has been adapted with K-singular value decomposition (K-SVD) to face the low-dose CT images.

### 15.4.2.3 Pre-processing for creating model

Most of the clinicians use medical images for diagnosing the disease to prevent patient's life. It is not applicable for any diagnostic system to use medical images as it is taken from the diagnostics tool. It must be converted into normal image format (jpeg). Only after the conversion, it may be given as an input to the model proposed. Picture archiving and communication system (PACS) is used to convert the medical images into the relevant data of the model. All the converted images must be put into a common training database. The proposed system is planned to use deep learning software, Santa Clara (NVIDIA Deep Learning GPU Training System) as training database.

### 15.4.2.4 System requirements

GPU specifications are:

- NVIDIA DIGITS for DL
- Augmented system with two GTX1080 Ti GPUs
- 11.34 T-Flops
- 484 GB per Sec size of bandwidth
- 11 Gigabyte of memory/board.

### 15.4.2.5 CPU specifications

- Single desktop with Intel i5-4590 Processor
- 3.3 GHz 6M Cache memory
- 16 GB Memory
- 500GB SATA HDD
- 10 GB Ethernet Card
- Python tool is used to design CNN. Jupyter IDE is used for code editing.
- Coding starts with including python libraries and then import the image data.

### 15.4.2.6 Evaluation procedure

The CNN model is evaluated based on the trained data. The overall accuracy of the model is evaluated using the true positive and true negative cases. The sensitivity (Se) and positive predictivity (PP) can be calculated based on the true positive (TP), true negative (TN), false positive (FP), and false negative (FN). Overall accuracy is acquired by the ratio between the numbers of correctly classified results in test images.

## 15.4.3 Architecture of proposed CNN model

Figure 15.2 illustrates the architecture of the proposed CNN model. The input dataset such as ECG signal and CT images are pre-processed, and the essential knowledge has been extracted from the clinical trials. It has been

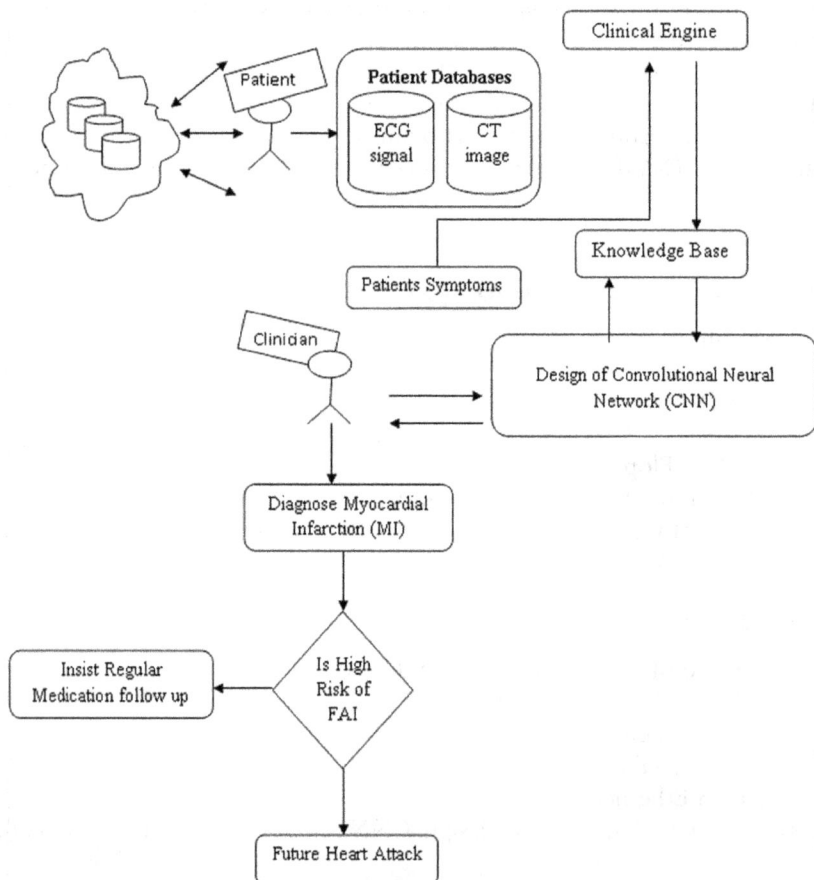

Figure 15.2 Architecture of automated diagnosis of myocardial infarction (MI).

kept in the knowledge base. The same is given as an input to the proposed CNN model. It has been trained with the past history of the patient's database to find the risk factor of MI. If the risk is found to be high with FAI index, then the model classifies it as the patient is identified with MI else the patient is classified as normal.

### 15.4.4 Training the model

Because the online databases have only limited set of CT images, it is not enough for training and testing the network model. So, before doing training process, the data must be augmented in order to have larger amount of data. Now, the database contains more images that are essential to build the CNN to train with a huge volume of data. The entire burden is made in the training phase itself so that it is easy for the model to test the new data to classify it exactly. Bootstrap aggregation is the technique used for data augmentation, which doubles the dataset by doing some minor changes on the existing data like flip left or right and make it a large dataset. More data are given as input to train the model as robust for accurate classification.

Some portion of an image is given as input to convolution (ConV) layer. The pixel of an image is taken into feature extraction with suitable filter/kernel. The low-level features are extracted pixel-by-pixel with suitable filter/kernel. The same operation is performed until all the pixels of the image are read. All the pixels/images are translated into a matrix format with digits. Subsequently, the convolved image is given to the pooling layer. This layer is capable of minimizing the dimensions of an image. Last layer is a fully connected layer in which every neuron of each layer is connected with every other neuron.

Overall 80% of the data from visual lab repository are considered to train the model. From the cardiac-fat database CT, 80% of data from each database is taken into account for training the model. Specifically, around 750 images from Ground Truth – (Fat Range[–200, –30]) database, Ground Truth – (Higher Range [–200, 500]), Ground Truth – (Combined [–200, –30] and [–200, 500]) were examined to do the process of training the model.

### 15.5 RESULTS AND DISCUSSIONS

The prognostic value of FAI is tested to validate the robustness of the network. Many statistical analysis tests are available for validating the system. In this work, the Mann–Whitney U-test is used to test the prognostic value of FAI along with the categorical variables of two groups. Mann–Whitney U-test is a kind of test for the independent sample t-test. Usually, it compares means of two samples derived from the similar population and is applied to check whether two sample means look identical or not. Generally, the Mann–Whitney U-test is applied when the data are ordinal.

The proposed system considers only the four attributes that predominantly help in validating the network in the sequence of diagnosing the disease.

Four statistical performance measures are applied and their formulae are given below for calculating the measures of the proposed system. The performance indicators are accuracy, precision, recall, F1-score. These parameters are defined using four measures TP, TN, FP, and FN.

The performance is analyzed using the following parameters:

**Precision** – It is the proportion of rightly predicted positive outcome to the total predicted positive outcomes

$$\Pr ecision = \frac{TP}{TP + FP} \tag{15.1}$$

**Recall** – This indicates the percentage of real beats that were rightly predicted by the model.

$$\operatorname{Re} call = \frac{TP}{TP + FN} \tag{15.2}$$

**F1 Score** – It is the weighted average of precision and recall. It takes both FP and FN for calculation.

$$F1Score = \frac{2^{*} \left( \operatorname{Re} call^{*} \Pr ecision \right)}{\operatorname{Re} call + \Pr ecision} \tag{15.3}$$

The overall accuracy of the model is evaluated based on the below-mentioned formula:

$$Acuuracy = \frac{TP + TN}{TP + TN + FP + FN} * 100 \tag{15.4}$$

According to these formulae, precision, recall, F1 score, and accuracy are calculated and the result of the comparison is shown in Table 15.1.

Table 15.1 depicts the performance measures of CNN with three kinds of training and testing split-up. The dataset is taken from the online visual lab Cardiac Fat Database – CT. Totally, there are 125 subjects from which the observations were considered. From each patient's dataset, there were about 25 images of heart that correspond to the risk factors of carotid stiffness, coronary artery calcification, and atrial fibrillation by taking into evaluation the performance measures. The proposed CNN model with FAI index gives better accuracy to this cardiac fat database when compared with other CNN models. The experimental result indicates that the proposed method will help doctors to predict the cardiac mortality as early as possible. Figure 15.3 illustrates the overall accuracy of the proposed CNN model.

Table 15.1 Performance measures for coronary artery of the heart (N = 125) using CNN

| Ratio of training and testing | Type of the class | Precision | Recall | F1 score | Accuracy |
|---|---|---|---|---|---|
| 90:10 | Normal artery | 0.77 | 0.76 | 0.80 | 78.5 |
| | Blockage artery | 0.79 | 0.78 | 0.78 | 78.5 |
| | Average | 0.78 | 0.77 | 0.79 | 78.7 |
| 80:20 | Normal artery | 0.77 | 0.80 | 0.78 | 79.2 |
| | Blockage artery | 0.76 | 0.78 | 0.81 | 79.1 |
| | Average | 0.77 | 0.79 | 0.79 | 78.7 |
| 70:30 | Normal artery | 0.80 | 0.80 | 0.77 | 79.4 |
| | Blockage artery | 0.81 | 0.76 | 0.79 | 78.9 |
| | Average | 0.80 | 0.78 | 0.78 | 79 |

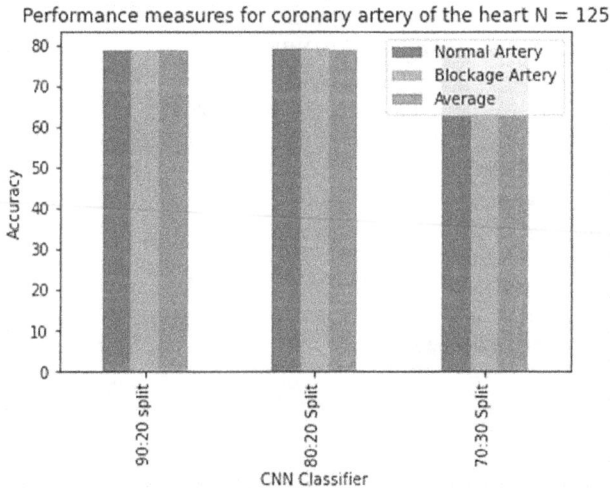

Figure 15.3 Overall accuracy of proposed CNN model.

## 15.6 CONCLUSION

Cardiac diseases are very much harmful to the human society that result in the increase of mortality rate. It is very much necessary to detect and prevent cardiac diseases as early as possible. Most of the existing technologies can diagnose heart-related diseases [70]. The proposed system gives much better results in diagnosing future fatal heart attack so many years before it happens. The experimental result is also more accurate because it uses FAI biomarker for the prediction. Furthermore, there is no pre-processing held because the dataset itself is denoised with Gaussian filters. Nevertheless, the error propagate rate is minimized because of this deep learning approach [71–73] that is reliable and optimized [74, 75, 76]. It helps the medical practitioners to predict heart attack earlier so that the patients need not go for further noninvasive tests.

## REFERENCES

[1] Ng, J. Y.-H., Hausknecht, M., Vijayanarasimhan, S., Vinyals, O., Monga, R., & Toderici, G. (2015). Beyond short snippets: Deep networks for video classification. In *Proceedings of the IEEE Conference on Computer Vision and Pattern Recognition* (pp. 4694–4702). IEEE.

[2] Chen, Y., Yin, X., Shi, L., Shu, H., Luo, L., Coatrieux, J. L., & Toumoulin, C. (2013). Improving abdomen tumor low-dose CT images using a fast dictionary learning based processing. *Phys. Med. Biol.* 58(16), 5803–5820.

[3] Liang, M., & Hu, X. (2015). Recurrent convolutional neural network for object recognition. In *Proceedings of the IEEE Conference on Computer Vision and Pattern Recognition* (pp. 3367–3375).

[4] De Mulder, W., Bethard, S., & Moens, M.-F. (2015). A survey on the application of recurrent neural networks to statistical language modeling. *Computer Speech & Language*, 30(1), 61–98.

[5] Poudel, R. P., Lamata, P., & Montana, G. (2016). Recurrent fully convolutional neural networks for multi-slice MRI cardiac segmentation. In *Reconstruction, Segmentation, and Analysis of Medical Images* (pp. 83–94). Springer.

[6] Litjens, G., Kooi, T., Bejnordi, B. E., Setio, A. A. A., Ciompi, F., Ghafoorian, M., van der Laak, J. A., van Ginneken, B., & Snchez, C. I. (2017). A survey on deep learning in medical image analysis. *Medical Image Analysis*, 42(Supplement C), 60–88.

[7] Sindhwani, N., Verma, S., Bajaj, T., & Anand, R. (2021). Comparative analysis of intelligent driving and safety assistance systems using YOLO and SSD model of deep learning. *International Journal of Information System Modeling and Design (IJISMD)*, 12(1), 131–146.

[8] Zreik, M., Lessmann, N., van Hamersvelt, R. W., Wolterink, J. M., Voskuil, M., Viergever, M. A., Leiner, T., & Išgum, I. (2018). Deep learning analysis of the myocardium in coronary CT angiography for identification of patients with functionally significant coronary artery stenosis. *Medical Image Analysis*, 44, 72–85.

[9] Xie, S., & Tu, Z. (2015). Holistically-nested edge detection. In *Proceedings of the IEEE International Conference on Computer Vision* (pp. 1395–1403).

[10] Zreik, M., Van Hamersvelt, R. W., Wolterink, J. M., Leiner, T., Viergever, M. A., & Išgum, I. (2018). A recurrent CNN for automatic detection and classification of coronary artery plaque and stenosis in coronary CT angiography. *IEEE Transactions on Medical Imaging*, 38(7), 1588–1598.

[11] Richardson, W. S., Glasziou, P., Polashenski, W. A., & Wilson, M. C. (2000). A new arrival: Evidence about differential diagnosis. *BMJ Evidence-Based Medicine*, 5(6), 164–165.

[12] Oikonomou, E. K., Marwan, M., Desai, M. Y., Mancio, J., Alashi, A., Centeno, E. H., ... & Antoniades, C. (2018). Non-invasive detection of coronary inflammation using computed tomography and prediction of residual cardiovascular risk (the CRISP CT study): A post-hoc analysis of prospective outcome data. *The Lancet*, 392(10151), 929–939.

[13] Ma, J., Huang, J., Feng, Q., Zhang, H., Lu, H., Liang, Z. and Chen, W. (2011). Low-dose computed tomography image restoration using previous normal-dose scan. *Medical Physics*, 38(10), 5713–5731.

[14] Raff, G., Abidov, A., Achenbach, S., Berman, D., Boxt, L., Budoff, M., Cheng, V., DeFrance, T., Hellinger, J., & Karlsberg, R. (2009). SCCT guidelines for the interpretation and reporting of coronary computed tomographic angiography. *Journal of Cardiovascular Computed Tomography*, 3(2), 122–136.

[15] Achenbach, S. (2018). Can CT detect the vulnerable coronary plaque? *The International Journal of Cardiovascular Imaging (formerly Cardiac Imaging)*, 24(3), 311–312.

[16] Raff, G. L., Abidov, A., Achenbach, S., Berman, D. S., Boxt, L. M., Budoff, M. J., ... & Karlsberg, R. P. (2009). SCCT guidelines for the interpretation and reporting of coronary computed tomographic angiography. *Journal of Cardiovascular Computed Tomography*, 3(2), 122–136.

[17] van Hamersvelt, R. W., Zreik, M., Voskuil, M., Viergever, M. A., Išgum, I., & Leiner, T. (2019). Deep learning analysis of left ventricular myocardium in CT angiographic intermediate-degree coronary stenosis improves the diagnostic accuracy for identification of functionally significant stenosis. *European Radiology*, 29(5), 2350–2359.

[18] Nguyen, U. T., Bhuiyan, A., Park, L. A., & Ramamohanarao, K. (2013). An effective retinal blood vessel segmentation method using multi-scale line detection. *Pattern Recognition*, 46(3), 703–715.

[19] Fu, H., Xu, Y., Lin, S., Wong, D. W. K., & Liu, J. (2016). Deepvessel Retinal vessel segmentation via deep learning and conditional random field. In *International Conference on Medical Image Computing and Computer-Assisted Intervention* (pp. 132–139).

[20] Wu, D., Wang, X., Bai, J., Xu, X., Ouyang, B., Li, Y., Zhang, H., Song, Q., Cao, K., & Yin, Y. (2019). Automated anatomical labeling of coronary arteries via bidirectional tree LSTMs. *International Journal of Computer Assisted Radiology and Surgery*, 14(2), 271–280.

[21] Cassar, A., Holmes Jr, D. R., Rihal, C. S., & Gersh, B. J. (2009). Chronic coronary artery disease: Diagnosis and management. *Mayo Clinic Proceedings*, 84(12), 1130–1146.

[22] Feruglio, P. F., Vinegoni, C., Gros, J., Sbarbati, A., & Weissleder, R. (2010). Block matching 3D random noise filtering for absorption optical projection tomography, *Physics in Medicine and Biology*, 55(18), 5401–5415.

[23] Kang, D., Slomka, P., Nakazato, R., Woo, J., Berman, D. S., Kuo, C. C. J., & Dey, D. (2013). Image denoising of low-radiation dose coronary CT angiography by an adaptive block-matching 3D algorithm. In *Proceeding SPIE 8669, Medical Imaging 2013: Image Processing* (p. 86692G).

[24] Tian, C., Xu, Y., Fei, L., & Yan, K. (2018). Deep learning for image denoising: A survey. *arXiv preprint arXiv:1810.05052*.

[25] Maninis, K. K., Pont-Tuset, J., Arbel_aez, P., & Van Gool, L. (2016). Deep retinal image understanding. In *International Conference on Medical Image Computing and Computer-Assisted Intervention* (pp. 140–148).

[26] Melin_s_cak, M., Prenta_si_c, P., & Lon_car_ic, S. (2015). Retinal vessel segmentation using deep neural networks. In *VISAPP 2015 (10th International Conference on Computer Vision Theory and Applications)*.

[27] Andermatt, S., Pezold, S., & Cattin, P. (2016). Multi-Dimensional Gated Recurrent Units for the Segmentation of Biomedical 3D-Data. In *Deep Learning and Data Labeling for Medical Applications* (pp. 142–151). Springer.

[28] Xue, W., Brahm, G., Pandey, S., Leung, S., & Li, S. (2018). Full left ventricle quantification via deep multitask relationships learning. *Medical Image Analysis*, 43, 54–65.

[29] Chen, H., Zhang, Y., Zhang, W., Liao, P., Li, K., Zhou, J., & Wang, G. (2017). Low-dose CT via convolutional neural network. *Biomedical Optics Express*, 8(2), 679–694.

[30] Li, Z., Yu, L., Trzasko, J. D., Lake, D. S., Blezek, D. J., Fletcher, J. G., McCollough, C. H., & Manduca, A. (2014). Adaptive nonlocal means filtering based on local noise level for CT denoising. *Medical Physics*, 41(1), 011908.

[31] Aharon, M., Elad, M., & Bruckstein, A. (2016). K-SVD: An algorithm for designing overcomplete dictionaries for sparse representation. *IEEE Transactions on Signal Processing*, 54(11), 4311–322.

[32] Karpathy, A., & Fei-Fei, L. (2015). Deep visual-semantic alignments for generating image descriptions. In *Proceedings of the IEEE Conference on Computer Vision and Pattern Recognition* (pp. 3128–3137).

[33] Ricci, E., & Perfetti, R. (2007). Retinal blood vessel segmentation using line operators and support vector classification. *IEEE Transactions on Medical Imaging*, 26(10), 1357–1365.

[34] Soares, J. V., Leandro, J. J., Cesar, R. M., Jelinek, H. F., & Cree, M. J. (2006). Retinal vessel segmentation using the 2-d gabor wavelet and supervised classification. *IEEE Transactions on Medical Imaging*, 25(9), 1214–1222.

[35] Zhang, B., Zhang, L., Zhang, L., & Karray, F. (2010). Retinal vessel extraction by matched filter with first-order derivative of gaussian. *Computers in Biology and Medicine*, 40(4), 438–445.

[36] Anand, R., Singh, B., & Sindhwani, N. (2009). Speech perception & analysis of fluent digits' strings using level-by-level time alignment. *International Journal of Information Technology and Knowledge Management*, 2(1), 65–68.

[37] Becker, C., Rigamonti, R., Lepetit, V., & Fua, P. (2013). Supervised feature learning for curvilinear structure segmentation. In *International Conference on Medical Image Computing and Computer-Assisted Intervention* (pp. 526–533). Springer.

[38] Ronneberger, O., Fischer, P., & Brox, T. (2015). U-net: Convolutional networks for biomedical image segmentation. In *International Conference on Medical Image Computing and Computer-Assisted Intervention* (pp. 234–241). Springer.

[39] Anand, R., Shrivastava, G., Gupta, S., Peng, S. L., & Sindhwani, N. (2018). Audio Watermarking with Reduced Number of Random Samples. In *Handbook of Research on Network Forensics and Analysis Techniques* (pp. 372–394). IGI Global.

[40] He, K., Zhang, X., Ren, S., & Sun, J. (2016). Deep residual learning for image recognition. In *Proceedings of the IEEE Conference on Computer Vision and Pattern Recognition* (pp. 770–778).

[41] Fu, H., Xu, Y., Lin, S., Wong, D. W. K., & Liu, J. (2016). Deepvessel: Retinal vessel segmentation via deep learning and conditional random field. In *International Conferenceon Medical Image Computing and Computer-Assisted Intervention* (pp. 132–139). Springer.

[42] Xie, S., & Tu, Z. (2015). Holistically-nested edge detection. In *Proceedings of the IEEE, International Conference on Computer Vision* (pp. 1395–1403).

[43] Goodfellow, I., Pouget-Abadie, J., Mirza, M., Xu, B., Warde-Farley, D., Ozair, S., Courville, A., & Bengio, Y. (2014). Generative adversarial nets. In *Advances in Neural Information Processing Systems* (pp. 2672–2680).

[44] Chen, Y., Yang, Z., Hu, Y., Yang, G., Zhu, Y., Li, Y., Chen, W., & Toumoulin, C. (2012). Thoracic low-dose CT image processing using an artifact suppressed large-scale nonlocal means. *Physics in Medicine and Biology*, 57(9), 2667–2688.

[45] Bakshi, G., Shukla, R., Yadav, V., Dahiya, A., Anand, R., Sindhwani, N., & Singh, H. (2021). An optimized approach for feature extraction in multi-relational statistical learning. *Journal of Scientific & Industrial Research*, 80, 537–542.

[46] Deepa, T., Sathiyabhama, B., Akilandeswari, J., & Gopalan, N. P., (2014). Action fuzzy rule based classifier for analysis of dermatology databases. *International Journal of Biomedical Engineering and Technology*, 15(4), 360–379.

[47] Poplin, R., Varadarajan, A. V., Blumer, K., Liu, Y., McConnell, M. V., Corrado, G. S., Peng, L., & Webster, D. R. (2018). Prediction of cardiovascular risk factors from retinal fundus photographs via deep learning. *Nature Biomedical Engineering*. DOI: 10.1038/s41551-018-0195-0.

[48] Ting, D. S., Peng, L., Varadarajan, A. V., & Liu, T. Y. A. (2019). Novel Retinal Imaging in Assessment of Cardiovascular Risk Factors and Systemic Vascular Diseases. In *Diabetic Retinopathy and Cardiovascular Disease* (Vol. 27, pp. 106–118). Karger. DOI: 10.1159/000486269.

[49] Krishnan, M. N. (2012). Coronary heart disease and risk factors in India – On the brink of an epidemic?. *Indian Heart Journal*, 64(4), 364–367. DOI: 10.1016/j.ihj.2012.07.001.

[50] Vinodhini, V., Sathiyabhama, B., Sankar, S., & Somula, R. (2020). A deep structured model for video captioning. *International Journal of Gaming and Computer-Mediated Simulations (IJGCMS)*, 12(2), 44–56.

[51] Sennan, S., Balasubramaniyam, S., Luhach, A. K., Ramasubbareddy, S., Chilamkurti, N., & Nam, Y. (2019). Energy and delay aware data aggregation in routing protocol for internet of things. *Sensors*, 19(24), 5486.

[52] Sankar, S., & Srinivasan, P. (2019). Fuzzy sets based cluster routing protocol for internet of things. *International Journal of Fuzzy System Applications (IJFSA)*, 8(3), 70–93.

[53] Raff, G. L., Abidov, A., Achenbach, S., Berman, D. S., Boxt, L. M., Budoff, M. J., Cheng, V., DeFrance, T., Hellinger, J. C., & Karlsberg, R. P., SCCT guidelines for the interpretation and reporting of coronary computed tomographic angiography. *Journal of Cardiovascular Computed Tomography*, 3(2), 122–136.

[54] Donahue, J., Anne Hendricks, L., Guadarrama, S., Rohrbach, M., Venugopalan, S., Saenko, K., & Darrell, T. (2015). Long-term recurrent convolutional networks for visual recognition and description. In *Proceedings of the IEEE Conference on Computer Vision and Pattern Recognition* (pp. 2625–2634).

[55] Cassar, A., Holmes Jr, D. R., Rihal, C. S., & Gersh, B. J. (2009). Chronic coronary artery disease: diagnosis and management. In *Mayo Clinic Proceedings* (Vol. 84, No. 12, pp. 1130–1146). Elsevier.

[56] Wu, D., Wang, X., Bai, J., Xu, X., Ouyang, B., Li, Y., Zhang, H., Song, Q., Cao, K., & Yin, Y. (2019). Automated anatomical labeling of coronary arteries via bidirectional tree LSTMs. *International Journal of Computer Assisted Radiology and Surgery*, 14(2), 271–280.

[57] Akinyemi, A., Murphy, S., Poole, I., & Roberts, C. (2009, August). Automatic labelling of coronary arteries. In *2009 17th European Signal Processing Conference* (pp. 1562–1566). IEEE.

[58] Raff, G. L., Abidov, A., Achenbach, S., Berman, D. S., Boxt, L. M., Budoff, M. J., ... & Karlsberg, R. P. (2009). SCCT guidelines for the interpretation and reporting of coronary computed tomographic angiography. *Journal of Cardiovascular Computed Tomography*, 3(2), 122–136.

[59] Juneja, S., & Anand, R. (2018). Contrast Enhancement of an Image by DWT-SVD and DCT-SVD. In *Data Engineering and Intelligent Computing* (pp. 595–603). Springer, Singapore.

[60] Choudhary, P., & Anand, M. R. (2015). Determination of rate of degradation of iron plates due to rust using image processing. *International Journal of Engineering Research*, 4(2), 76–84.

[61] Saini, P., & Anand, M. R. (2014). Identification of defects in plastic gears using image processing and computer vision: A review. *International Journal of Engineering Research*, 3(2), 94–99.

[62] Vyas, G., Anand, R., & Holê, K. E. Implementation of advanced image compression using wavelet transform and SPHIT algorithm. *International Journal of Electronic and Electrical Engineering*.

[63] Juneja, S., Juneja, A., & Anand, R. (2020). Healthcare 4.0-digitizing healthcare using big data for performance improvisation. *Journal of Computational and Theoretical Nanoscience*, 17(9–10), 4408–4410.

[64] Kohli, L., Saurabh, M., Bhatia, I., Shekhawat, U. S., Vijh, M., & Sindhwani, N. (2021). Design and development of modular and multifunctional UAV with amphibious landing module. In *Data Driven Approach Towards Disruptive Technologies: Proceedings of MIDAS 2020* (pp. 405–421). Springer, Singapore.

[65] Revathi, T. K., Sathiyabhama, B., & Sankar, S. (2021). A deep learning based approach for diagnosing coronary inflammation with multi-scale coronary response dynamic balloon tracking (MSCAR-DBT) based artery segmentation in coronary computed tomography angiography (CCTA). *Annals of the Romanian Society for Cell Biology*, 25(6), 4936–4948.

[66] Kohli, L., Saurabh, M., Bhatia, I., Sindhwani, N., & Vijh, M. (2021). Design and Development of Modular and Multifunctional UAV with Amphibious Landing, Processing and Surround Sense Module. In *Unmanned Aerial Vehicles for Internet of Things (IoT): Concepts, Techniques, and Applications* (p. 207).

[67] Saini, M. K., Nagal, R., Tripathi, S., Sindhwani, N., & Rudra, A. (2008). PC interfaced wireless robotic moving arm. In *AICTE Sponsored National Seminar on Emerging Trends in Software Engineering* (Vol. 50).

[68] Revathi, T. K., Sathiyabhama, B., & Sankar, S. (2021). Diagnosing cardio vascular disease (CVD) using generative adversarial network (GAN) in retinal fundus images. *Annals of the Romanian Society for Cell Biology*, 2563–2572.

[69] Vinodhini, V., Sathiyabhama, B., Sankar, S., & Somula, R. (2020). A deep structured model for video captioning. *International Journal of Gaming and Computer-Mediated Simulations (IJGCMS)*, 12(2), 44–56.

[70] Singh, H., Rehman, T. B., Gangadhar, C., Anand, R., Sindhwani, N., & Babu, M. (2021). Accuracy detection of coronary artery disease using machine learning algorithms. *Applied Nanoscience*, 1–7.

[70] Malsa, N., Singh, P., Gautam, J., Srivastava, A., & Singh, S. P. (2020). Source of Treatment Selection for different States of India and Performance Analysis Using Machine Learning Algorithms for Classification. In *Soft Computing: Theories and Applications*.

[71] Jain, S., Kumar, M., Sindhwani, N., & Singh, P. (2021). SARS-Cov-2 detection using deep learning techniques on the basis of clinical reports. In *2021 9th International Conference on Reliability, Infocom Technologies and Optimization (Trends and Future Directions) (ICRITO)* (pp. 1–5). DOI: 10.1109/ICRITO51393.2021.9596455.

[72] Ratnaparkhi, S. T., Singh, P., Tandasi, A., & Sindhwani, N. (2021). Comparative analysis of classifiers for criminal identification system using face recognition. In *2021 9th International Conference on Reliability, Infocom Technologies and Optimization (Trends and Future Directions) (ICRITO)* (pp. 1–6). DOI: 10.1109/ICRITO51393.2021.9596066.

[73] Sindhwani, N. (2017). Performance analysis of optimal scheduling based firefly algorithm in MIMO system. *Optimization*, 2(12), 19–26.

[74] Juneja, S., Juneja, A., & Anand, R. (2019, April). Reliability modeling for embedded system environment compared to available software reliability growth models. In *2019 International Conference on Automation, Computational and Technology Management (ICACTM)* (pp. 379–382). IEEE.

[75] Sindhwani, N., Bhamrah, M. S., Garg, A., & Kumar, D. (2017, July). Performance analysis of particle swarm optimization and genetic algorithm in MIMO systems. In *2017 8th International Conference on Computing, Communication and Networking Technologies (ICCCNT)* (pp. 1–6). IEEE.

[76] Anand, R. & Chawla, P. (2022). Bandwidth Optimization of a Novel Slotted Fractal Antenna Using Modified Lightning Attachment Procedure Optimization. In *Smart Antennas, Latest Trends in Design and Application*, pp. 379–392. DOI: 10.1007/978-3-030-76636-8_28.

Chapter 16

# Wireless networks and communication-based optimization algorithms for smart healthcare devices

*N. Srikanth*
Annamalai University, Chidambaram, India

*T. Shankar*
GCE, Trichy, India

*G. Yamuna*
Annamalai University, Chidambaram, India

## CONTENTS

## 16.1 INTRODUCTION

Wireless sensor network (WSN) is assuring its dominance for developing smart healthcare devices, due to its complexity and effectiveness of use. The role of WSN [1] is to track the area of interest and to collect and rely on some information for postanalysis [2, 3]. The efficient algorithms are appropriate and well suited for a few diverse application scenarios. WSN designers, in particular, need to fix some basic issues identified with data

DOI: 10.1201/9781003239888-16

accumulation, data replication, limitation, node grouping, energy-awareness routing, fault detection, or security. WSN typically consists of a sensor, controller, and communication system. If the communication is with each node, then it is called as WSN machine learning (ML). It is a learning technique using a computer to learn and act like human and learning over time in an autonomous fashion, by collecting and processing large data using sensor nodes, feeding and collecting the information to form of observation and real-world interaction [4].

ML [5–7] is a computer-based statistical field that encompasses a range of algorithms and methods that learn from datasets and are able to predict the performance of networks. ML was developed in the late 1950s, over a long time its emphasis changed, turning more to computationally viable and robust algorithms. These methods have been widely used in healthcare devices and applications, like classification, regression, and density prediction. The adoption of statistical methods to enhance computer efficiency by identifying and defining training data consistencies and patterns is employed. Developing computational models and offering solutions for improving the present system standards are quite common. It also includes internet of things (IoT) [8, 9], cyber-physical systems (CPS), and machine to machine (M2 M) integration [10].

The first step in a wireless network is to collect the data by the sensor nodes and collector sensor, which is to sense the environmental condition, and then the collector after collecting the data forwards it to the base station of the WSN and subsequently the data are sent to communicate. Then, ML technique and algorithm come into the picture as the data collected are to be arranged in proper format which is easily readable by the machine and hence some preprocessing is performed on that data and noise is removed from the data. After that, data is divided into two sections: training and testing. The first step is to apply the learning algorithms on trained data to predict the category of classification as output and after that the same technique is applied on testing data and these two data are compared depending on their properties and a decision is taken based on that data properties. By applying different ML algorithms, a proper decision is taken that is applicable for WSNs system. In this process, the data are transmitted, processed, and received by the base stations of wireless network which limit the computation because of the limited energy source and bandwidth of WSNs system. To train the data, communicate, and distribute on WSN, WSN ML Implementation in Routing plays an important role in improving network performance. Sensor network dynamic behavior includes complex routing algorithms to optimize the performance of the system. The objective is to include a detailed review on the use of ML techniques in sequence to enhance the routing protocol output in WSNs for smart health devices. WSNs have many other difficult issues, such as centralized medium access, translation, optimum location, and distribution. Growing network lifetime is a major problem in WSNs to execute the tasks energy costs. We assume that these dynamic distributed problems can be solved effectively, including routing and clustering. Early survey explains algorithms in their implementations.

The memory and computing demands of ML methods are greater than the conventional WSN approaches. This chapter provides a large selection of effective, up-to-date ML algorithms to compare their strengths and weaknesses in WSNs for smart health applications. Rest of the chapter is organized as follows. Section 16.2 presents different types of ML. Section 16.3 explains the related work of ML techniques to WSN routing protocols used for healthcare devices. The subsequent section specifies the major difficulties in routing layer. The next section outlines about the application of ML in WSN for health devices followed by the comparison of different ML techniques and computational intelligence (CI) techniques to evaluate the optimization in the next section. The last section draws the conclusion.

## 16.2 MACHINE LEARNING TECHNIQUES

MLL is a method of analysis and prediction of data and predicting the feature outcome and building a model using different algorithms and techniques to get an output. Simply, it is a technique in which a relationship between input and output is identified and patterns and trends are employed to make a perfect decision with minimum human interference. In this section, we discuss some popular ML techniques for future health devices and their uses, advantages, and disadvantages in WSNs [11]. There are basically three types of ML techniques used to design a WSN: supervised, unsupervised, and reinforcement ML. The supervised learning describes a problem class that includes using a model to learn the mapping between example input and goal variable. There are two major categories of supervised learning; (a) classification and (b) regression.

Unsupervised learning describes a series of problems for defining or extracting data relationships. In reinforcement learning, a set of challenges working in an environment need to learn and to use the input to work.

### 16.2.1 Supervised learning

Supervised learning is a technique used in ML. In this learning, both input and output are provided to the machine that finds the relation between the input and output variables to identify the pattern between them. During training, the most important feature of supervised learning is to find the relation between the input features and forecasting output. Supervised learning solves the various problems in WSNs for smart health devices. Localization in a sensor node refers to finding the geographical area to locate the sensor node of WSN. In simple WSN technique, it requires more time to find each location physically identifying the sensor nodes. In some situations, it is required to reprogram the architecture of WSNs network. Because of these problems, applying ML algorithm in such situations improves the accuracy of the location of the node. The algorithms are classified between the anchor node in WSN and unknown nodes in the network [12].

Mobile sensor nodes progressively and continuously change their situations/positions in WSNs and hence the capability to distinguish the exact location requires more time but it is quick with ML approaches. Using ML algorithm in WSNs, coverage and connectivity are increased and the number of sensor nodes connected can be found rapidly in WSN. In this method, the machine model is constructed using a specified training set (i.e., predefined data and labels). This model is employed to describe the various parameters like input, output, and device. The use of these algorithms is to address the numerous problems in WSNs, like identification and target tracking.

*Logistic Regression (LR)*: Logistic regression is a classification technique. Decision boundary (generally linear) based on the probability interpretation results in a nonlinear optimization for parameter estimation. The goal of LR is given as a new data point, predicting the data point that is likely to be originated and identifying a category belonging to the previous data with known categories. When the number of categories is two, it becomes a binary classification problem. Input features can be both qualitative and quantitative. If the inputs are qualitative, then there has to be a systematic way of converting them to quantities. Binary input like a "Yes" or "No" can be encoded as "1" and "0". Binary classification can be evaluated depending on the side of the half-plane it falls in.

*Modeling as probabilities*: Probability of "Yes" or "No" gives a better information of the sample's membership to a particular category. Estimating the binary outputs from the probabilities is straight forward through simple thresholding. Binary output for new samples can now be easily predicted.

To prevent over-fitting, we need to penalize the coefficients. Regularization helps in building noncomplex models that avoid capturing noise in the model due to over-fitting. The objective becomes regularization and helps the model work better on test data.

**k-NN algorithm:** The k-nearest neighbor (k-NN) algorithm uses both the labeled and unlabeled data used for classification and regression. It is a learning algorithm where all the computations are deferred until classification completes. It performs explicit generalization where the function is approximated. KNN does not show any operation on the training data. It is used when the boundaries between the data set are nonlinear; it is used in the large data set and also when the data set is categorical. The KNN has used data points of the nearest location. The parameter k is selected based on data and distance matrix is to define the distance between the data points. The distance is measured by using different distance-measuring techniques like Euclidean distance. These algorithms do not make any sense about underlying data distribution.

## 16.2.2 Unsupervised learning

It is a technique in which no labeling of output data associated with input is there. The main approach of unsupervised learning is to detect a pattern in a cluster. The main advantage of unsupervised learning is to solve many problems like anomaly detection, routing, and data aggregation. Anomaly detection is improved using an unsupervised ML technique as it minimizes the complexity and communication problems. It has also advantages of fault-detection attack and outliers detection in WSNs in supervised methods using past and previous data sets. It is possible to adjust the parameters of sensor nodes dynamically. Routing [13] is the most important parameter as routing adopts the changes in the environment without physically reprogramming. In optimal routing, there are low earning communication overhead and delay-awareness, etc. Data aggregation is a process of collecting the data to sensor nodes. Data aggregation affects the various parameters of the WSNs system like communication overhead units and power memory loss. By using the ML unsupervised algorithm, this problem can be reduced. It is used in dimension reduction of the node level and therefore it reduces the communication overhead in the network. This reduces the delay in the network nodes. It also reduces the dimensions of the sensor node using environmental condition. This is called unsupervised learning without a teacher. It's mostly related to the concept of using a series of gathered or clustered findings from a sample. This learning methodology differs from the supervised learning methodology in that there is no output vector and this method does not require an input label.

*K-means Clustering:* It is a technique to divide the N observations data points into K clusters, where K and N are based on the nearest mean. Clustering is one of the most straightforward and essential unsupervised learning techniques. Hence, like every other problem, it deals with finding the unlabeled data.

## 16.2.3 Reinforcement learning

Reinforcement learning (RL) is an ML technique in which the trial–error principal is to find the best possibilities out in the search space. RL is learning continuously through the environment and gathering the data from sensor nodes to take appropriate action. RL algorithm has maximized the performance by learning to the environment, and it also provides good results because there is no need to store the large data set used. In Q learning, each agent gathers the data to the environment and generates a sequence of observations. Based on the previous observation, it will take a proper decision, and therefore, reinforcement learning provides a very good result in WSNs system. It is used in communication range control of sensor network. RL basically consists of the parts like environment, state, reward, action, and agent. In WSNs, the environment consists of many small sensors which collect the data and information is passed on to agent through the State. State plays the mediator role between the environment and agent. After collecting the information, data agent takes the proper decision and gives the rewards to the environment. Depending on that rewards, the agent takes the action. If the environment is changed rapidly, then the agent is able to take proper action. It also makes changes depending on previous data but depends on the environmental situation. Therefore, it is able to take proper decision instantly and hence its speed and decision-making capability are optimal. Q learning provides good accuracy and hence RL is one of the important ML techniques used in WSNs system. RL works on the sensor node to interpret process and communicate data with its context. The agent must acquaint himself in this ML approach to take the necessary measures. This technique for ML depends purely on two measures: trial and error; check and delayed.

## 16.3 RELATED WORK

The authors in Ref. [14] explored implementations of three standard ML algorithms at all communication levels in the WSNs (i.e., decision trees, neural networks, and reinforcement learning). In comparison, targeted surveys were also published about learning, in particular, WSN challenges. The authors in Ref. [15, 16] discussed the creation of effective outer detection methods out of which some methods depend on ML principles. In Ref. [17], the author addressed the techniques of artificial intelligence to tackle the problems in WSNs, for example, routing, data collection and convergence, work management, optimum delivery, and localization. This computational intelligence is a subset of ML that concentrates on the biologically inspired method [18]. The zone-based energy-efficient routing (ZEEP) protocol is developed for mobile sensor networks in Ref. [19] using a fuzzy method. ZEEP uses the fuzzy inference system (FIS) to pick a range of channels (CHs) based on the parameters like mobility, energy, and distance, including neural networks, fuzzy structures, and evolutionary algorithms. In Ref. [20], a routing protocol based on deep learning has been presented, with the base station being used as an interface. It indicates the path which the base station has preserved, allocated, and retrieved. The suggested deep learning–based algorithm utilizes dynamic routing in a sensor network. Firstly, the base station generates a set of simulated routing routes and determines the best path from them. For WSNs, ant colony optimization (ACO)–based routing algorithm has been implemented in Ref. [21]. The various criteria, such as a node's residual energy, transmission frequency, transmission direction, and the most precise route from the source nodes to the base station, have been considered to determine the optimum routing. This algorithm achieves low energy loss and lengthens the network lifetime. As seen, there are many advantages in ML technique but there are some limitations also using these ML algorithms. ML algorithms are not able to produce an instant result and accurate prediction because ML algorithm first trains a large amount of historical data. If the data size is large, then more energy is consumed because of the high complexity of the ML algorithm. Also, the validation and prediction of the real-time data is a very difficult task in WSN because the data from the sensor are not in a proper format and it also changes when the condition of the environment changes. Also, the size of the sensor is very important in WSNs [22]. When the size changes, then the amount of data also changes and is very difficult in some situations to predict the proper accuracy. Sometimes, it is very difficult to select a good ML technique for the complex issues in WSN system.

## 16.4 ROUTING LAYER

The routing applied is a fundamental question regarding movement of a data packet from one node to another when there is no direct node connection in the network. This is also referred to as multi-hop routing, which means that many intermediate nodes usually transfer the data packets to their destination. A routing protocol specifies the series of intermediate nodes to guarantee the packet distribution. There is a distinction between unicast and multicast routing protocols. The data packets routed from a single source to a unique destination come under the unicast routing protocol. The data packets concurrently routed to multiple destinations come under the multicast routing protocol. These protocols remain a vast deal of literature on routing concerning WSNs and wireless ad hoc networks in general. The problem is to handle the weak transmission connections, node crashes, and node stability and, most significantly, to allow the effective use of resources. With the computational intelligence, an attempt to produce energetic routing and prolong the network lifetime is the primary concern of the author [14, 22].

## 16.5 APPLICATIONS OF MACHINE LEARNING IN ROUTING

ML methods can be used by approximating the sensor data with so many algorithms to reduce interaction. In the area of WSNs for healthcare devices, the main objective of learning strategies is to minimize the amount of energy used by sensor nodes by limiting the amount of contact with the node. ML techniques are attractive in sensor networks for the four reasons. There is generally an amount of consistency of data from the sensor network. Redundancy derives that sensors nearby are likely to obtain the identical measurements and measurements taken at two different instants are strongly related as well. The exact measurement is rarely important and generally the observer will accept the approximations. Lesser the accuracy, the more versatile are the learning models and hence large communication gains are possible. This makes it possible to design the strategies for data collection which results in energy precision. It is associated with the involvement of software agents in an atmosphere to optimize the idea of cumulative prizes. The method elects a standard action and at specific action earns a credit. However, the right or successful move is not decided in advance. Therefore, the program carries out the various actions and learns from the experience [20]. Applications of ML techniques in routing protocol are most common in mobile ad-hoc network (MANET) and WSN distributed problems like routing, timing, medium access control, and network positioning.

## 16.6 ROUTING IN WSN

When a node is required to transmit a data packet, a nearby node may be chosen as per the values contained in its routing tables. As far as routing algorithm is concerned, the action is to greedily select the neighboring node, including the best value of the routing table. The routing algorithms have some specific guidelines for the ML that enables a sensor network to learn from the past interactions, to implement appropriate routing decisions, to respond to the changing environment, to estimate the cost functions, and to update the routing tables at execution time. ML reduces the difficulty of a standard routing issue by grouping it into more easy routing problems. The nodes in each problem are formed by the formations of the graph, including their immediate close neighbors; a low-cost, reliable, and present-time routing is therefore accomplished. In order to meet Quality of Service Routing task specifications, we use fairly basic computational methods and classifiers.

*Distributed Regression Framework*: This framework is an efficient and general framework in network sensor data modeling. Within this context, the sensor network nodes cooperate to match each of their local measurement optimally with a global function. The algorithm is based on linear regression of the kernel. This model takes the weighted sum of the local dependent functions [23]. The kernel functions map the training observations to a certain function space to allow data analysis. The proposed system exploits the assumption that multiple sensor readings are strongly correlated. It would reduce the overhead for contact. It identifies the sensor structure data. These findings act as an essential step in the creation of the distributed wireless network using different ML techniques and algorithms. The benefit of using these methods is very strong fitting performance and low computing overheads.

*Artificial Neural Networks (ANNs)*: Energetically effective and reliable artificial neural network routing scheme for WSNs is referred to as Energy-efficient Low Duty Circle (ELDC). In this methodology, the network remains focused on enormous data collection that includes almost all the scenarios to make the system very useful and environmentally efficient. ELDC technique is exceptionally energy-efficient and capable of rising the lifetime of the sensor nodes. An artificial neural network creates dominant threshold values for choosing the chief node of a system, and a cluster head depends upon the technique of back propagation. ANN is used for the training of the protocol by considering the appropriate parameters like remaining capacity, node distance from CH, distance from the border node and to base station (BS), the traffic load on the current link and the likelihood of insurance status of the given network [24].

The architecture of an ANN is shown in Figure 16.1.

*Data Routing using Self-Organizing Map (SOM)*: The artificial intelligence (AI) techniques in WSN for healthcare devices use SOM that uses the concept of self-organization. It is based on unsupervised learning to find the efficient routing strategies, which are called Sensor Intelligence Routing (SIR). SIR makes a minor improvement to the Dijkstra's algorithm to build the foundation of the smallest paths from a base station to any node on the network. The second-layer neurons engage with each other during route learning to assign the high weights within the learning chain. The weights of the winning neuron are then modified to match the input patterns. The training process is a highly analytical method with the goal of constructing neural networks [2]. SOM consists of two phases, including the learning phase and the execution phase. The learning phase arranges a two-dimensional map of the neurons, and it is done within a resourceful central station. The execution phase runs on network nodes. Each sensor node calculates the quality of service (QoS) of its connections. Each node gathers the input samples and runs the algorithm of the winning neuron election. The complexity and the learning methods are the key challenges to implement this type of algorithm, whether the topology and structure of the network change [2, 24].

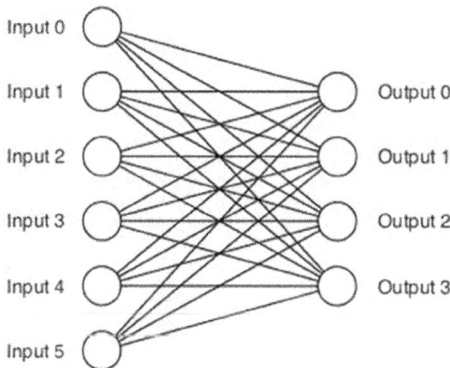

*Figure 16.1* Architecture of ANN.

The use of AI technologies (e.g., neural networks) in WSNs is declared to be a valuable method for optimizing the network performance. The tremendous work of applying a SOM method on a sensor node implies that the usage of AI technologies will boost the efficiency of the WSNs in smart health devices.

*Q-Learning*: Q-learning is a simple and effective algorithm [25] that does not require any environment model. It is also used for online feature learning. It is very easy to execute and has good memory. In our multiple-sink example, each sensor node is an infinite learning agent and actions are options for the next hop(s) into a subset of sinks using separate neighbors. A simple solution is to greedily choose the best (lowest) Q-value for the operation. The flexibility of the Q-learning methodology and the prospect of enhancing current Q-learning protocols have been there. There are different types of Q-routing: distributed routing, Q-routing with compression, Q-probabilistic routing (Q-PR), and geography-based routing.

*Routing enhancement using reinforcement learning (RL)*: This learning falls within the requirement of the algorithms of ML; meanwhile, an agent goes through the encounters with the environment learning. The main purpose is to understand the method of optimizing incentives to identify the appropriate policies. An RL agent knows what action by itself will lead to optimality.

A hierarchical algorithm has been used in this learning model for opportunistic routing schemes. Figure 16.2 shows multicast routing in which a node transfers the identical message to the numerous recipients. Multiagent reinforcement learning (MARL) is appropriate for the network distribution where multiple agents still exist. Two types of MARL are there, namely single-hop and multi-hop [26].

*Feedback Routing for Optimizing Multiple Sinks (FROMS) in WSNs with RL*: This protocol depends on Q-learning, and it operates on the mechanism to exchange the local knowledge of a node to other nearby nodes as inputs without creating any overhead network. The network used to

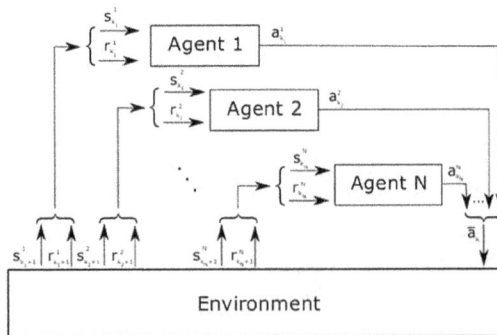

*Figure 16.2* Multiagent reinforcement learning (MARL) scheme.

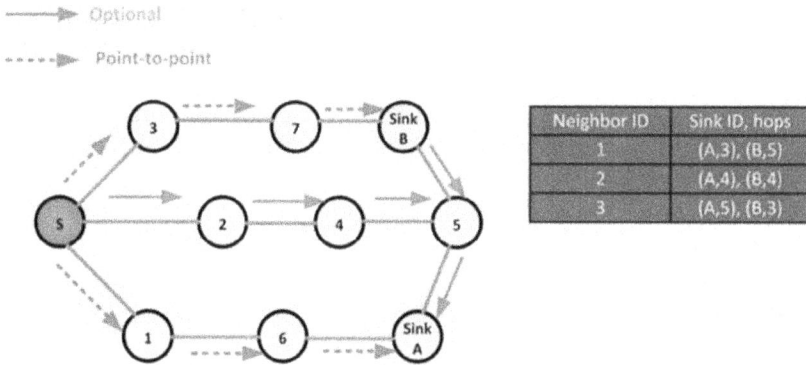

*Figure 16.3* Routing scenario in FROMS.

implement this protocol is architecture in multi-sink form. The best thing about this routing system is to consider both the techniques of discovery and development to find an optimal route. The only extraction will lead to a local optimum solution and unnecessary overhead exploration can prolong the time discovery of path.

Figure 16.3 shows a routing scenario in FROMS which consists of one source node and two sink nodes. The solid line represents the best shared route and dashed line indicates point-to-point routes. The exceptional commitment of this protocol is that multiple sinks are taken into account in network architecture and using multiple sink nodes greatly decreases the network overheads. Even if any node fails, FROMS will have a recovery mechanism. On the other hand, FROMS is vulnerable to node failure and instability leads to errors in the routing setup process [27].

Table 16.1 shows the routing algorithms for WSNs for smart devices based on ML technique.

*Table 16.1* Routing algorithms for WSNs for smart devices based on ML technique

| Machine learning techniques | Topology | Routing protocol | Complexity | QOS | Environment |
|---|---|---|---|---|---|
| K-Means | Hybrid/Tree | Distributed regression framework | Low/moderate | No | Distributed |
| ANN | Tree | ELDC | High/moderate | No/yes | Centralized/ distributed |
| Q-Learning | Flat/Multi-hop | Data routing using SOM | Low | No | Distributed |
| Q-Learning | Flat/Multi-hop | MARL | Moderate | Yes | Distributed |
| Q-Learning | Flat/Multi-hop | FROMS | High | No | Distributed |

## 16.7 COMMUNICATION-BASED OPTIMIZATION (CBO) ALGORITHMS

The key drawback of routing algorithms focused on reinforcement learning is the restricted awareness to potential knowledge. The algorithms are thus not appropriate for the extremely complicated conditions because it takes a long time to acquire the optimal paths. A study of the improvement strategies that alter or encourage the smart actions in diverse and dynamic environments lead to CBO algorithms [28]. Such structures represent the concepts that possess a potential for informing or adapting to new things, generalizing, abstracting, exploring, and associating. CBO is illustrated because method descriptions and information resources that can specifically position the actual sensory statistical expertise have accurate and timely responses and endure high tolerance to faults. The CBO frameworks are responsive to WSN's complex design for smart healthcare devices. The following subsections explain briefly several CBO paradigms used in WSN clustering [12, 29].

*Genetic Algorithm*: Genetic algorithm (GA) is an adaptive heuristic search algorithm that models the genetic, biological evolution. It is shown that a robust optimizer is looking for a community of solutions and demonstrating versatility in addressing complex issues. Several NP-hard problems have been solved successfully. A key challenge in genetic algorithm (GA) problem is the translation of the problem into a series of chromosomes, while each of these chromosomes constitutes a solution of the problem. A fitness function measures the position of each chromosome. The main feature of GA [30, 31] is to find an optimization solution for the search route [32, 33]. To seek the global optima, it retains a search frontier and solves the problems of multi-criterion optimization. However, GA's capability to describe rule-based, permutation-based, and proactive approaches to the various pattern recognition and ML problems is a more precise benefit. GA-Routing Method for creating an aggregation tree that covers every sensor node is used for homogeneous and small networks. It prolongs the lifetime of the node and improves the node energy output. GA-EECP technique works to build the clusters that are energy efficient. The cluster size, relative size to the base station, energy flow, average cluster distance variance, and the number of communications are the determining variables. It builds on large scale networks [34].

*Ant Colony Optimization*: The ACO algorithm [35] is derived from the real action of the ants that interact with each other via a medium designated as a pheromone [36]. During the walk, the ants lay a chemical signal on the space and detect the pheromone's current intensity for guidance. At first, no pheromone is accumulated on the branches, and the ants do not know the length of the branches. However, if a shorter version is detected, it will be given at a higher rate. By contrast, pheromone is limited to a fixed area. Prematurity and instability can be easily avoided in this situation, but the convergence speed is slowed down. Second, at least, all of the connections have identical pheromone; the ants roam with no warning, spontaneously. The list would remain inaccurate, and the other is misguided. Third, any mistake in route selection or pheromone updating will affect the final optimization in the ACO process. Some of the ACO-based routing protocols choose the routing route by the allocation of probabilities. Many different paths are built in this protocol. It is ideal for smart healthcare applications and essential where the priority is on the sink node, and ordinary nodes need to retain the robust connectivity to the sink [37]. Another protocol energy efficient ant base routing (EEABR) [37] proposes that simulation tests show that it minimizes the contact load in various WSNs in smart device situations and maximizes energy consumption, which stresses the increased lifespan of the network.

*Particle Swarm Optimization*: Swarm intelligence (SI) is one of the emerging approaches for these heuristic computation challenges from the bioinspired computation. James Kennedy and Russell Eberhart developed particle swarm optimization (PSO) in 1995. It is a strong nonlinear stochastic optimization strategy focused on swarm's mobility applied to WSNs in healthcare devices designing. It is based on birds' social behavior, where a group of birds is looking for food in an environment by chasing the closest bird to the food. It blends the local search methods. It is a population-based stochastic optimization beginning with a randomly generated population group. It has fitness attributes for assessing the population, and with random processes, it refines the population and aims for the maximum. PSO does vary from GA in that there is no overlap and mutation [38, 39]. Its particles do not die while their internal velocities are modified. Finally, the structure of knowledge exchange in PSO is noticeably different. In a multidimensional space, every particle is viewed as a point and adjusts its location, determined by two components: the cognitive component and the social component arising from neighbor contact [40].

*Artificial Immune System*: The artificial immune system is primarily motivated by the natural or actual immune systems, and certain features of immune systems are modeled. The human immune system (HIS) has tremendous ability to suit the sequences. It is used to discriminate among the alien cells that join the body (antigenic or nonself) and those that belong to the body (self). HIS combats the antigens and stores its structure. The networks depend on the idea that the system is using a typical network of interconnected B cells – a part of the adaptive immune system to recognize the antigen. The ability of the two B cells to interconnect is directly proportionate to the bond they participate in. A population of B cells holds two groups of subpopulation's original population and the cloned population. If the excellent binding is accomplished, the B cell is cloned and mutated, resulting in several antibodies. Once a B cell generates, it connects to the closest B cells in the network. Unless the new cell cannot be inserted, the population is discarded. If all bindings fail, a B cell is produced utilizing the antigen as a template and then included in the artificial immune network, pattern recognition problems, smart healthcare devices, telemedicine for health systems, classification, clustering, anomaly detection, and computer virus detection [41].

*Fuzzy Logic*: A fuzzy logic (FL) [42, 43] is an arrangement of mathematics developed to describe theoretical human reasoning. Unlike the traditional set theory, which requires components to either be incorporated in a set or not, it can set the average values based on semantic variables and rules of inference. In other words, in a fuzzy package, a particular entity is authorized to have an influenced membership, which is in the range (0,1). There are two parts in FL:

I.  To determine the membership which corresponds to a given value of a linguistic attribute, a fuzzy membership function is set. The membership function may be programmed to represent the optimal goodness actions of a target in a versatile manner, depending on specific needs.

II. FL provides a floating aggregation operator, ordered weighted averaging (OWA), as an alternative to weighted numbers, to develop a multiobjective cost function.

FL was successfully implemented in designing smart healthcare devices, optical image processing systems [44, 45], pattern recognition systems, and control systems such as automotive motor controls, power systems, home appliances, and elevators. However, FL is ideal for applying the heuristics clustering and improving routing to accomplish the various goals simultaneously. This algorithm generates nonoptimal solutions, however, fuzzy rules upon topology modifications tend to be relearned [46]. The FL protocols incorporate the heuristics clustering or routing optimization to accomplish several entities simultaneously. Fuzzy color histogram (FCH) sees capacity, focus, and centrality as three linguistic factors in order to assess the probability of being the head of the cluster. In terms of the first description, it was confirmed to achieve a significant improvement in network lifespan. Fuzzy multiobjective routing characteristics are applied to achieve several WSN routing goals in healthcare applications.

*Cuckoo Search*: The suggested algorithm for multicast routing is built on the Cuckoo Search (CS) algorithm, which relies upon the environment concerning the cuckoo species [46]. The algorithm takes into account three rules:

I.   The bird lays one egg at a time, which is a solution, on a probable selected host nest.

II.  The high-quality egg or the best-fit solution is the algorithm.

III. The host bird leaves the poor quality alien egg when picking the best with some probability.

The newly developed fitness functions in the CS algorithm solution automate the multicast routing. Pb (probability of egg discovery) has values between zero and 1. Eu is derived from a regular normal distribution with zero mean and standard deviation of unity. It can further be practiced as a Levy Flight distribution and holds a random step-length walk that depends on the current position plus a chance of transition [47].

*Adaptive Critic Design*: A dynamic optimization referred to as a novel action-dependent adaptive critical design (ACD) is created. The suggested combination of an optimization-based particle swarm actor and a neural network critique are illustrated by complex sleep scheduling of wireless sensor nodes [48, 49] for smart healthcare devices. The adaptive critical approach deters the optimal control laws for a system by integrating two subsystems, an agent (dispensing feedback signals) and a critic (learning the ideal output index for the functions associated with the program) [50]. The ACD determines integrated sleep pattern in high-quality data collection and enhances energy efficiency. One possible way for this research to be expanded is to explore the lightweight types of PSO and compact neuronal structures. In addition, there is room for investigating the use of the ACD in collective multinode sleep scheduling in WSNs for healthcare industry.

## 16.8 CONCLUSION AND FUTURE SCOPE

ML and communication-based optimization algorithms for smart healthcare devices can improve WSN capability in response to the wireless network constraints [51]. Analysis of CBO algorithms, which act as a reference for practicing CBO algorithms for WSNs in smart health devices, is provided. An innovative CBO methodology known as adaptive critical design aims to provide realistic, optimal/suboptimal solutions to the problem of dispersed sensor scheduling. In this chapter, a thorough analysis and current investigation of wireless networks and CBO techniques in WSNs for smart healthcare devices has been presented. The research work carried in this chapter may be considered as a scope for the future research work [52–58]. In this chapter, only flaws in some existing methods are pointed out to resolve the flaws of these existing methods. Some new methods are also proposed to meet the future scope requirements.

## REFERENCES

[1] Meelu, R., & Anand, R. (2010 November). Energy efficiency of cluster based routing protocols used in wireless sensor networks. In *AIP Conference Proceedings* (Vol. *1324*, No. 1, pp. 109–113). American Institute of Physics.
[2] Kumar, D. P., Amgoth, T., & Annavarapu, C. S. R. (2019). Machine learning algorithms for wireless sensor networks: A survey. *Information Fusion*, *49*, 1–25.

[3] Rawat, P., Singh, K. D., Chaouchi, H., & Bonnin, J. M. (2014). Wireless sensor networks: A survey on recent developments and potential synergies. *The Journal of Supercomputing, 68*(1), 1–48.

[4] Guestrin, C., Bodik, P., Thibaux, R., Paskin, M., & Madden, S. (2004, April). Distributed regression: An efficient framework for modeling sensor network data. In *Proceedings of the 3rd International Symposium on Information Processing in Sensor Networks* (pp. 1–10).

[5] Sindhwani, N., Verma, S., Bajaj, T., & Anand, R. (2021). Comparative analysis of intelligent driving and safety assistance systems using YOLO and SSD model of deep learning. *International Journal of Information System Modeling and Design (IJISMD), 12*(1), 131–146.

[6] Singh, H., Rehman, T. B., Gangadhar, C., Anand, R., Sindhwani, N., & Babu, M. (2021). Accuracy detection of coronary artery disease using machine learning algorithms. *Applied Nanoscience*, 1–7.

[7] Bakshi, G., Shukla, R., Yadav, V., Dahiya, A., Anand, R., Sindhwani, N., & Singh, H. (2021). An optimized approach for feature extraction in multi-relational statistical learning. *Journal of Scientific & Industrial Research, 80*, 537–542.

[8] Gupta, A., Srivastava, A., Anand, R., & Tomažič, T. (2020). Business Application Analytics and the Internet of Things: The Connecting Link. In *New Age Analytics* (pp. 249–273). Apple Academic Press.

[9] Anand, R., Sinha, A., Bhardwaj, A., & Sreeraj, A. (2018). Flawed Security of Social Network of Things. In *Handbook of Research on Network Forensics and Analysis Techniques* (pp. 65–86). IGI Global.

[10] Akyildiz, I. F., Su, W., Sankarasubramaniam, Y., & Cayirci, E. (2002). Wireless sensor networks: A survey. *Computer Networks, 38*(4), 393–422.

[11] Babu, D. M., & Ussenaiah, M. (2020). Cuckoo search and M-tree-based multi-constraint optimal multicast Ad hoc on-demand distance vector routing protocol for MANETs. *International Journal of Recent Technology and Engineering, 8*(2S3), 876–879.

[12] Prajapati, J., & Jain, S. C. (2018, April). Machine learning techniques and challenges in wireless sensor networks. In *2018 Second International Conference on Inventive Communication and Computational Technologies (ICICCT)* (pp. 233–238). IEEE.

[13] Alwakeel, S. S., & Al-Nabhan, N. A. (2012, December). A cooperative learning scheme for energy efficient routing in wireless sensor networks. In *2012 11th International Conference on Machine Learning and Applications* (Vol. 2, pp. 463–468). IEEE.

[14] Förster, A., & Murphy, A. L. (2010). Machine learning across the WSN layers. *Emerging Communications for Wireless Sensor Networks*, 165–183.

[15] Zhang, Y., Meratnia, N., & Havinga, P. (2010). Outlier detection techniques for wireless sensor networks: A survey. *IEEE Communications Surveys & Tutorials, 12*(2), 159–170.

[16] Hodge, V., & Austin, J. (2004). A survey of outlier detection methodologies. *Artificial Intelligence Review, 22*(2), 85–126.

[17] Kulkarni, R. V., Förster, A., & Venayagamoorthy, G. K. (2010). Computational intelligence in wireless sensor networks: A survey. *IEEE Communications Surveys & Tutorials, 13*(1), 68–96.

[18] Swagatam, D. A. S., Abraham, A., & Panigrahi, B. (2010). *Foundations, Perspectives and Recent Trends, Intelligence and Pattern Analysis in Biological Informatics*.

[19] Srivastava, J. R., & Sudarshan, T. S. B. (2015). A genetic fuzzy system based optimized zone based energy efficient routing protocol for mobile sensor networks (OZEEP). *Applied Soft Computing*, 37, 863–886.

[20] Lee, Y. (2017). Classification of node degree based on deep learning and routing method applied for virtual route assignment. *Ad Hoc Networks*, 58, 70–85.

[21] Sun, Y., Dong, W., & Chen, Y. (2017). An improved routing algorithm based on ant colony optimization in wireless sensor networks. *IEEE Communications Letters*, 21(6), 1317–1320.

[22] Förster, A., & Murphy, A. L. (2010). Machine learning across the WSN layers. *Emerging Communications for Wireless Sensor Networks*, 165–183.

[23] Barbancho, J., León, C., Molina, J., & Barbancho, A. (2006, January). SIR: A new wireless sensor network routing protocol based on artificial intelligence. In *Asia-Pacific Web Conference* (pp. 271–275). Springer, Berlin, Heidelberg.

[24] Barbancho Concejero, J., León de Mora, C., Molina Cantero, F. J., & Barbancho Concejero, A. (2007). Using artificial intelligence in routing schemes for wireless networks. *Computer Communications*, 30(14–15), 2802–2811.

[25] Watkins, C. J. C. H. (1989). Learning from delayed rewards. Ph.D. Thesis, University of Cambridge, England.

[26] Arya, A., Malik, A., & Garg, R. (2013). Reinforcement learning based routing protocols in WSNs: A survey. *International Journal of Computer Science Engineering and Technology*, 4, 1401–1404.

[27] Habib, M. A., Arafat, M. Y., & Moh, S. (2018). Routing protocols based on reinforcement learning for wireless sensor networks: A comparative study. *Journal of Advanced Research in Dynamical and Control Systems*, 14, 427–435.

[28] Juneja, S., Juneja, A., & Anand, R, (2020). Health care 4.0 –Digitizing healthcare using big data for performance improvisation, *Journal of Computational and Theoretical Nanoscience*, 17(9–10), 4408–4410.

[29] Yang, W., Wang, X., Song, X., Yang, Y., & Patnaik, S. (2018). Design of intelligent transportation system supported by new generation wireless communication technology. *International Journal of Ambient Computing and Intelligence (IJACI)*, 9(1), 78–94.

[30] Singh, L., Saini, M. K., Tripathi, S., & Sindhwani, N. (2008). An intelligent control system for real-time traffic signal using genetic algorithm. In *AICTE Sponsored National Seminar on Emerging Trends in Software Engineering* (Vol. 50).

[31] Sindhwani, N., & Singh, M. (2014). Transmit antenna subset selection in MIMO OFDM system using adaptive mutation Genetic algorithm. *arXiv preprint arXiv:1410.6795*.

[32] Kadam, K., & Srivastava, N. (2012, March). Application of machine learning (reinforcement learning) for routing in Wireless Sensor Networks (WSNs). In *2012 1st International Symposium on Physics and Technology of Sensors (ISPTS-1)* (pp. 349–352). IEEE.

[33] Das, S. K., Samanta, S., Dey, N., & Kumar, R. (Eds.). (2020). *Design Frameworks for Wireless Networks*. Springer, Singapore.

[34] Meelu, R., & Anand, R. (2011). Performance evaluation of cluster-based routing protocols used in heterogeneous wireless sensor networks, *International Journal of Information Technology and Knowledge Management*, 4(1), 227–231.

[35] Sindhwani, N., & Singh, M. (2017, March). Performance analysis of ant colony based optimization algorithm in MIMO systems. In *2017 International Conference on Wireless Communications, Signal Processing and Networking (WiSPNET)* (pp. 1587–1593). IEEE.

[36] Gao, W. (2007, August). Study on immunized ant colony optimization. In *Third International Conference on Natural Computation (ICNC 2007)* (Vol. 4, pp. 792–796). IEEE.

[37] Camilo, T., Carreto, C., Silva, J. S., & Boavida, F. (2006, September). An energy-efficient ant-based routing algorithm for wireless sensor networks. In *International Workshop on Ant Colony Optimization and Swarm Intelligence* (pp. 49–59). Springer, Berlin, Heidelberg.

[38] Paliwal, K. K., Israna, P. R. A., & Garg, P. (2011). Energy efficient data collection in Wireless sensor network-a survey. In *International Conference on Advanced Computing, Communication and Networks' II*.

[39] Sindhwani, N., Bhamrah, M. S., Garg, A., & Kumar, D. (2017, July). Performance analysis of particle swarm optimization and genetic algorithm in MIMO systems. In *2017 8th International Conference on Computing, Communication and Networking Technologies (ICCCNT)* (pp. 1–6). IEEE.

[40] De, D., Mukherjee, A., Das, S. K., & Dey, N. (Eds.). (2020). *Nature Inspired Computing for Wireless Sensor Networks*. Springer.

[41] Solaiman, B., & Sheta, A. (2013). Computational intelligence for wireless sensor networks: Applications and clustering algorithms. *International Journal of Computer Applications*, 73(15), 1–8.

[42] Malik, S., Saroha, R., & Anand, R. (2012). A simple algorithm for reduction of blocking artifacts using SAWS technique based on fuzzy logic. *International Journal of Computational Engineering Research*, 2(4), 1097–1101.

[43] Malik, S., Singh, N., & Anand, R. (n.d.) Compression artifact removal using saws technique based on fuzzy logic. *International Journal of Electronics & Electrical Engineering*, 2(9), 11–20.

[44] Saini, P., & Anand, M. R. (2014). Identification of defects in plastic gears using image processing and computer vision: A review. *International Journal of Engineering Research*, 3(2), 94–99.

[45] Choudhary, P., & Anand, M. R. (2015). Determination of rate of degradation of iron plates due to rust using image processing. International *Journal of Engineering Research*, 4(2), 76–84.

[46] Guo, W., & Zhang, W. (2014). A survey on intelligent routing protocols in wireless sensor networks. *Journal of Network and Computer Applications*, 38, 185–201.

[47] Yang, X. S., & Deb, S. (2010). Engineering optimisation by cuckoo search. *International Journal of Mathematical Modelling and Numerical Optimisation*, 1(4), 330–343.

[48] Kohli, L., Saurabh, M., Bhatia, I., Shekhawat, U. S., Vijh, M., & Sindhwani, N. (2021). Design and development of modular and multifunctional UAV with amphibious landing module. In *Data Driven Approach Towards Disruptive Technologies: Proceedings of MIDAS 2020* (pp. 405–421). Springer, Singapore.

[49] Kohli, L., Saurabh, M., Bhatia, I., Sindhwani, N., & Vijh, M. (2021). Design and Development of Modular and Multifunctional UAV with Amphibious Landing, Processing and Surround Sense Module. In *Unmanned Aerial Vehicles for Internet of Things (IoT): Concepts, Techniques, and Applications* (p. 207).

[50] Kulkarni, R. V., & Venayagamoorthy, G. K. (2010). Adaptive critics for dynamic optimization. *Neural Networks, 23*(5), 587–591.

[51] Singh, P., Pareek, V., & Ahlawat, A. K. (2017). Designing an energy efficient network using integration of KSOM, ANN and data fusion techniques. *International Journal of Communication Networks and Information Security (IJCNIS), 9*(3), 466–474.

[52] Singh, P., Raw, R. S., Khan, S. A., Mohammed, M. A., Aly, A. A., & Le, D. N. (2021). W-GeoR: Weighted geographical routing for VANET's health monitoring applications in urban traffic networks. *IEEE Access*. DOI: 10.1109/ACCESS.2021.3092426.

[53] Singh, P., Raw, R. S., & Khan, S. A. (2021). Link risk degree aided routing protocol based on weight gradient for health monitoring applications in vehicular ad-hoc networks. *Journal of Ambient Intelligence Humanized Computing*. DOI: 10.1007/s12652-021-03264-z.

[54] Rana, K., Tripathi, S., & Raw, R. S. (2019). Fuzzy logic-based directional location routing in vehicular ad-hoc network. In *Proceedings of the National Academy of Sciences, India Section A: Physical Sciences Springer*.

[55] Aliyu, A., Abdullah, A. H., Kaiwartya, O., Cao, Y., Usman, M. J., Kumar, S., Lobiyal, D. K., & Raw, R. S. (2017). Cloud computing in VANETs: Architecture, taxonomy and challenges. *IETE Technical Review, 35*, 523–547.

[56] Kumar, S., & Raw, R. S. (2020). Health Monitoring Planning for On-Board Ships Through Flying Ad Hoc Network. In *Advanced Computing and Intelligent Engineering* (pp. 391–402). Springer. ISBN: 978-981-15-1483-8.

[57] Kumar, A., Tripathi, S., & Raw, R. S. (2016). Bringing healthcare to doorstep using VANETs. In *3rd IEEE International Conference as INDIACom-2016*, Delhi, India (pp. 4747–4750).

[58] Singh, P. (2020). Vehicle Monitoring and Surveillance through Vehicular Sensor Network. In *Cloud-Based Big Data Analytics in Vehicular Ad-Hoc Networks*. IGI Global. https://www.igi-global.com/book/cloud-based-big-data-analytics/237840.

# Chapter 17

# An IoT approach of managing smart healthcare services

*Deena Nath Gupta and Rajendra Kumar*
Jamia Millia Islamia, New Delhi, India

## CONTENTS

## 17.1 INTRODUCTION

The healthcare industry handles the manufacturing of goods to be used for medical purposes. In the healthcare industry, the focused entity is patient. Healthcare industry provides many services for the rehabilitation of the patient. Medicines are the product of the healthcare industry. These medicines are used to treat a patient. Doctors in the healthcare industry act as the service provider. Doctors perform their duties to cure or prevent the patients from some possible diseases. This, however, can be seen as an industry that can directly affect the economy of a country and is also known as health economy. Healthcare industry is an integration of different entities such as doctors, nurses, and hospitals. Some providers of diagnostics and health insurance firms can also be included under the healthcare industry [1]. Therapeutic, remedial, and preventive services and pharmaceutical manufacturers are also part of the healthcare industry [2, 3].

Like other industries, healthcare industry also affects the gross domestic product (GDP) of a country. With the proper handling of the manufacturing and services under this industry, a country can enhance its export status, employment, and capital investments. The focus of the entire hospital team should be on patients rather than on staff or service providers, if a country really wants to do well in this industry. A country can establish a whole team of healthcare providers under its law. They may include doctor of medicine, podiatrist, psychologist, nurse practitioner, midwife, or any one from social work background. An extension may be given to the social worker by the law for performing some medical practice under some domain [4, 5].

The U.S. Bureau of Labor Statistics divided the healthcare industry into nine fields. The first and the most important is the hospital. Hospitals can offer a variety of services under one roof. Some of the actors under the hospital system are nurses, psychiatrists, physicians, social workers, therapists, administrative clerks, and building maintenance workers. Second most important entity of the healthcare industry is residential care facility or nursing facility. Round the clock hours, a lot of work is needed in case of some critical patient conditions. Some of the centers providing round-the-clock-hours services are rehabilitation centers, convalescent homes, and nursing homes. Workers under these facilities include home health aides, psychiatrists, and nurses. Next come the physicians. Physicians can either work separately or with other physicians in office. The same applies to dentists too. Dentists can work with dental assistants, administrative clerks, and dental hygienists [6, 7].

Personal aids and personal assistants are also included in the healthcare industry with the flexibility of caring outpatients at their home. Occupational therapists, chiropractors, psychologists, optometrists, and physical therapists are also included as health practitioners in the list. Outpatient care centers include emergency health clinics, abuse rehab centers, and mental health rehab centers. Next is an ambulatory service. Ambulatory service includes emergency medical technicians, ambulance drivers, paramedics, and attendants. The last one in the list is known as medical and diagnostic laboratory. Diagnostic laboratory includes radiologists, medical assistants, surgical equipment preparers, and medical transcription specialists [8, 9].

The rest of the chapter is structured as follows. Study about wearable devices is presented in section 17.2. The application of internet of things (IoT) in healthcare is elaborated in section 17.3. Communication protocol for seamless transfer of data and information is discussed in section 17.4. It is concluded that IPv6 is best suitable for the purpose. Section 17.5 presents a discussion on quality of service (QoS) needed for wearable and healthcare devices. Some common threats are listed in section 17.6. All the discussion about the presented manuscript and final conclusion is drawn in section 17.7.

## 17.2 WEARABLE DEVICES

These are sensor-enabled medical equipment specially designed for specific patients. Wearable devices are available nowadays from many manufacturers. Accenture surveyed customers using wearable devices. Earlier, in 2014, only 9% of the consumers opted for wearable devices. The survey shows that the usage rises to more than four multiple in just four years. In 2018, there were 33% consumers who were using these wearable devices. A global savings of nearly $200 billion is estimated in the next 25 years by enabling wearable devices with big data, machine learning, cloud computing, and artificial intelligence (AI) [10, 11].

According to GlobeNewswire, the market of wearable devices in India will grow with a compound annual growth rate (CAGR) of nearly 26% by 2024. From 4.72 million in 2019, it will reach 16.22 million in 2024. The most popular wearable healthcare device in India is the wrist watch having nearly 48% of market share followed by ear-worn devices capturing nearly 44% of market share. Top player in the field of wearable devices in Indian market is Xiaomi Technologies India Private Limited, a Chinese multinational company. Other prominent players are GOQii Technologies Private Limited, Titan Company Limited, Fitbit India Private Limited, Fossil India Private Limited, and Samsung India Electronics Private Limited [2, 3].

Some examples of top healthcare wearable products include AVA, AliveCor, TEMPTRAQ, BioScarf, Blinq, SmartSleep, Bio-Patch, Smart Glasses, Smart Hearing Aids, and Wireless Patient Monitoring. AVA mainly focuses on the health of women by tracking period cycles. The overall health of women, including their fertility and pregnancy, is tracked by AVA. It also helps a pregnant woman to get her weight, sleep, and stress level with utmost accuracy. AliveCor, a portable device, acts as a personal electrocardiogram (EKG) for its users. It detects atrial fibrillation, bradycardia, tachycardia, or normal heart rhythm in just 30 seconds and delivers it to a smartphone and medical professionals. TEMPTRAQ monitors the temperature of babies and children continuously without interrupting them in their comfort/sleep in any illness. A soft patch includes a Bluetooth sensor that measures the temperature of a baby body continuously and informs at different time intervals. BioScarf is a trendy alternative to the regular air pollution masks. Almost 99.75% of the airborne pollutants (e.g., pet dander, pollen, smoke, and pm2.5 among others) are filtered by this scarf. Blinq, a wearable ring, is a combination of class and function. The wearable smart rings look like aesthetic jewels and fit within the limit of these fine jewelries. Blinq is water resistant and has a battery life of more than 48 hours. Philip's SmartSleep, soft headbands with sensors, provides the solution for individuals' sleeping needs. Audio tones embedded [12] in the device help people improve the depth and duration of rapid eye movement (REM) sleep. Bio-Patches are the latest, noninvasive wearables that can help medical professionals monitor and measure the patients' heart rate, electrocardiogram (ECG), heart rate variability, respiration rate, and activity. Augmented reality eyewear for point-of-view (POV) video sharing is the next innovation in smart glasses. Vuzix's Smart Glasses is eyeing to integrate these features to produce a new kind of telehealth. Livio AI, a product from Starkey Hearing Technologies, selectively filters noises and focuses on some very specific sources of sound. The sensors and AI fitted in the wearable make it possible to keep a track of some important health metrics like physical activities and are built to measure the heart rate in the future. Leaf Patient Monitoring System prevents many pressure-related injuries and assists caregivers to enhance the safety of their patients. It results in 79% reduction in specialty rental beds. Leaf Healthcare offers wireless patient monitoring [13–15].

## 17.3 INTERNET OF HEALTHCARE THINGS (IOHT)

Technology changes lives. Some technologies use the models for treatment. There are therapies for depression or anxiety disorder used across the globe. The use of virtual and augmented reality in the healthcare industry is also well known. Because this is the era of globalization, no country can isolate itself. Each one is depending on the findings of others in many ways. The networking makes the task simple. If everyone will be connected, the information about a particular disease will be shared to everyone in case of some medical emergency. The chance of finding a quick cure will be high in this way. People can find doctors from the mobile app. With networking, we can add different stakeholders in one platform for fast action. If a patient is registered over the network, the network will have all the information about the patient illness. Doctors from all over the world may suggest necessary cures in advance so that patients can be saved from the extreme condition. If needed, patients will be directed to the local services to get an appointment with an urgent treatment center. Medicines can be sent to the patients in emergency from the nearest pharmacy as well.

Digitization plays a very important role in the healthcare industry. Women can check their maternity records digitally, and this will help them take leave from their workplace. They just need to link their record with the companies they are working for and hence there will be no need to produce the documents and get them attested by their doctors. The digital version of the record about their child will help the parents in many ways. In this way, a digital personal health record can be built about an individual right from his/her birth. Every node is connected in an IoT network, every hospital will have information about a patient undergoing treatment in any other hospital. In case of transfer of hospital, no patient has to look for the referrals from the hospital in which his treatment was going on. Every detail of the patient will be automatically transferred to the new hospital before the arrival of the patient. The doctors can prepare with all the instruments in

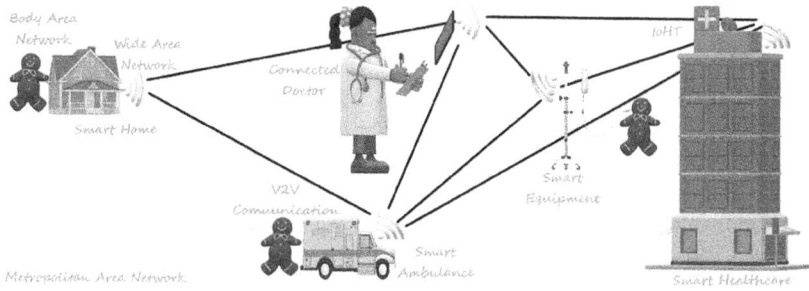

*Figure 17.1* IoT in healthcare.

advance in the case of an emergency. An illustration of the possible scenario of IoHT is presented in Figure 17.1.

In IoT [16–18], technically every single entity is treated as nodes. There will be many types of nodes in healthcare IoT such as the patient node, the doctor node, the hospital node, and the nurse node. A patient can be taken care of individually. Nutrition plans can be personalized for an individual node. There will be sensors attached to the body of the patient in forms of wearable or implantable health monitoring devices. These sensors will collect the data from the patient's body parts. With the help of these data, the dietician can formulate an exact plan for the patient. This plan will suit the patient's unique DNA and metabolism. The future of healthcare can be seen from here. The prediction about the health of a child can be seen from birth. A healthcare roadmap will be generated for gene therapies, surgeries, and custom vaccines to avoid some serious health issues in future. The implantable health monitoring devices will also reduce the administrative burden and empowers clinicians [19–22].

In this new environment, where everyone will be connected, only the best practice using the AI techniques will be applied on the patients for fast and best treatment. Sometimes, it is seen that a particular local area got infected by some virus, for example, the recent COVID-19 (The CoronaVirus) [23]. In this case, a predictive technique should be used to support local health systems from the experts of any region worldwide. A patient need not be admitted to the hospital; the team of doctors can take care of the patient by using the data received from the wearable devices and can offer them some guidance digitally.

The symptoms of the disease can be recognized earlier that will help the patient avoid extreme harmful conditions in future. Video calling and web chat can be used as important tools for remote treatment. Patients can get virtual consultation using these techniques. The drone [24, 25] technology can also play a vital role in this advancement. Drones can be used to take the biosamples from the home of a patient in case the patient finds himself/herself not able to visit the nearby clinic. In automated laboratories [26, 27], AI will be used to produce the results within minutes so that disease will be diagnosed earlier [28, 29].

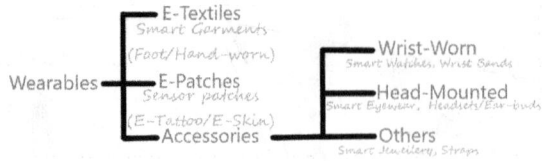

*Figure 17.2* Categories of wearable devices.

Some of the important examples of IoHT include glucose monitoring and insulin pens, connected inhalers, apple watch that monitors depression, connected contact lenses, hearing aid, wearable external devices, implanted medical devices, and automated treatment devices. The US Food and Drug Administration approved the first glucose monitoring devices in 1999. A smart continuous glucose monitoring (CGM), Freestyle Libre, sends blood glucose levels to its users at regular intervals. Propeller Health, a leading producer of connected inhalers, connects its sensor with Bluetooth spirometer to provide the allergen forecasts to the patients. AI in healthcare is provided by the Takeda Pharmaceuticals and the Cognition kit limited. Some popular categories of wearable devices are shown in Figure 17.2.

## 17.4 COMMUNICATION PROTOCOL

IPv4 is a well-known protocol used for the communication between different devices under a computing environment. Almost all the communication inside a network followed the IPv4 protocol suite before the IoT came into existence. Some limitations of IPv4 are discovered in an IoT environment. These limitations open the window for a new version of this communication protocol known as IPv6. In this section, the authors will talk about the limitations of IPv4 in an IoHT environment, suitability of IPv6 in an IoHT environment, and the comparison between the two [30].

### 17.4.1 Limitations of IPv4

The main limitations of IPv4 for managing the smart healthcare services are discussed as follows:

(i) Scarcity of IPv4 Addresses
   The IPv4 addressing scheme uses a 32-bit address space. This 32-bit address space is classified to further A, B, and C classes. The 32-bit address space allows 4,294,967,296 IPv4 addresses, but the previous and current IPv4 address allocation schemes limit the number of available public IPv4 addresses. The addresses which are allocated to the organizations were not used many times and this created the scarcity

of IPv4 addresses. So, the scarcity of IPv4 addresses is a major limitation of the IPv4 addressing system. For managing the smart healthcare services, the networking embodies a drawback because end-to-end services are hard to configure [31].

(ii) Private addressing and translation

To solve the issue caused by the scarcity of IPv4 and to save public addresses, people started using private addresses for intranets. Private IP addressing uses addresses from the class C range reserved for network address translation (NAT) (192.168.0.0 – 192.168.255.255) because private addresses cannot be routed on public IP networks. By using NAT, we can map many internal private IPV4 addresses to a public IPv4 address which helps in preserving IPv4 addresses. NAT also has many shortfalls. NAT does not support network layer security standards and it does not support the mapping of all the upper layer protocols. In some cases, NAT also creates some network problems when two hospitals communicate with the same private IPv4 address ranges [32].

(iii) IP configuration

To overcome the scarcity of IPv4, most of the existing IPv4 operations must be either manually configured or using a dynamic host configuration protocol (DHCP). DHCP is a standardized network protocol based on transmission control protocol/internet protocol (TCP/IP) networks. A DHCP server can enable the computers to request IP addresses and networking constraints automatically from the internet service provider (ISP), dropping the need for a network administrator or a user to manually assign internet protocol (IP) addresses to all network devices.

(iv) Security-related issues

Internet protocol security (IPsec) is a protocol suite that enables network security [33] by protecting the data being sent over the network from external attacks. Confidential communications over a public medium such as the internet requires security services that shield the data being sent from being sniffed, viewed, or modified in transportation. Even though there is a standard for IPv4 security such as IPsec, some implementations of it are proprietary and require consumers to spend more money for the license fee to use this security suite on the client site [34].

(v) *Suitability of IPv6*

There are several arguments to show that IPv6 will be a key enabler for managing the smart healthcare services in the IoHT[35, 36]. These are described below.

(vi) *Adoption is just a matter of time*

For any internet connection, it is necessary to have the IP. Internet data transfer is addressed using this scheme. A shift from IPv4 to IPv6 is inevitable because of its limited size.

(vii) *Scalability*

There is no addressing scheme as scalable as IPv6. It has $3.4 \times 10^{38}$ addresses, which is equal to $2^{128}$ unique addresses provided. Almost any present-day or future communication device will be able to take advantage of it [37].

## 17.4.2 Solving the NAT barrier

A trick, the NAT, was needed in order to cope with the unplanned expansion of IPv4. In NAT, one public IP address can be shared by several users and devices. However, two tradeoffs must be made for this solution to work.

✓ IP addresses are borrowed and shared by NAT users. In that case, they do not have their own public IP address, leaving them homeless on the internet. Despite their access to the internet, they cannot be directly accessed via the internet.

✓ The end-to-end connection is broken and authentication is seriously compromised as a result.

## 17.4.3 Strong security enablers

An end-to-end connection, also called end-to-end IPv6, is a distributed routing technology. Also, IPv6 is supported by a huge user and researcher community that is actively working on improving its security features.

## 17.4.4 Tiny stacks available

There is a long history of research in IPv6 and the IoHT. An IPv6 compressed version 6LoWPAN has been developed by the research community. The compressed address size is a simple and efficient method of reducing IPv6 address length for constrained devices, whereas border routers are able to translate the compressed addresses into regular IPv6 addresses. Meanwhile, tiny stacks, such as Contiki, have been developed such that they only consume 11.5 kB.

## 17.4.5 Enabling the extension of the internet to the web of things

Any device and service can connect to the internet with IPv6. Many experiments have proven that IPv6 addresses cannot only be used for small deployments of sensors, but even for large-scale deployments like smart buildings, smart cities, and even hospitals. In addition, the CoAP protocol allows the constrained devices to behave as web services, providing easy access and compliance with the REST architecture [38].

## 17.4.6 Mobility

With IPv6, both end-nodes and routing nodes can be mobile because they provide strong features and solutions to support them.

## 17.4.7 Address self-configuration

Address autoconfiguration is provided by IPv6 (stateless mechanism). There is a great deal of autonomy in how the nodes define their addresses. The configuration effort and cost are reduced drastically as a result.

## 17.4.8 Fully internet compliant

It is fully compliant with IPv6; IPv6 is an essential component of the internet. One can, therefore, use a global network of connected smart healthcare objects to build one's own smart healthcare network or to interconnect one's own smart healthcare device with the rest of the world.

## 17.4.9 Comparison between IPv4 and IPv6

IPv4 and IPv6 are the versions of internet protocol where IPv6 is the enhanced version of IPv4. There are various differences between IPv4 and IPv6 protocols. For example, IPv4 has 32-bit address length, whereas IPv6 has 128-bit address length. IPv4 addresses represent the binary numbers in decimals. On the other hand, IPv6 addresses express binary numbers in hexadecimal. IPv6 uses end-to-end fragmentation, whereas IPv4 requires an intermediate router to fragment any datagram that is too large. Header length of IPv4 is 20 bytes. In contrast, the header length of IPv6 is 40 bytes. IPv4 uses checksum fields in the header format for handling error checking. On the contrary, IPv6 removes the header checksum field. In IPv4, the base header does not contain a field for header length, and a 16-bit payload length field replaces it in the IPv6 header. The option fields in IPv4 are employed as extension headers in IPv6. The Time to live field in IPv4 is referred to as Hop limit in IPv6. The header length field which is present in IPv4 is eliminated in IPv6 because the length of the header is fixed in this version. IPv4 uses broadcasting to transmit the packets to the destination computers while IPv6 uses multicasting and any-casting. IPv6 provides authentication and encryption, but IPv4 does not [38, 39]. The comparison between IPv4 and IPv6 is provided in Table 17.1.

*Table 17.1* The comparison between IPv4 and IPv6

| Properties | IPv4 | IPv6 |
|---|---|---|
| Address configuration | Supports manual and DHCP configuration | Supports autoconfiguration and renumbering |
| End-to-end connection integrity | Unachievable | Achievable |
| Address space | $2^{32}$ unique addresses | $2^{128}$ unique addresses |
| Security features | Security is dependent on application | IPSEC is inbuilt in the IPv6 protocol |
| Address length | 32 bits (4 bytes) | 128 bits (16 bytes) |
| Address representation | In decimal | In hexadecimal |
| Fragmentation performed by | Sender and forwarding routers | Only by the sender |
| Packet flow identification | Not available | Available and uses flow label field in the header |
| Checksum field | Available | Not available |
| Message transmission scheme | Broadcasting | Multicasting and any-casting |

## 17.5 QOS FOR IOHT NETWORK

There are various challenges while developing an IoHT network. One of the main challenges is QoS requirements in terms of data drop, data quality sensing, resource consumption, etc. The QoS handles all the parameters that can influence the network's reliability, availability, and performance directly or indirectly. In this category, some points considered by the European Commission in 2014 are bandwidth, cost efficiency, capacity and throughput, latency, resource optimization [40], trustworthiness, and scalability [41, 42].

## 17.6 OTHER CHALLENGES FOR IOHT NETWORK

(i) Secure Communication
   The communication channel linking different communicating nodes, such as cloud services and the IoHT devices, must be secured against any attack. In most cases, data sent by IoHT devices without encryption is an easy target for different network attacks. Therefore, by using an appropriate encryption method or separate networks for separator devices and creating private communication channels, such attacks can be reduced.
(ii) System Resilience
   The system should be able to defend other network nodes from any attack if an IoHT device is compromised [43–48]. Therefore, system resilience plays a significant role in the system's ability to respond to unforeseen attacks/situations without receding.

(iii) Complex System

The numerous heterogeneous devices interact together in the IoHT system. With the increase of interfaces, interactions, people, and devices in the IoT system, the risks of security breaches are increasing as well. Consequently, achieving the high security required to manage the large-scale network is a very difficult task due to time, memory, and energy limitations.

(iv) Common threats to IoHT

The IoHT connects everything to the network. In the case of the healthcare industry, every patient will have their unique identification over the network. The doctors, also having their unique identification, of different hospitals can get the information about the patient. The information should not be revealed to any third person. The information related to a particular disease of a patient is very critical. An adversary can hack the hospital network to obtain the data about the patient or doctor or some particular disease or some particular cure [49–52].

*Unauthorized access*: A malicious node can be injected into the hospital network to gain the authoritative permissions. If this node, anyhow, gets access to the network, it will be able to communicate with any of the nodes in the network. This malicious node will then be able to communicate with the other nodes on the network. It can send the information received from doctor node or patient node to some other hospital network or it can use this information in any desired way [53].

*Denial of services*: A malicious node, by using the ID of a patient node, can send the wrong information about the patient's health to the hospital network. This may cause a stampede. A warning about the patient's health will be issued to the doctors. The doctor may hurry to the patient for some emergency treatment [54]. Much resources of the hospital will be allocated for the emergency treatment of the patient. But all these efforts will go in the bin when the doctors will find the patient in all the right situations. They will come to know that the patient has no idea about what is happening with his ID.

*Side channel attack*: An outsider node may learn some pattern of communication. An ill-fitted node may try to replace the instructions from doctor node to patient node by his own instruction. If the patient will receive some forged instruction, he may go through some dangerous situation. A single replacement of yes to no may cause blunder. This scenario is very likely to be possible when the doctor from outside the hospital wants to instruct the patient. Note that the hospital cannot guarantee the outside network [55].

*Cybercrime*: A set of systems works together in isolation to produce them as a trusted and verified hospital network. A new patient may trust this network as the original hospital network and may produce all of its details to this forged network. They ask the questionnaire in such a way that a new patient has much possibility to produce their sensitive information to them. These networks can use the record of patients to blackmail them in public if the patient is infected with such a disease that is not acceptable in public. These networks sometimes steal the information about a patient's bank details. These networks can act as a middleware for seeking the payments from the patient to the hospital [56, 57].

*Advanced persistent threats*: An injected node may reside in the network for a very long period of time. This node may record every communication within the network as long as it wishes. It may find some useful patterns in the communication between doctor nodes and patient nodes. It may use the information of one hospital network to sell to another hospital network, for example, research data. In an IoT scenario, a large volume of data is transferred among the nodes. One can peacefully record all the data for some future work. Suppose a health insurance company is watching the development of a patient, it may then make its plan according to the current situation of the patient [58].

*Remote recording*: A corrupt node may control the security devices of a hospital network from outside the network. Suppose an outsider gains control of the security camera installed inside the hospital, it will see every movement inside the organization. The person may stop the camera for some particular movement. If a person gets access to security gates, then he may do any harm to the hospital. Suppose a device is constantly recording the lock pattern of different users from the hospital's entry gate, in that case it can make it simple for anyone to get access to the hospital in future. A person sitting outside the hospital will know everything about the hospital such as number of patient visits, prominent business partners, any VIP visit, and prominent doctors [59].

*Cloud storage*: In the industrial IoT framework, a huge number of sensors are used to collect data. Sometimes, the edge devices are not able to handle this large amount of data at their level. To store the large volume of data, we need some storage outside the hospital network. There may be some unnecessary or irrelevant data that exists, for example, temperature of the room for every second. Although we need the data about room temperature, we may not find anything relevant from these data at the end of the day. So, there will be no benefit of storing these data for long. Industrial internet of things (IIoT) uses cloud storage and hence there is much security associated with this cloud storage. There are many types of cloud storage such as private cloud and public cloud. Many industries can share one single cloud storage sometimes. This can cause a problem for secure storage [60–63].

## 17.7 DISCUSSION AND CONCLUSION

In this chapter, the authors have presented an emerging application of IoT known as IoHT. The growth of IoHT is very crucial for an individual as well as for a country. Currently, almost all the hospitals are working in isolation.

This sometimes restricts the findings of an ongoing survey or research project about the current pandemic or epidemic. The recent example of such a mistake happening is COVID-19. Almost every country faces the challenge of collaborative research. So, the need for networking in healthcare is very important. Keeping the current trend of computer science in mind, the authors advocate the networking of hospitals in an IoT way. This gives birth to the IoHT. The authors talked about different actors involved in a healthcare industry, the possible communication between the constrained and unconstrained devices, and security challenges in order to achieve a seamless and secure transfer of information.

The communicating wearable devices need to be compliant with the IoT environment. The rising number of sensing devices require log bit addressing and hence IPv4 seems not be able to solve the purpose. Hence, a new addressing mechanism comes into existence, i.e., IPv6. IPv6 is having four times more address space than IPv4. The 128-bit addressing can accumulate simultaneously all the IoT devices present on the earth till date. QoS also needs to be maintained. All the communicating wearable devices should take care of the protocol. Also, there are many threats and attacks existing on the way of secure communication. All these need a lightweight mechanism to handle because of the constrained nature of wearable devices.

If a hospital network wants to cope up with the above-mentioned threats, it should adopt some cyber-security measures. Cyber-security professionals can develop some mechanism as per the requirement of the hospital network. The cyber-security professionals use modern technologies such as big data, block chain, and AI to protect the IoT-enabled networks. Industries have their own industrial control system (ICS). These industrial control systems include distributed control system (DCS), programmable logic controllers (PLC), supervisory control and data acquisition (SCADA), and human machine interface (HMI). Because the adaptations of these systems are based on internet protocol, these are prone to cyber-attack mostly. Because each device in the network is communicating, the risk of man-in-the-middle attack is high. By using some of the methods, we can reduce the risk of attack [64, 65].

If we are going to apply IoT over our existing healthcare system, we should be careful in the naming of the devices [66]. Because hospitals serve the public, they have to communicate to different public devices as well. The naming of the devices should be done keeping in mind the names used by the outside world. Physically unclonable functions (PUF) are used to provide names to the devices. This provides unique naming by including some hardware characteristics of the devices, for example, MAC addresses.

In an IoT environment, the prime concern is communication security. Because any number of devices can request for communication with any other device at a time, the network should keep an eye on the communication between devices. A central key issuing authority should be there to issue the key for each communication. Any outsider device from the edge of the network can present itself as one of the devices of the network by stealing the information of the victim device and can establish the connection. Random binary bit sequences can be used as digital signatures for the mutual authentication between the devices. The server should ask some questionnaires to both of the devices that want to communicate for authentication before allowing them to communicate.

Encryption is an all-time proven method of security. Although the computer industry has a handful of methods of encryption, not every method is suitable for all the applications. RSA, DES, AES, and ECC are well-known cryptographic ciphers. These are using different mechanisms like, Feistel structure, S-box, P-box, and quadratic equations. Also, these are based on a large number of rounds and long key bits or on complex computation. Both of the conditions are not suitable for an IoT environment. Modern cryptographic algorithms are based on the requirement of constrained devices. The developers of modern cryptographic algorithms need to take care of two things: (1) NIST test suite for randomness [67], and (2) EPC Global standard for constrained devices [68, 69].

## REFERENCES

[1] Juneja, S., Juneja, A., & Anand, R. (2020). Healthcare 4.0-digitizing healthcare using big data for performance improvisation. *Journal of Computational and Theoretical Nanoscience*, 17(9–10), 4408–4410.

[2] Firouzi, F., Chakrabarty, K., & Nassif, S. (Eds.). (2020). *Intelligent Internet of Things: From Device to Fog and Cloud*. Springer Nature.

[3] Peng, S. L., Pal, S., & Huang, L. (Eds.). (2020). *Principles of Internet of Things (IoT) Ecosystem: Insight Paradigm*. Springer International Publishing.

[4] Jin, C., Xu, C., Zhang, X., & Zhao, J. (2015). A secure RFID mutual authentication protocol for healthcare environments using elliptic curve cryptography. *Journal of medical systems*, 39(3), 1–8.

[5] Ishida, M., Ushioda, S., Nagasawa, Y., Komuroa, Y., Tang, Z., Hu, L., ... & Sakatani, K. (2020). Development of an IoT-based monitoring system for healthcare: A preliminary study. In *Oxygen Transport to Tissue XLI* (pp. 291–297). Springer, Cham.

[6] Sinha, D. M., & Fukey, D. L. N. (n.d.) Smart wearable healthcare devices: Personal Health care companion, current and future consumer adoption status. In *PBME* (p. 28).

[7] Selvaraj, S., & Sundaravaradhan, S. (2020). Challenges and opportunities in IoT healthcare systems: a systematic review. *SN Applied Sciences*, 2(1), 1–8.

[8] Gupta, P., Pandey, A., Akshita, P., & Sharma, A. (2020). IoT based healthcare kit for diabetic foot ulcer. In *Proceedings of ICRIC 2019* (pp. 15–22).

[9] Rani, D. J., & Roslin, S. E. (2016, November). Light weight cryptographic algorithms for medical internet of things (IoT)-a review. In *2016 Online International Conference on Green Engineering and Technologies (IC-GET)* (pp. 1–6). IEEE.

[10] Sindhwani, N., Verma, S., Bajaj, T., & Anand, R. (2021). Comparative analysis of intelligent driving and safety assistance systems using YOLO and SSD model of deep learning. *International Journal of Information System Modeling and Design (IJISMD)*, 12(1), 131–146.

[11] Singh, H., Rehman, T. B., Gangadhar, C., Anand, R., Sindhwani, N., & Babu, M. (2021). Accuracy detection of coronary artery disease using machine learning algorithms. *Applied Nanoscience*, 1–7.

[12] Juneja, S., Juneja, A., & Anand, R. (2019, April). Reliability modeling for embedded system environment compared to available software reliability growth models. In *2019 International Conference on Automation, Computational and Technology Management (ICACTM)* (pp. 379–382). IEEE.

[13] Lucero, S. (2016). IHS TECHNOLOGY IoT platforms: Enabling the internet of things. technology.ihs.com, 5.

[14] Vermesan, O., & Friess, P. (Eds.). (2014). *Internet of Things-From Research and Innovation to Market Deployment* (Vol. 29). River Publishers, Aalborg.

[15] Forrest, E., Marinchak, C. M., & Hoanca, B. (2021). Intelligent Assistants and the Internet of Things as the Next Marketing Landscape. In *Encyclopedia of Organizational Knowledge, Administration, and Technology* (pp. 2070–2084). IGI Global.

[16] Anand, R., Sinha, A., Bhardwaj, A., & Sreeraj, A. (2018). Flawed Security of Social Network of Things. In *Handbook of Research on Network Forensics and Analysis Techniques* (pp. 65–86). IGI Global.

[17] Gupta, A., Srivastava, A., Anand, R., & Tomažič, T. (2020). Business Application Analytics and the Internet of Things: The Connecting Link. In *New Age Analytics* (pp. 249–273). Apple Academic Press.

[18] Gupta, R., Shrivastava, G., Anand, R., & Tomažič, T. (2018). IoT-Based Privacy Control System through Android. In *Handbook of E-business Security* (pp. 341–363). Auerbach Publications.

[19] Nautiyal, S., & Devi, R. (2020). Design and development of IoT-enabled portable healthcare device for rural health workers. In *International Conference on Intelligent Computing and Smart Communication 2019* (pp. 1509–1523). Springer, Singapore.

[20] Basu, S., Ghosh, M., & Barman, S. (2020). Raspberry PI 3B+ based smart remote health monitoring system using IoT platform. In *Proceedings of the 2nd International Conference on Communication, Devices and Computing* (pp. 473–484). Springer, Singapore.

[21] Almulhim, M., & Zaman, N. (2018, February). Proposing secure and lightweight authentication scheme for IoT based E-health applications. In *2018 20th International Conference on Advanced Communication Technology (ICACT)* (pp. 481–487). IEEE.

[22] Fernandes, E., Rahmati, A., Eykholt, K., & Prakash, A. (2017). Internet of things security research: A rehash of old ideas or new intellectual challenges?. *IEEE Security & Privacy*, 15(4), 79–84.

[23] Jain, S., Kumar, M., Sindhwani, N., & Singh, P. (2021). SARS-Cov-2 detection using deep learning techniques on the basis of clinical reports. In *2021 9th International Conference on Reliability, Infocom Technologies and Optimization (Trends and Future Directions) (ICRITO)* (pp. 1–5).

[24] Kohli, L., Saurabh, M., Bhatia, I., Shekhawat, U. S., Vijh, M., & Sindhwani, N. (2021). Design and development of modular and multifunctional UAV with

amphibious landing module. In *Data Driven Approach Towards Disruptive Technologies: Proceedings of MIDAS 2020* (pp. 405–421). Springer, Singapore.

[25] Kohli, L., Saurabh, M., Bhatia, I., Sindhwani, N., & Vijh, M. (2021). Design and Development of Modular and Multifunctional UAV with Amphibious Landing, Processing and Surround Sense Module. In *Unmanned Aerial Vehicles for Internet of Things (IoT): Concepts, Techniques, and Applications* (p. 207).

[26] Saini, M. K., Nagal, R., Tripathi, S., Sindhwani, N., & Rudra, A. (2008). PC interfaced wireless robotic moving arm. In *AICTE Sponsored National Seminar on Emerging Trends in Software Engineering* (Vol. 50).

[27] Singh, L., Saini, M. K., Tripathi, S., & Sindhwani, N. (2008). An intelligent control system for real-time traffic signal using genetic algorithm. In *AICTE Sponsored National Seminar on Emerging Trends in Software Engineering* (Vol. 50).

[28] Shaila, S. G., Vadivel, A., & Naksha, V. (2020). Introduction to the World of Artificial Intelligence. In *Handbook of Research on Applications and Implementations of Machine Learning Techniques* (pp. 359–379). IGI Global.

[29] Malsa, N., Singh, P., Gautam, J., Srivastava, A., & Singh, S. P. (2020). Source of Treatment Selection for different States of India and Performance Analysis using Machine Learning Algorithms for Classification. In *Soft Computing: Theories and Applications*. http://www.springer.com/series/11156.

[30] Narendra, P., Duquennoy, S., & Voigt, T. (2015, October). BLE and IEEE 802.15.4 in the IoT: Evaluation and Interoperability Considerations. In *International Internet of Things Summit* (pp. 427–438). Springer, Cham.

[31] Galis, A., & Gavras, A. (2013). *The Future Internet: Future Internet Assembly 2013: Validated Results and New Horizons* (p. 369). Springer Nature.

[32] Ali, A. N. A. (2012). Comparison study between IPV4 & IPV6. *International Journal of Computer Science Issues (IJCSI)*, 9(3), 314.

[33] Anand, R., Shrivastava, G., Gupta, S., Peng, S. L., & Sindhwani, N. (2018). Audio Watermarking With Reduced Number of Random Samples. In *Handbook of Research on Network Forensics and Analysis Techniques* (pp. 372–394). IGI Global.

[34] Chandra, D. G., Kathing, M., & Kumar, D. P. (2013, April). A comparative study on IPv4 and IPv6. In *2013 International Conference on Communication Systems and Network Technologies* (pp. 286–289). IEEE.

[35] Al-Kashoash, H. A., & Kemp, A. H. (2016). Comparison of 6LoWPAN and LPWAN for the Internet of Things. *Australian Journal of Electrical and Electronics Engineering*, 13(4), 268–274.

[36] Qiu, Y., & Ma, M. (2016). A mutual authentication and key establishment scheme for m2m communication in 6lowpan networks. *IEEE Transactions on Industrial Informatics*, 12(6), 2074–2085.

[37] Paul, H. C., & Bakon, K. A. (2016). A study on IPv4 and IPv6: The importance of their co-existence. *International Journal of Information System and Engineering*, 4(2).

[38] Feldner, B., & Herber, P. (2018). A qualitative evaluation of IPv6 for the industrial internet of things. *Procedia Computer Science*, 134, 377–384.

[39] Sarvaiya, M. S. B., & Satange, D. N. (2021). *Transition from IPv4 to IPv6 Network in IoT Security Based Upon Transition Methods*.

[40] Sindhwani, N. (2017). Performance analysis of optimal scheduling based firefly algorithm in MIMO system. *Optimization*, 2(12), 19–26.

[41] Duan, R., Chen, X., & Xing, T. (2011, October). A QoS architecture for IOT. In *2011 International Conference on Internet of Things and 4th International Conference on Cyber, Physical and Social Computing* (pp. 717–720). IEEE.

[42] Awan, I., Younas, M., & Naveed, W. (2014, September). Modelling QOS in IOT applications. In *2014 17th International Conference on Network-Based Information Systems* (pp. 99–105). IEEE.

[43] Singh, P., Raw, R. S., Khan, S. A., Mohammed, M. A., Aly, A. A., & Le, D. -N. (2021). W-GeoR: Weighted geographical routing for VANET's health monitoring applications in urban traffic networks. *IEEE Access*. DOI: 10.1109/ACCESS.2021.3092426.

[44] Singh, P., Raw, R. S., & Khan, S. A. (2021). Link risk degree aided routing protocol based on weight gradient for health monitoring applications in vehicular ad-hoc networks. *Journal of Ambient Intelligence Humanized Computing*. DOI: 10.1007/s12652-021-03264-z.

[45] Aliyu, A., Abdullah, A. H., Kaiwartya, O., Cao, Y., Usman, M. J., Kumar, S., Lobiyal, D. K. and Raw, R. S. (2018). Cloud computing in VANETs: Architecture, taxonomy and challenges. *IETE Technical Review*, 35, 523–547.

[46] Kumar, S., & Raw, R. S. (2020). Health Monitoring Planning for On-Board Ships Through Flying Ad Hoc Network. *Advanced Computing and Intelligent Engineering* (pp. 391–402). Springer, ISBN: 978-981-15-1483-8.

[47] Kumar, A., Tripathi, S. and Raw, R. S. (2016). Bringing healthcare to doorstep using VANETs. In *3rd IEEE International Conference as INDIACom-2016*, Delhi, India (pp. 4747–4750).

[48] Singh, P. (2020). Vehicle Monitoring and Surveillance through Vehicular Sensor Network. In *Cloud-Based Big Data Analytics in Vehicular Ad-Hoc Networks*. IGI Global. https://www.igi-global.com/book/cloud-based-big-data-analytics/237840.

[49] Rana, K., Tripathi, S., & Raw, R. S. (2019). Fuzzy logic-based directional location routing in vehicular ad-hoc network. In *Proceedings of the National Academy of Sciences, India Section A: Physical Sciences Springer.*

[50] Langiu, A., Boano, C. A., Schuß, M., & Römer, K. (2019, July). UpKit: An open-source, portable, and lightweight update framework for constrained IoT devices. In *2019 IEEE 39th International Conference on Distributed Computing Systems (ICDCS)* (pp. 2101–2112). IEEE.

[51] Jindal, V., & Singhal, D. (2021). Implementing Information Security Using Multimodal Biometrics. In *Handbook of Research on Cyber Crime and Information Privacy* (pp. 338–355). IGI Global.

[52] Da Veiga, A. (2019). Achieving a Security Culture. In *Cybersecurity Education for Awareness and Compliance* (pp. 72–100). IGI Global.

[53] Gupta, D. N., & Kumar, R. (2019). Lightweight cryptography: An IoT perspective. *Trivium*, 80(1), 2580.

[54] Gupta, D. N., & Kumar, R. (2021). Distributed Key Generation for Secure Communications Between Different Actors in Service Oriented Highly Dense VANET. In *Cloud and IoT-Based Vehicular Ad Hoc Networks* (pp. 221–232).

[55] Gupta, D. N., & Kumar, R. (2020, June). Generating Random Binary Bit Sequences for Secure Communications between Constraint Devices under the IOT Environment. In *2020 International Conference for Emerging Technology (INCET)* (pp. 1–6). IEEE.

[56] Pospisil, B., Huber, E., Quirchmayr, G., & Seboeck, W. (2020). Modus Operandi in Cybercrime. In *Encyclopedia of Criminal Activities and the Deep Web* (pp. 193–209). IGI Global.

[57] Rehman, T. U. (2020). International Context of Cybercrime and Cyber Law. In *Encyclopedia of Criminal Activities and the Deep Web* (pp. 412–423). IGI Global.

[58] Hudson, B. (2014). *Advanced Persistent Threats: Detection, Protection and Prevention*. Sophos Ltd.

[59] Bala, D. Q., Maity, S., & Jena, S. K. (2017, February). A lightweight remote user authentication protocol for smart e-health networking environment. In *2017 International Conference on I-SMAC (IoT in Social, Mobile, Analytics and Cloud)(I-SMAC)* (pp. 10–15). IEEE.

[60] Sahu, S. N., Moharana, M., Prusti, P. C., Chakrabarty, S., Khan, F., & Pattanayak, S. K. (2020). Real-Time Data Analytics in Healthcare Using the Internet of Things. In *Real-Time Data Analytics for Large Scale Sensor Data* (pp. 37–50). Academic Press.

[61] Tuli, S., Basumatary, N., Gill, S. S., Kahani, M., Arya, R. C., Wander, G. S., & Buyya, R. (2020). HealthFog: An ensemble deep learning based Smart Healthcare System for Automatic Diagnosis of Heart Diseases in integrated IoT and fog computing environments. *Future Generation Computer Systems*, *104*, 187–200.

[62] Moharana, S. R., Jha, V. K., Satpathy, A., Addya, S. K., Turuk, A. K., & Majhi, B. (2017, May). Secure key-distribution in IoT cloud networks. In *2017 Third International Conference on Sensing, Signal Processing and Security (ICSSS)* (pp. 197–202). IEEE.

[63] Bonomi, F., Milito, R., Zhu, J., & Addepalli, S. (2012, August). Fog computing and its role in the internet of things. In *Proceedings of the First Edition of the MCC Workshop on Mobile Cloud Computing* (pp. 13–16).

[64] Ng, J., Keoh, S. L., Tang, Z., & Ko, H. (2018, February). SEABASS: Symmetric-keychain encryption and authentication for building automation systems. In *2018 IEEE 4th World Forum on Internet of Things (WF-IoT)* (pp. 219–224). IEEE.

[65] Ng, J., Keoh, S. L., Tang, Z., & Ko, H. (2018, February). SEABASS: Symmetric-keychain encryption and authentication for building automation systems. In *2018 IEEE 4th World Forum on Internet of Things (WF-IoT)* (pp. 219–224). IEEE.

[66] Anand, R., Sindhwani, N., & Saini, A. (2021). Emerging Technologies for COVID-19. In *Enabling Healthcare 4.0 for Pandemics: A Roadmap Using AI, Machine Learning, IoT and Cognitive Technologies* (pp. 163–188).

[67] Kirichenko, V. V. (2015). Information security of communication channel with UAV. *Electronics and Control Systems*, *3*, 23–27.

[68] Wang, Z., & Edwards, R. M. (2020, March). An enhanced road vehicle positioning method using roadside furniture with radio frequency identity tags and the EPC Gen2 standard. In *2020 14th European Conference on Antennas and Propagation (EuCAP)* (pp. 1–4). IEEE.

[69] Thiesse, F., & Michahelles, F. (2006). An overview of EPC technology. *Sensor Review*, *26*, 101–105.

# Index

For Product Safety Concerns and Information please contact our EU
representative GPSR@taylorandfrancis.com
Taylor & Francis Verlag GmbH, Kaufingerstraße 24, 80331 München, Germany

9 781032 145488